**The Fifth Decade
of Cardiac Pacing**

This book is dedicated to the memory of
Jacques Mugica MD, pioneer in cardiac pacing

The Fifth Decade of Cardiac Pacing

EDITED BY

S. Serge Barold, MD, FRACP, FACP, FACC, FESC

Professor of Medicine
University of South Florida College of Medicine
and J.A. Haley VA Medical Center
Tampa, Florida, USA

AND

Jacques Mugica, MD†

Pacemaker Center
Centre Chirurgical Val d'Or
St Cloud-Paris, France

Blackwell
Publishing

Futura, an imprint of Blackwell Publishing

© 2004 by Futura, an imprint of Blackwell Publishing

Blackwell Publishing, Inc./Futura Division, 3 West Main Street, Elmsford, New York 10523, USA
Blackwell Publishing, Inc., 350 Main Street, Malden, Massachusetts 02148-5020, USA
Blackwell Publishing Ltd, 9600 Garsington Road, Oxford OX4 2DQ, UK
Blackwell Publishing Asia Pty Ltd, 550 Swanston Street, Carlton, Victoria 3053, Australia

04 05 06 07 5 4 3 2 1

ISBN: 1-4051-1644-7

The fifth decade of cardiac pacing / edited by S. Serge Barold and
Jacques Mugica. — 1st ed.
     p. ; cm.
Includes bibliographical references and index.
  ISBN 1-4051-1644-7
  1. Cardiac pacing
  [DNLM: 1. Cardiac Pacing, Artificial—methods. 2.
Arrhythmia—prevention & control. 3. Heart Failure,
Congestive—prevention & control. 4. Pacemaker, Artificial. WG 168
F469 2004] I. Barold, S. Serge. II. Mugica, Jacques.
  RC684 .P3F535 2004
  617 .4'120645—dc22

2003019456

A catalogue record for this title is available from the British Library

Acquisitions: Jacques Strauss
Production: Julie Elliott
Typesetter: Graphicraft Limited, Hong Kong
Printed and bound by CPI Bath, Bath, UK

For further information on Blackwell Publishing, visit our websites:
www.futuraco.com
www.blackwellpublishing.com

Notice: The indications and dosages of all drugs in this book have been recommended in the
medical literature and conform to the practices of the general community. The medications
described do not necessarily have specific approval by the Food and Drug Administration for use
in the diseases and dosages for which they are recommended. The package insert for each drug
should be consulted for use and dosage as approved by the FDA. Because standards for usage
change, it is advisable to keep abreast of revised recommendations, particularly those concerning
new drugs.

Contents

Colour plate section falls between pp. 84 and 85

List of Contributors

S. Serge Barold, MD, FRACP, FACP, FACC, FESC
Professor of Medicine, University of South Florida College of Medicine, and J. A. Haley VA Medical Center, Tampa, Florida, USA ssbarold@aol.com

Peter H. Belott, MD, FACC
Director, Cardiac electrophysiology laboratory, Grossmont Hospital, San Diego, CA pbelmd@msn.com

David G. Benditt, MD, FACC, FRCP(C)
Co-Director, Cardiac Arrhythmia Center, Department of Medicine, Cardiovascular Medicine, University of Minnesota Medical School, Minneapolis, MN bendi001@umn.edu

David A. Casavant, MS
Medtronic, Inc., Minneapolis, MN
dave.casavant@medtronic.com

Jacques Clémenty MD
Professor of Cardiology, University of Bordeaux; Hôpital Cardiologique du Haut Lévêque, Bordeaux-Pessac, France

Andrea Colella, MD FESC
Assistant Professor of Cardiology, Institute of Internal Medicine and Cardiology, University of Florence, Florence, Italy

Eugene Crystal, MD
Assistant Professor of Medicine, Schulich Heart Center, Department of Medicine, University of Toronto, Toronto, Ontario, Canada

Gabriele Demarchi, MD
Cardiology Fellow, Institute of Internal Medicine and Cardiology, University of Florence, Florence, Italy

Michael Eldar, MD, FACC, FESC
Professor of Cardiology, Sackler Faculty of Medicine, Tel Aviv University, Tel Aviv, Israel; Director, Heart Institute, Sheba Medical Center, Tel Hashomer, Israel

Ignacio Gallardo, MD, FACC
Florida Cardiovascular Institute and Tampa General Hospital, Tampa, FL

Stéphane Garrigue, MD, MS
Assistant Professor, Clinical Cardiac Pacing and Electrophysiology Department, University of Bordeaux, Hôpital Cardiologique du Haut Lévêque, Bordeaux-Pessac, France stephane.garrigue@chu-bordeaux.fr

Michael R. Gold, MD, PhD, FACC
Professor of Medicine and Director, Division of Cardiology, Medical University of South Carolina, Charleston, SC goldmr@musc.edu

Greg Hauck, BSEE
St. Jude Medical Cardiac Rhythm Management Division, Sylmar, CA

David L. Hayes, MD, FACC
Professor of Medicine and Chair of Cardiovascular Diseases, Mayo Clinic, Rochester, MN dhayes@mayo.edu

Carsten W. Israel, MD
Department of Cardiology, Division of Cardiac Electrophysiology, J. W. Goethe University Hospital, Frankfurt, Germany C.W.Israel@em.uni-frankfurt.de

Emmanuel M. Kanoupakis, MD
Senior Registrar, Department of Cardiology, Heraklion University Hospital, Heraklion, Greece

David A. Kass, MD, FAHA
Professor of Medicine, Johns Hopkins School of Medicine, Cardiology Division, Johns Hopkins Hospital, Baltimore, MD dkass@jhmi.edu

Mark Kroll, PhD
Vice President, Technology, St. Jude Medical Cardiac Rhythm Management Division, Sylmar, CA

Chu-Pak Lau, MD, FRCP, FRACP, FACC
Professor of Medicine and Chief, Cardiology Division, Queen Mary Hospital, University of Hong Kong, Hong Kong cplau@hkucc.hku.hk

Arnaud Lazarus, MD
InParys, Saint Cloud, France lazarus@inparys.com

Kathy Lai-Fun Lee, MBBS, MRCP
Honorary Clinical Assistant Professor, Cardiology Division,
Queen Mary Hospital, University of Hong Kong, Hong Kong

Paul A. Levine, MD, FACC.
Vice President and Medical Director, St. Jude Medical, Cardiac
Rhythm Management Division, Sylmar, CA; Clinical Professor
of Medicine, Loma Linda University School of Medicine, Loma
Linda, CA plevine@sjm.com

Charles J. Love, MD, FACC
Associate Professor, Director, Arrhythmia Device Services,
Division of Cardiology, The Ohio State University, Columbus,
OH Love-2@medctr.osu.edu

Mary E. McGrory-Usset, BS, MBA
Medtronic, Inc., Minneapolis, MN

Rick McVenes, BS
Bakken Fellow, Director of Leads Research, Cardiac Rhythm
Management, Therapy Delivery Division, Medtronic, Inc.,
Minneapolis, MN rick.mcvenes@medtronic.com

Antonio Michelucci MD, FESC
Associate Professor of Cardiology, Institute of Internal
Medicine and Cardiology, University of Florence, Italy

Jacques Mugica, MD†
Pacemaker Center, Centre Chirurgical Val d'Or, Saint Cloud,
France

I. Eli Ovsyshcher, MD, PhD, FESC, FACC
Professor of Medicine/Cardiology, Faculty of Health Sciences,
Ben Gurion University of the Negev, BeerSheva, Israel
eliovsy@bgumail.bgu.ac.il

Luigi Padeletti MD, FESC
Professor of Cardiology, Director of Post-Graduate School of
Cardiology (Electrophysiology), University of Florence, Italy
elettrofisiologia@dfc.unifi.it

Paolo Pieragnoli, MD
Cardiology Fellow, Institute of Internal Medicine and
Cardiology, University of Florence, Florence, Italy

Sergio L. Pinski, MD
Head, Section of Cardiac Pacing and Electrophysiology,
Cleveland Clinic Florida, Weston, FL pinskis@ccf.org

Maria Cristina Porciani, MD FESC
Assistant Professor of Cardiology, Institute of Internal
Medicine and Cardiology, University of Florence, Florence,
Italy

Alessandra Sabini, MD
Cardiologist, Institute of Internal Medicine and Cardiology,
University of Florence, Florence, Italy

Balakrishnan Shankar, BSE (Biomedical Engineering)
Director, Operations, St. Jude Medical Cardiac Rhythm
Management Division, Sylmar, CA

Robert E. Smith Jr., BSEE
Senior Scientist, St. Jude Medical Cardiac Rhythm
Management Division, Sylmar, CA

Jeffrey Snell, MSEE
St. Jude Medical Cardiac Rhythm Management Division,
Sylmar, CA

Roland X. Stroobandt MD, PhD
Associate Professor of Cardiology, University Leuven, Leuven,
Belgium; Head, Department of Cardiology, AZ Damiaan
Hospital, Oostende, Belgium

Cristina Tosti Guerra, BS
Research Scientist, Institute of Internal Medicine, University
of Florence, Florence, Italy

Hung-Fat Tse, MD, FACC
Associate Professor in Medicine, Cardiology Division, Queen
Mary Hospital, University of Hong Kong, Hong Kong

Panos E. Vardas, MD, PhD (London), FACC, FESC
Professor and Chief of Cardiology, Department of Cardiology,
Heraklion University Hospital, Heraklion, Greece
cardio@med.uoc.gr

André Walker, MSEE
Vice President, Electrical Engineering, St. Jude Medical
Cardiac Rhythm Management Division, Sylmar, CA

†Deceased.

Jacques Edmond Mugica, MD (1933–2002)

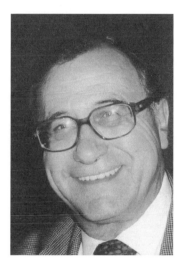

Dr Mugica graduated from the University of Paris, France in 1965, and subsequently trained in cardiopulmonary medicine. He then joined the Val d'Or Medical Center in St Cloud, a suburb of Paris, where he stayed for the rest of his career. In the early years he practiced pulmonary medicine, cardiology and intensive care. In 1968, Dr Mugica established the first multi-disciplinary, free standing pacemaker center in the world. Starting with 60 implantations a year, the numbers grew rapidly to over 1000 a year and the Val d'Or soon became one of the most important pacemaker centers in the world. It provided advanced care, teaching, research and attracted many international students for post-graduate training. Dr Mugica recruited a superb medical and technical team that like himself, quickly established a reputation for creativity, innovation and scientific achievements.

Dr Mugica created the well-known CARDIO-STIM organization when he realized that progress in pacing required a closer collaboration of physicians with industry for the proper clinical application of new technology. The first CARDIOSTIM symposium was held in 1978 in Paris. It soon became one of the most important regular international meetings in pacing and electrophysiology. Indeed, over 5000 participants converged to Nice, France from all over the world for CARDIOSTIM 2002. Over the years CARDIOSTIM never lost sight of its original mission. The refreshing participation of medical experts side-by-side with industry scientists, and the futuristic themes of many of the sessions have made CARDIO-STIM unique. Indeed, many consider CARDIO-STIM the premier meeting in the field. The importance of CARDIOSTIM is reflected by the regular publication of its best papers in a special issue of Pacing and Clinical Electrophysiology (PACE) since 1982 and later in two supplements to accommodate implantable cardioverter-defibrillators. A number of books (including this one) also originated from CARDIOSTIM symposia. The success of CARDIOSTIM has fostered other CARDIOSTIM meetings in Russia, Latin America and the Mediterranean countries under Dr Mugica's leadership and philosophy.

Dr Mugica lectured all over the world, and was a leading authority on many aspects of pacing, especially leads for which he gathered the largest computerized database in the world from a single center. He pioneered a number of important developments in pacing. He was the first to conceive of the benefit of a diagnostic pacemaker. His work also included a pacemaker with automatic threshold detection, screw-in leads, the concept of the fully automatic pacemaker and multichamber pacing in dilated cardiomyopathy with heart failure. The first implantation of a biventricular pacemaker in the world (actually a four-chamber device in a patient with additional interatrial conduction block) was successfully performed by the Val d'Or team in 1994 with meticulous documentation of the result. This remarkable milestone should not be surprising considering Dr Mugica's unrelenting drive for scientific excellence, iconoclastic thinking and leadership that he exhibited throughout his professional life. Dr Mugica had a special gift of predicting future developments in pacemaker technology. In this respect, he predicted the astounding developments that have taken place in the last 20 years published in a relatively short but remarkable article in 1984 on the future of stimulation [1].

Dr Mugica served on the editorial boards of five journals, including PACE. He published over 250 articles and 12 books plus this volume. His 1992 book on Cardiac Pacing in French remains a classic.

Dr Mugica received many awards for his contributions to cardiology. These include the Medal of the City of Paris, the Merci Prize from the French Hospital Association, the prestigious Gold Medal from the Société d'Encouragement au Progrès, and many others from international societies including the Distinguished Service Award from the North American Society of Pacing and Electrophysiology (NASPE) in 1995.

The CARDIOSTIM organization and Dr Mugica's superb medical team will continue to flourish as his legacy. His infectious enthusiasm, vision, courage, enormous energy coupled with the ability to get things done, warm personality and friendship will be missed. It has been a privilege for me over 25 years to have had Dr Mugica as a friend, colleague and collaborator in a number of articles and books.

S. Serge Barold

---

[1] Mugica J, Ripart A, Torresani J. La stimulation du futur. In: *La Stimulation Cardiaque Physiologique*. Maloine, 1984: 235–238.

Preface

The last of an ongoing series of CARDIOSTIM monographs was published six years ago. Since then, cardiac pacing has undergone spectacular progress. Thus, we felt it was time for another another CARDIOSTIM monograph to review the remarkable advances in the field. The book is devoted solely to cardiac pacing with emphasis on biventricular pacing for the treatment of congestive heart failure. We are grateful to the contributors who worked so hard to complete their manuscripts on time. Unfortunately my coauthor Dr Jacques Mugica passed away in December 2002 soon after completion of the book which is dedicated to his memory.

Working with the publishers, especially Julie Elliott was a real pleasure. Their patience, courtesy and efficiency are very much appreciated.

S. Serge Barold

PART I
Implantation and Explantation

CHAPTER 1

Implantation Techniques for Cardiac Resynchronization Therapy

Peter H. Belott

Introduction

Cardiac resynchronization therapy has clearly demonstrated hemodynamic benefit in patients with advanced congestive heart failure (CHF) [1–7]. Successful stimulation of the left ventricle (LV) is critical to this new pacing modality. This can be accomplished by either an epicardial or endocardial approach. The endocardial approach involves access to the LV endocardium transatrially through a patent foramen ovale or a direct transseptal puncture, but this technique is considered potentially dangerous because of the risk of thromboembolism and stroke [8]. The epicardium of the LV can be accessed by direct placement of pacing leads via thoracic surgery or a thoracoscopic approach. The direct placement of electrodes via thoracotomy in patients with advanced CHF is a relatively high-risk procedure. The LV epicardium may also be accessed transvenously by passing a lead via the coronary sinus to a posterolateral branch of the coronary sinus on the LV free wall [9]. The coronary sinus has been used for atrial and ventricular pacing for many years [10–14]. Permanent LV pacing via the great cardiac vein was initially reported by Bai *et al.* in an unusual situation where there was no right ventricular (RV) access [15]. In 1994, Bakker reported the benefits of biventricular pacing in CHF by using an endocardial RV lead and an epicardial LV lead, both connected to the ventricular channel of a pacemaker [16]. In that same year, Cazeau and coworkers reported the benefit of four-chamber pacing in a patient with end-stage dilated cardiomyopathy [17]. Leads were placed transvenously to the left atrium, right atrium and RV apex, with the LV lead placed on the epicardium via thoracotomy. Subsequently, Daubert and coworkers clearly demonstrated the feasibility and safety of acute and long-term LV pacing using leads inserted transvenously into coronary veins over the LV free wall [9]. The transvenous approach is now favored and biventricular pacing can be accomplished using conventional pacing hardware with only minor adaptations compared to the thoracotomy approach associated with poor lead reliability (sensing and chronic pacing thresholds), as well as increased morbidity and mortality.

Anatomic considerations

A complete understanding of the gross and radiographic cardiac anatomy is essential for successful cardiac resynchronization. Appreciation of the right atrial anatomy is necessary for coronary sinus cannulation. It is also important to understand that the right atrial and coronary sinus anatomy can be quite variable, especially in patients with advanced CHF where the heart is usually extremely dilated and the normal cardiac anatomic structures are distorted.

Right atrium

In the frontal plane, the right atrial cavity is located to the right and anteriorly. The left atrium is located to the left and mainly posterior to the interatrial septum. When viewed in the transverse plane, it runs obliquely from a left anterior position to a right posterior position. The right atrium is somewhat larger than the left but its walls are somewhat thinner. Traditionally, the right atrium is considered to consist of two parts: a posterior smooth-walled part into which the superior and inferior vena cavae

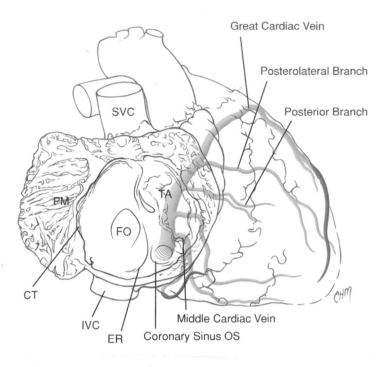

Great Cardiac Vein

Posterolateral Branch

Posterior Branch

SVC

PM

TA

FO

CT

IVC

ER

Middle Cardiac Vein

Coronary Sinus OS

Figure 1.1 Heart rotated into the right anterior oblique projection with the right atrial cavity exposed demonstrating the superficial and deep anatomy of the right heart in relation to the coronary sinus and its branch tributaries.

enter, and a very thin-walled, trabeculated part located anterolaterally [18]. The two parts of the atrium are separated by a muscular ridge called the crista terminalis. This ridge consists of muscle which is more prominent superiorly and tapers as it moves in an inferolateral direction. Externally, the crista terminalis corresponds to a seam known as the sulcus terminalis. The pectinate muscles run laterally in a parallel fashion from the crista terminalis along the right atrial free wall. The atrial wall between the pectinate muscle bundles is almost paper thin and translucent. The right atrial appendage is the triangular-shaped superior portion of the right atrium. It is filled with pectinate muscles. The eustachian valve is a fold of tissue that guards the anterior border of the inferior vena caval ostium. In humans it demonstrates considerable variability and may even be absent. Occasionally, it is perforated and even fenestrated, forming a lace-like network known as the network of Chiari. Anterior and medial to the eustachian valve, the coronary sinus enters the right atrium. The Thebesian valve is a valve-like fold of tissue that guards the orifice of the coronary sinus. The interatrial septum forms the posterior medial wall of the right atrium. Its central, ovoid portion is thin and fibrous and forms a shallow depression known as the fossa ovalis. The remainder of the septum is

muscular, forming a ridge known as the limbus fossa ovalis (Figure 1.1).

The recent developments in interventional electrophysiology techniques and resynchronization therapy mandate a better understanding of atrial anatomy. Contemporary anatomists Ho and Anderson have led the way to a better understanding of anatomy as it relates to cardiac electrophysiologic interventions [19,20]. Ho considers the right atrium as consisting of three components, the appendage, a venous part, and the vestibule (Plate 1.1, facing p. 84). The interatrial septum, a fourth component, is shared by the right and left atrium. Viewed from the epicardium, the atrial appendage is a triangular-shaped structure located anteriorly and laterally. The sulcus terminalis, corresponding to the crista terminalis, can be seen running along the lateral wall as a fat-filled groove. Epicardially, the sinus node is located in this groove adjacent to the superior vena cava–atrial junction. The right atrial musculature extends from the superior vena cava externally and terminates at the entrance of the inferior vena cava. When viewed externally, the pectinate muscles, as previously noted, can be seen radiating from the terminal crest. The pectinate muscles spread throughout the entire wall of the atrial appendage, extending to the lateral and inferior walls of the atrium. The pectinate muscles never reach the orifice of the tricuspid valve. The vestibule is a smooth muscular rim that surrounds the tricuspid valve orifice (Plate 1.2, facing p. 84). The posterior smooth wall of the atrium composes the venous component. The terminal crest marks the division between the venous smooth and trabeculated parts of the atrium. The terminal crest is a muscular bundle that begins on the superior aspect of the medial wall and passes anteriorly and laterally to the orifice of the superior vena cava. It then descends obliquely along the lateral atrial wall. Its terminal portion consists of a number of smaller muscle bundles, extending to the vestibule and orifice of the inferior vena cava. As mentioned previously, the eustachian valve, a triangular flap of fibromuscular tissue, guards the entrance of the inferior vena cava. This valve inserts medially and forms the eustachian ridge or sinus septum, which is the border between the fossa ovalis and coronary sinus. The eustachian valve may at times be quite large and at other times fenestrated, perforated and delicate. The free border of the eustachian valve extends as a tendon that runs into the musculature of the sinus septum, forming the posterolateral border of Koch's triangle. The anterior border is marked by the hinge of the septal leaflet of the tricuspid valve. The vestibular portion of the right atrium that surrounds the valvular orifice is the common location for slow-pathway ablations of AV node reentrant tachycardia. The Thebesian valve is a small, flat, crescentic flap of fibrous tissue that guards the orifice of the coronary sinus. It also shows variability in size and thickness, and is occasionally fenestrated. The atrial wall inferior to the coronary sinus os often forms a pouch known as the subeustachian sinus. The coronary sinus is the terminal portion of the great cardiac vein and is located posteriorly in the left atrioventricular groove. It is frequently covered by muscular fibers of the left atrium. The coronary sinus receives the veins draining the LV, including the great cardiac vein, posterior cardiac vein, left cardiac vein and anterior cardiac veins. The coronary sinus terminates in the inferoposterior aspect of the right atrium between the inferior vena cava. The ostia of the veins draining into the coronary sinus may be guarded by unicuspid or bicuspid valves.

Angiographic anatomy

In addition to an understanding of the gross anatomy of the right atrium and coronary sinus, the radiologic and angiographic anatomy is crucial to success in cardiac resynchronization. There are few papers devoted to the angiographic anatomy of the coronary sinus and coronary veins [21,22]. In an attempt to better define the angiographic anatomy of the coronary sinus, Gilard *et al.* studied 110 consecutive patients [23]. The venous phase of left coronary angiography was analysed in the right anterior oblique 30°, anteroposterior (AP), and left anterior oblique 60° projections. The precise radio-anatomic descriptions of the number, dimensions, angulations, and tortuosity of tributaries of the coronary sinus were recorded. The diameter of the coronary sinus ostium was also measured. The tributaries of the coronary sinus were described as follows: the great cardiac vein, originating in the lower middle third of the interventricular sulcus, courses the sulcus and turns toward the left side of the atrioventricular groove, entering the coronary sinus at an approximately 180° angle. Frequently, the valve of Vieussens coincides with the great cardiac vein ostium. The middle cardiac vein has an origin at the cardiac apex and courses within the posterior interventricular groove and drains into the coronary sinus just prior to the coronary sinus ostium. The left posterior vein arises from the lateral and posterior aspects of the LV, draining into the great cardiac vein or coronary sinus. The left oblique vein of Marshall is a coronary vein that courses diagonally on the posterior surface of the left atrium and joins the great cardiac vein at a point where it becomes the coronary sinus. In the antero-posterior view, the coronary sinus has its ostium superimposed over the posterior portion of the thoracic vertebrae at the level of the diaphragm. Unfortunately, these landmarks are extremely variable and of little value in individual cases. Anatomically, the coronary sinus ends at the level of the Thebesian valve and the great cardiac vein ends in the coronary sinus at the level of the Vieussens valve. The middle cardiac vein consistently arises in the coronary sinus near the coronary sinus ostium at an angle of 60–90°, approximately 1 cm from the coronary sinus ostium. The great cardiac vein in the anteroposterior view demonstrates considerable variability, curving toward the atrioventricular groove. Past the curve, the great cardiac vein maintains an axis parallel to the coronary sinus. There is considerable variability with respect to tortuosity and diameter. The posterior

RAO Projection

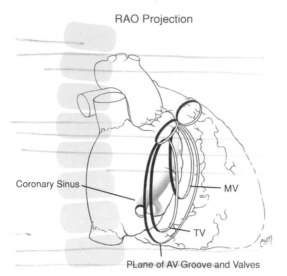

Figure 1.2 Heart rotated in the right anterior oblique view showing the relationship of the atrioventricular groove and spin.

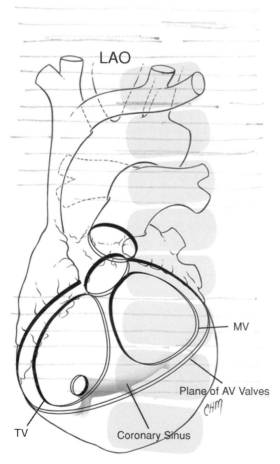

Figure 1.3 Heart rotated in the left anterior oblique view where the atrioventricular groove is tipped horizontally.

veins originate from the posterior and lateral aspects of the LV and join the coronary sinus or great cardiac vein. The posterior veins are highly variable in number, size and angulation. In general, this study demonstrated wide variation in the number and size of the left posterior veins. Occasionally, these veins were quite diminutive and even absent. In the frontal plane, the right ventricle occupies most of the cardiac silhouette as an anterior structure. The upper half of the right heart border is formed by the superior vena cava, while the lower portion is formed by the lateral wall of the right atrium. The plane of the lateral valve is sandwiched between the anterior right ventricle and posterior LV. It can be conceptualized as an oval ring tipped somewhat to the left. The coronary sinus is located at the inferior aspect of the cardiac silhouette at the level of the diaphragms, approximately in the midline. Cannulation of the coronary sinus in this view can be somewhat difficult. The 30–60° right anterior oblique projection, however, rolls the right ventricle to the left. In this projection, the superior and inferior vena cavae and right atrium become an anterior structure. The plane of the tricuspid and mitral valves becomes more vertical and perpendicular to the anteroposterior plane. The right ventricle is pushed to the left. In the frontal projection, the coronary sinus runs obliquely from a right inferior position to a left superior position in the cardiac silhouette. As the heart is rotated to the right anterior oblique projection, the coronary sinus is tipped more superiorly (Figure 1.2). In the left anterior oblique projection, the plane of the tricuspid and mitral valves becomes frontal, with the coronary sinus tipped in a more horizontal position, crossing over the spine as it courses to the left, crossing over the spine from right to left and turning superiorly along the left heart border (Figure 1.3). In the right and left anterior oblique projections, the os of the coronary sinus can be found at the inferior aspect of the cardiac silhouette at the level of the diaphragms just to the right of the spine. Rotating from the right anterior oblique to the left anterior oblique projection and back becomes extremely important when trying to cannulate the coronary sinus os. As a simple example, when in the frontal projection, the catheter may appear to be in the vicinity of the coronary sinus os with a trajectory pointing inferiorly and to the left, but when the image is rotated to the left anterior oblique projection, the catheter actually is 180° away from the coronary sinus os, pointing anteriorly and to the right. After adjusting the catheter to a posterior and leftward position, the right anterior oblique projection may show the catheter pointing laterally to the right, away from the coronary sinus os. Thus, the use of multiple views becomes essential for coronary sinus os cannulation.

Use of the left anterior oblique (LAO) projection is extremely important in defining the tributaries of the coronary sinus (Plate 1.3, facing p. 84). In the frontal and right anterior oblique projections, tributaries of the coronary sinus appear to run perpendicular to the coronary sinus obliquely from a superior to an inferior direction (Plate 1.4, facing p. 84). The branches appear to be parallel, and differentiation of anteroseptal, lateral and posterolateral branches is almost impossible. For simplicity and for the purpose of this discussion, branches or tributaries of the coronary sinus are described from their ostia in the coronary sinus. In the LAO projection, the great cardiac vein or anterior cardiac vein comes off the coronary sinus superiorly to the right. It then turns acutely, descending inferiorly and to the right in the interventricular septum. The lateral and posterolateral branches of the coronary sinus generally come off the superior aspect, but arc superiorly and inferiorly to the left, crossing over to the left of the spine. The posterior branches generally come off the coronary sinus at right or acute angles, directed inferiorly and to the left of the spine. Reporting on his cardiac resynchronization experience, Niazi has noted the importance of understanding the right atrial anatomy and pointed out the variations in the coronary sinus and its angulations [24]. It is noted that these directly relate to guiding catheter selection for catheterizing the coronary sinus os. In addition, further analysis of the coronary sinus anatomy has demonstrated considerable variation in the branch anatomy. When viewed from the outside, Niazi considers the right atrium a tubular structure as opposed to a simple sac joined by the inferior and superior vena cavae. The synchronization experience demonstrates the importance of understanding the presence of the Thebesian valve and the eustachian valve, as well as the valve of Vieussens. Valvular structures and fossae of the right atrium can usually be demonstrated by simple puffs of contrast from the guiding catheter. The puffs of contrast are extremely useful in distinguishing fossae from the

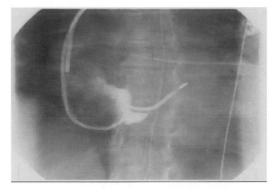

Figure 1.4 Puffs of contrast through the guiding catheter defining the coronary sinus os and lower right atrial anatomy. Image courtesy of Imran Niazi, MD.

coronary sinus os itself (Figure 1.4). It is important to distinguish the subeustachian fossa, the pouch beneath the eustachian ridge and the eustachian valve, as it can make coronary sinus cannulation extremely difficult. In patients presenting for resynchronization therapy, it was noted that the annulus of the tricuspid valve was extremely dilated and that the right atrial anatomy was considerably distorted. The tricuspid valve annulus was dilated, as well as the various fossae, and occasional muscular ridges were encountered. These distortions and alterations in the right atrium rendered coronary sinus ostial cannulation extremely difficult. Niazi's study of 82 patients with heart failure noted that the right atrial size varied between 20 and 53 mm [24]. Approximately 70% of the right atria were dilated and there was a 75% incidence of mild to moderate tricuspid regurgitation. As well as variations in the right atrial anatomy, coronary sinus os size, height of origin, shape, diameter and angulation as well as the presence of valves were also noted. The coronary sinus angulation varied from shallow to extreme superior angulation. The coronary sinus varied from very small to large, in addition to variations in angulation. Coronary sinus os variations were noted, from an extremely wide and funnel-shaped to a small coronary sinus os occasionally covered with the Thebesian valve. Niazi studied 52 patients with heart failure and noted that the diameter of the coronary sinus ranged between 2 and 22 mm [24]. The shape of the coronary sinus also varied from tubular to wafer or funnel (Figure 1.5a–c). In an evaluation of 48 patients, Niazi noted that 20% of the coronary sinus angulations were sharp superior,

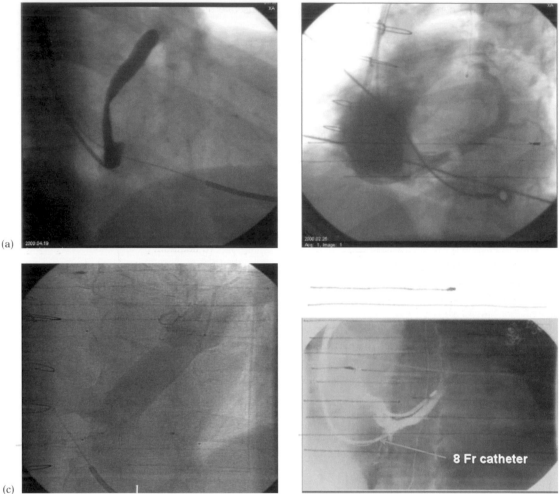

(a)
(b)
(c)
(d)

Figure 1.5 (a) Flat vertical coronary sinus (from [24] with permission). Image courtesy of Imran Niazi, MD. (b) Funnel-shaped coronary sinus. Image courtesy of Imran Niazi, MD. (c) Large superiorly angulated coronary sinus. Image courtesy of Imran Niazi, MD. (d) Small superiorly angulated coronary sinus. Image courtesy of Imran Niazi, MD.

40% moderately superior, 15% horizontal and 25% inferior [24]. It appears that the angulation of the coronary sinus directly relates to the planes of the tricuspid and mitral valves. If the mitral valve is in a higher plane than the tricuspid, coronary sinus angulation will generally be upwards. In addition, coronary sinus angulation is also related to the size of the mitral valve annulus. The larger the mitral valve annulus, the more posteriorly displaced the coronary sinus is from its origin. In the case of a small mitral valve annulus, the degree of curvature posteriorly of the coronary sinus generally appears to be somewhat less. In addition to variations to the coronary sinus and its os, considerable branch vari-

ation was also noted by Niazi. The branches have been noted to vary in angle of branch take-off, size, the presence of valves and extreme tortuosity. The experience of Niazi and others has underscored the need to be prepared for considerable variation in the coronary sinus os and coronary sinus vein anatomy. Transverse branches of the coronary sinus have been noted to have considerable variations, from shallow take-off to acute take-off.

Implantation

LV pacing has undergone considerable evolution in its short history. Initially, pacemaker electrodes were placed in the coronary sinus using a stylet-driven technique. This has evolved to the currently acceptable use of contrast venography with a guiding catheter for either a stylet-driven or some form of guidewire-assisted placement.

Preoperative planning

An echocardiogram can be very helpful in defining marked structural changes associated with advanced CHF. Marked LV hypertrophy, dilatation of tricuspid and mitral annuli, and extreme right atrial dilatation may alert the operator to possible structural changes in the coronary sinus os, and its location and size.

Coronary sinus lead placement often requires contrast venography. It is therefore important to check the blood urea nitrogen and creatinine levels before the procedure because CHF patients often have renal insufficiency. If renal function is impaired, the patient should be optimally hydrated, the volume of contrast material minimized and the contrast material diluted if necessary. In extremely advanced renal failure, premedication with flumazicon has proven helpful. The patient's fluid therapy during the procedure must be carefully monitored because patients can easily develop severe CHF and pulmonary edema.

In general, the support personnel required to carry out biventricular pacing are similar to those utilized for a permanent pacemaker or ICD procedure [25]. These include a nurse to administer drugs and deliver supplies to the surgical field, a scrub nurse or technician familiar with all the particular needs of the implanting physician, and a cardiovascular technician familiar with the operation of sophisticated radiologic equipment. The same individual can assist with the electrophysiologic measurements. Unlike a simple pacemaker procedure, it is recommended that an anesthesiologist be present to administer conscious sedation or general anesthesia. Patients requiring cardiac resynchronization are extremely ill and may require airway support by an anesthesiologist. Biventricular pacing systems from a variety of manufacturers are complex, with many components unique to particular manufacturers. A highly trained manufacturer's representative can occasionally be invaluable during the procedure. In addition, as the newer delivery systems for coronary sinus leads incorporate the tools of interventional cardiology, the support cardiovascular technician should be thoroughly familiar with the tools and techniques of interventional cardiology.

The cardiac catheterization laboratory is the ideal place for cardiac resynchronization procedures. It offers high-quality images and easily obtainable multiple projections required for coronary sinus lead placement. The cardiac catheterization laboratory is also the resource for a variety of catheters, guidewires, sheaths or angiographic material that may be required in any given situation. It is also the location of sophisticated physiologic recording and monitoring equipment.

The establishment of 12-lead electrocardiographic monitoring is often useful in determining LV capture. In addition, patient monitoring equipment should include an automated blood pressure cuff, continuous oxygen saturation monitoring, and intravascular arterial and venous pressure monitoring.

The procedure usually requires a minor surgical tray with a limited number of instruments. A simple pacemaker or implantable cardioverter defibrillator (ICD) surgical tray is more than adequate [26]. Today, most manufacturers offer a complete delivery system for implantation of their coronary sinus leads. These systems generally include a percutaneous lead introduction kit with needles, syringes and guidewires, peel-away introducers, an assortment of guiding catheters, adjustable hemostatic valve systems, coronary sinus lead, and an assortment of lead stylets. In the case of the over-the-wire lead system, multiple angioplasty stylets are available. An example of lead delivery components is shown in Table 1.1.

Table 1.1 Components of delivery system for coronary sinus cannulation.

1 Percutaneous introducer kit: sheath with hemostatic valve, multiple sizes
2 Guide catheters: multiple shapes and lengths
3 Hemostatic valves with optional flush system
4 Balloon catheters
5 Angiographic contrast material
6 Guidewires
7 Lead stylets
8 Interventional guidewires
9 Electrophysiologic catheters, preformed and deflectable
10 Angioplasty guidewires

The biventricular procedure may be performed with either general anesthesia or conscious sedation. Most centers recommend conscious sedation to avoid the risks of general anesthesia. There is a divergence of opinion with respect to the use of general anesthesia, and some groups consistently use general anesthesia with no untoward complications.

If a resynchronization patient is to undergo coronary angiography, the operator is encouraged to perform a forward angiogram demonstrating the venous or levo phase to localize the coronary sinus. The coronary venous anatomy is visualized during the levo phase after injection of the left main coronary artery in both the left anterior and right anterior oblique projections. Cine-angiography is continued through the visualization of the coronary system and then continued through the venous system, delineating the great cardiac vein, all major tributaries and the coronary sinus with its os. In addition, in anticipation of actually having to perform coronary angiography during the resynchronization procedure, in the case of extreme difficulty in cannulating the coronary sinus, the right groin should be prepped and draped in readiness.

Equipment and delivery systems

The initial placement of permanent pacemaker electrodes in tributaries of the coronary sinus was performed by a simple stylet-driven approach. This approach proved to be quite difficult because of the distorted anatomy of large dilated hearts and the variability in the coronary sinus anatomy. These problems led to the development of a number of delivery systems to expedite location, cannulation and coronary sinus lead placement [27]. Each manufacturer has developed a delivery system unique to its particular coronary sinus electrode (Figure 1.6). Most systems consist of an introducer kit for venous access, hemostatic valves, and an assortment of guiding catheters and guidewires. The guiding catheters are preformed in a number of shapes for rapid coronary sinus access. A number of sheaths with hemostatic valves are also used for guiding catheter stabilization and ease of manipulation. The delivery system also consists of a balloon catheter for the performance of venography within the coronary sinus (Figure 1.7). Hemostatic valve components of the delivery system are important, to prevent not only back-bleeding but also the aspiration of air and air embolization.

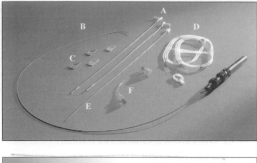

(a)

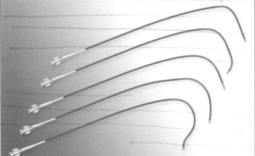

(b)

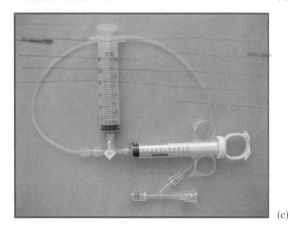

(c)

Figure 1.6 (a) Straight lead delivery sheaths with soft distal tips (A), steerable delivery system catheter (B), with slitters (C), guidewires (D), dilator (E) and hemostasis valve (F); Medtronic Model 6218. Courtesy of Medtronic, Inc. (b) Family of guiding catheters with multiple distal tip curves. (c) Hemostatic valve and flush system. Courtesy of Guidant Corporation.

Implantation procedure

The transvenous route is ideally performed in the cardiac catheterization laboratory. Although the operating room offers optimal sterility, the cardiac catheterization laboratory has all of the tools and equipment for both pacemaker and angioplastic procedures. The fluoroscopy should offer storage capability and readily available cine-angiography.

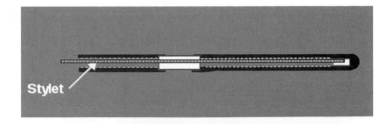

Figure 1.7 Diagram of a stylet-driven lead. Courtesy of Guidant Corporation.

Table 1.2 Endocardial approaches for coronary sinus left ventricular lead placement.

---

1 Free lead—stylet driven
2 Guiding catheter assisted with free lead—stylet driven
3 Free over-the-wire—guidewire driven without the use of a guide catheter
4 Guiding catheter-assisted, over-the-wire

A 12-lead electrocardiogram is essential so that proper LV lead placement and capture can be documented. Both pectoral areas and one groin are surgically prepped. A flush system should also be set up to allow for flushing of the delivery system and ease of delivery of contrast.

Table 1.2 lists the endocardial approaches for positioning of a lead in a tributary vein of the coronary sinus for LV pacing. The simplest approach uses a stylet-driven lead but this technique can be problematic. A more desirable approach employs a guiding catheter with a stylet-driven lead. Even with a guiding catheter for localization and cannulation of the coronary sinus os, the stylet-driven approach has proven somewhat difficult. The conventional stylet-driven approach for lead placement precludes the accessibility of distal coronary sinus branches, often necessary for successful LV pacing. Figure 1.8 shows an example of a simple stylet-driven electrode. The lead is preformed in a curve to facilitate placement of the lead tip in the appropriate branch of the coronary venous system. The curve also helps stabilize the lead in the coronary sinus branch to prevent dislodgement. Drawing on interventional and angioplasty techniques, pacemaker wires were adapted for an over-the-wire and side-wire approach [28]. A number of electrode designs incorporate different tip shapes and angulations for coronary sinus branch fixation. The monorail or side-wire lead design encorporates a small loop or ring on the lead tip that tracks over a guide wire. This design has been largely abandoned because

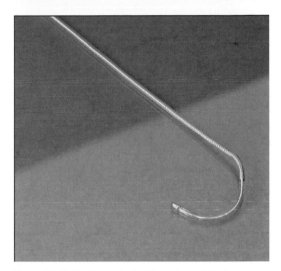

Figure 1.8 Stylet-driven lead with preformed tip for support in the coronary sinus

a tortuous anatomy requiring frequent wire exchanges makes repositioning of the guide wire through the loop or ring difficult. The over-the-wire design appears ideal at this time. Using angioplastic guidewires, distal tortuous branches of the coronary sinus can now be accessed with lead placement in a desired coronary sinus tributary (Figure 1.9).

Venous access

A number of venous access techniques are available for insertion of the multiple leads for biventricular pacing (Table 1.3). Venous access is required for three electrodes: the coronary sinus lead and its delivery system, an RV lead and a right atrial lead. One approach places up to three sheaths percutaneously with three separate venous access sites: repeated access to the subclavian or axillary vein carries the increased risk of pneumothorax and access failure. A combination procedure consists of a cut-down (for right atrial and RV leads) and a percutaneous approach (for the LV lead). Another approach uses two percutaneous punctures, one for

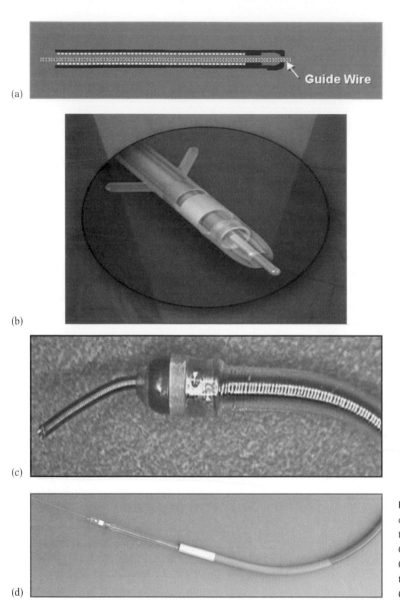

(a)

(b)

(c)

(d)

Figure 1.9 (a) Stylized drawing of over-the-wire lead design. Two over-the-wire leads: (b) EASY trak by Guidant Corporation and (c) Attain OTW by Medtronic. (d) Lead exiting the guiding sheath over the wire. Courtesy of Guidant Corporation.

RV and atrial electrode insertion, and a second for the coronary sinus lead and delivery system. More recently, a single axillary venous stick has been used based on the principles of the retained guidewire [29,30] for successful placement of all three electrodes.

A 4 or 5 French sheath is passed over the guidewire. The dilator is removed and the initial guidewire retained. A second 0.037-inch guidewire is passed down the sheath. The sheath is removed, thereby leaving two intravascular guidewires. One of the guidewires is secured to the drape for future use. A hemostatic sheath is then passed over the initial guidewire. The coronary sinus lead (stylet-driven) may be passed and positioned in a branch of the coronary sinus through this hemostatic sheath. Alternatively, a delivery system may be passed through the hemostatic sheath: guiding catheter and a coronary sinus lead (stylet-driven, or an over-the-wire system).

With regard to the sequence of lead placement, some operators prefer placing the RV electrode first for potential emergency RV pacing because of the risk of complete AV block related to trauma to the

Table 1.3 Venous access for biventricular pacing.

1 Three separate percutaneous sticks—multiple venous entry sites.

2 Combination of percutaneous sticks and cutdown with or without retaining the guidewire, resulting in multiple venous entry sites.

3 Single percutaneous venous puncture with retention of the guidewire for sequential placement of multiple sheaths.

4 Single venous entry via cutdown. The vein is cannulated with a guidewire and sheath (Ong–Barold technique). The retained guidewire technique is used for sequential placement of multiple sheaths.

right bundle branch during lead manipulation in patients with left bundle branch block. Other operators prefer to place the coronary sinus lead first and, if necessary, depend on rate support via a temporary transvenous pacemaker placed via the femoral vein. The issue of a possible unsuccessful LV procedure favors placing the coronary sinus lead first. Should the LV procedure fail and the right-sided electrodes have been already placed, a pacing system will have been implanted without an indication, unless of course a future second attempt is contemplated. The possibility of placing a right-sided system without a clear indication has become less problematic in view of the MADIT II criteria for prophylactic ICD implantation [31].

Locating and cannulating the coronary sinus os

Locating the coronary sinus os can be problematic in the case of distorted anatomy. Table 1.4 outlines the techniques devised to cannulate the coronary sinus. With a simple stylet-driven lead coronary sinus placement, the coronary sinus access depends on the operator's skill and knowledge of the anatomy for safe and reliable placement. Localization of the coronary sinus os is much easier with a guiding

Table 1.4 Locating the coronary sinus os.

1 Puffs of contrast material in the right atrium through guiding catheter
2 Direct cannulation with guiding catheter
3 Electrophysiologic catheter through guiding catheter
4 0.035-inch guidewire through guiding catheter
5 Levophase coronary angiogram
6 Femoral vein coronary sinus cannulation

catheter delivery system. The operator simply selects the guiding catheter that best fits a given anatomy and attaches a hemostatic valve. A flush system is also incorporated for delivery of contrast. As the guiding catheter is positioned in the low right atrium, puffs of contrast may be injected to define the anatomy in the vicinity of the eustachian valve and even the location of the coronary sinus os (Figure 1.10). A popular technique for locating and cannulating the coronary sinus os uses an electrophysiologic (EP) catheter specifically designed for this purpose (Figure 1.11). This catheter comes with either a preformed or a deflectable tip. An alternative approach utilizes a 0.035-inch guidewire passed via the guide catheter in an attempt to locate and cannulate the coronary sinus os. The guidewire technique is often successful and is safe. The use of a deflectable EP catheter offers the capability of adjusting catheter shape to accommodate the right atrium. The EP catheter can also provide electrical confirmation of successful coronary sinus placement. An EP catheter provides excellent support for the guiding catheter because it has more consistency than a guidewire. However, the EP catheter carries the risk of dissection. When the guiding catheter is used for locating the coronary sinus os, the use of contrast puffs in the right atrium frequently demonstrates retrograde flow from the coronary sinus os producing an angiographic pattern that assists in its localization. Occasionally, the guiding catheter itself will pass directly into the coronary sinus because of favorable anatomy and selection of the correct tip curve of the deflecting catheter. After locating the coronary sinus os, the guide catheter may be simply advanced directly into the coronary sinus. If the guide catheter fails to cannulate the coronary sinus, a guidewire or EP catheter should be used. The guidewire or EP catheter is passed down the guiding catheter and manipulated into the coronary sinus. After coronary sinus cannulation, the guiding catheter is gently advanced over the guidewire or EP catheter, stabilizing its position in the coronary sinus. Once the guiding catheter is positioned some distance in the coronary sinus, the guidewire or EP catheter is removed. Standard angiographic catheters with and without a guidewire have also been used for the above maneuver. Once the guiding catheter is in place, its location within the coronary sinus is confirmed by the injection of puffs of contrast material.

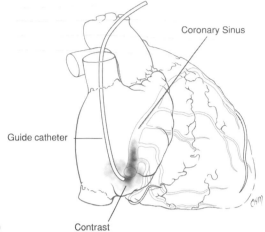

Coronary Sinus

Guide catheter

(a)   Contrast

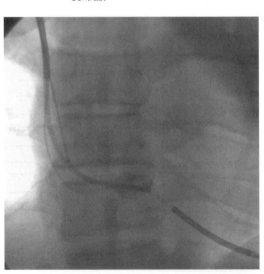

(b)

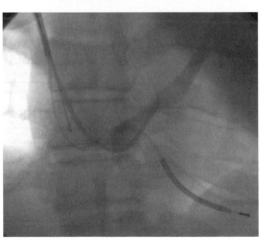

(c)

Occasionally irritation may cause coronary sinus spasm and constriction. In this case, coronary sinus cannulation should be attempted with an 0.035-inch guidewire instead of the deflectable EP catheter.

The coronary sinus may be guarded by or contain valves that may interfere with cannulation. In extreme circumstances, the coronary sinus may be catheterized via the femoral vein. The femoral catheter may then be used to hold the valve open while the guiding catheter is introduced into the coronary sinus from above.

Finally, as a general rule, if cannulation of the coronary sinus os proves very difficult, it is important to consider alternative catheters and methodology within a reasonable period of time. No more than 15 or 20 min should be spent on any given approach. In extreme instances, if a left-sided venous access proves unsuccessful for coronary sinus cannulation, switching to right-sided venous access may be useful.

Contrast venography

Contrast venography is performed to visualize the anatomy of the coronary venous system, tributaries and target branch [32]. The operator must be completely familiar with the fluoroscopic coronary venous anatomy in multiple projections. The AP projection is least helpful in defining the coronary sinus branch anatomy.

A venogram is usually obtained by using an occlusive balloon catheter to prevent washout of contrast caused by venous flow into the right atrium. The occlusive venogram provides good visualization of distal vein branches. Small puffs of contrast should be used for localization of the balloon tip. Caution is required to prevent balloon overinflation and possible vascular dissection. The initial balloon inflation should be approximately half to assess the required level of inflation for total occlusion. Visualization also ensures that the balloon catheter tip is not against a vessel wall or in a tributary. The balloon catheter should be positioned in the middle

Figure 1.10 (*left*) (a) A puff of contrast through the guide catheter helps locate the coronary sinus (CS) os by outlining the anatomy of the lower right atrium and CS os. (b) Radiograph showing the guide catheter in the lower right atrium. The puff of contrast outlines the fossa close to the CS os. (c) The contrast puff shows that the guide catheter has now engaged the CS os. Courtesy of Guidant Corporation.

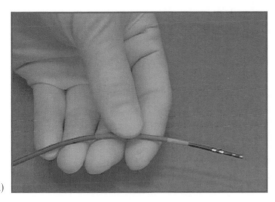
(a)

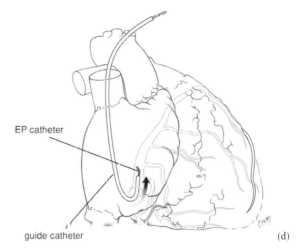
(b)

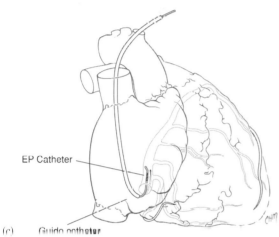
(c)   Guide catheter

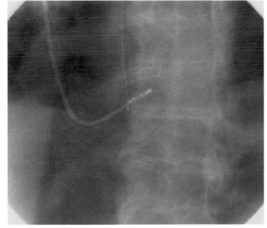

(e)

Figure 1.11 (a) Electrophysiology (EP) catheter for passing down guiding sheath. (b) Alternative method using a 0.037-inch guidewire down the guiding catheter. (c) EP catheter passed down the guiding sheath and engagement of the coronary sinus (CS). (d) Guiding catheter advanced over the EP catheter into the CS. (e) Radiograph of EP catheter in the CS through the guiding catheter. (a), (b) and (e), Courtesy of Guidant Corporation.

of the coronary sinus to optimize branch definition. If the balloon catheter is advanced too distally, contrast may be injected beyond the desirable lateral or posterior branches, precluding their visualization (Figure 1.12). Venograms should be performed in both the right anterior oblique and left anterior oblique projections (Figure 1.13a,b). Occasionally, a minor dissection may occur. This is usually caused by a forceful injection of contrast into the vessel wall. A minor dissection appears as transient staining. Minor dissections are considered benign and of no clinical consequence and the procedure can be

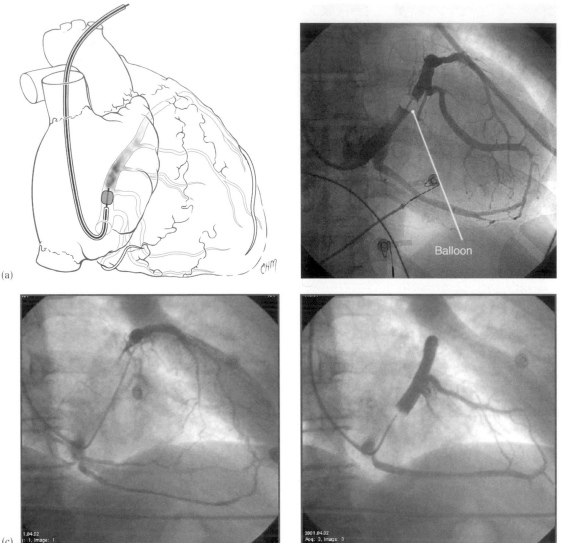

(a)

(b)

(c)

Figure 1.12 (a) Coronary sinus (CS) balloon catheter through guiding catheter. (b) Contrast venography using inflated balloon. (c) The venogram in the right panel with the balloon catheter advanced too distally conceals the more desirable proximal posterolateral branches. In the left panel the balloon catheter was positioned more proximally, revealing the lateral branches. (c) Courtesy of Guidant Corporation.

continued. A persistent large area of staining may indicate a larger dissection and the operator may choose to discontinue the procedure.

Right-sided lead placement

The RV and right atrial leads are placed using standard techniques. Initial right-sided placement offers pacing in case of complete AV block, assists in locating the coronary sinus os and precludes manipulation that could dislodge the coronary sinus lead. On the other hand, initially placed right heart leads are vulnerable to dislodgement during cannulation of the coronary sinus.

Lead positioning

With the guiding catheter safely positioned in the coronary sinus and the target coronary sinus tributary identified, the coronary sinus lead is positioned. If a stylet-driven approach is used, success depends on operator experience and skill, coronary sinus

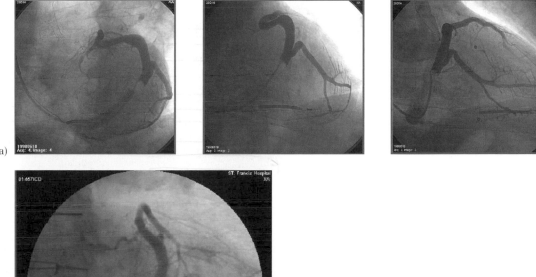

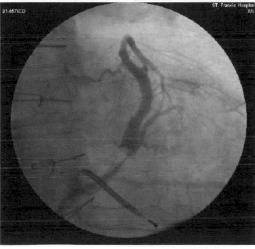

Figure 1.13 (a) Venogram of the coronary sinus (CS). Left anterior oblique, anteroposterior and right anterior oblique projections from right to left. (b) Venogram of the CS demonstrating the marked variability of the CS. In this example there are no true left lateral or posterolateral branches. Courtesy of Guidant Corporation.

anatomy, lead stylet selection and stylet management. Stylet management refers to the configuration or shape of the distal stylet and the firmness of the stylet itself. Most manufacturers offer a spectrum of stylet flexibility, but even in the best of circumstances, successful positioning is directly dependent upon coronary sinus anatomy. Success depends on the correct selection of lead, stylet and curve configuration. With the over-the-wire approach, appropriate guidewire selection and handling are essential. The operator must be familiar with guidewire design and selection, the indications for use, and the benefits of each type of guidewire. These skills are currently possessed by the interventional cardiologist and now are essential to the electrophysiologist. The variations in the coronary sinus anatomy necessitate the use of guidewires of different designs to navigate the vasculature and reach desirable locations. Today, there is a constellation of guidewires designed for the over-the-wire technique (Figure 1.14). In essence, they range from extremely flexible to less flexible or rigid. The tips of the guidewires can be curved and shaped to negotiate the turns of the desired tributary of the coronary sinus. These guidewires allow the lead to advance easily to the coronary sinus branches. Appropriate guidewire selection offers support for lead delivery and strengthens the force of the lead through the desired vein. The curve applied to the tip of the guidewire enables the wire to navigate acute angles and prolapse across coronary sinus venous valves. Both the over-the-wire and guidewire-directed coronary sinus leads are passed into the guiding catheter through a hemostatic valve. In the over-the-wire technique, the lead is advanced over the guidewire and lodged into the desired tributary branch. With the over-the-wire technique, a torquing device on the guidewire assists in the selection and penetration into the appropriate vein. Occasionally, when advancing the guidewire and/or lead, the guiding catheter dislodges from the coronary sinus. Therefore, it is important during lead positioning to observe lead movement, guidewire stability, and position of the guiding catheter simultaneously. If

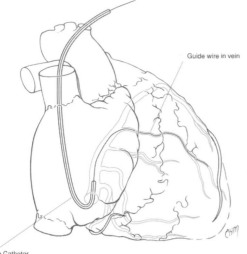

(a) Guide Catheter

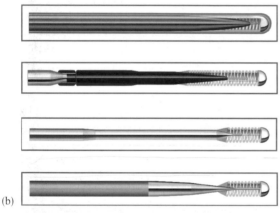

(b)

Figure 1.14 (a) Guidewire in a posterolateral branch of the coronary sinus. (b) Example of the various angioplasty guidewires for use in over-the-wire lead techniques for lead implantation.

the guiding catheter retracts, forward pressure and lead advancement should be stopped. The guidewire should always be positioned in the most distal possible position in the desired vein branch before advancing the lead over it. Like the stylet and lead in the stylet-driven system, the over-the-wire technique is a learned skill, and the operator will develop his or her own technique for appropriate lead advancement, and guidewire management. Initial placement calls for a posterolateral vein but another branch can be used if the posterolateral vein is unattainable (Figure 1.15). Adequate lead position, as verified by electrical performance, should be undertaken with partial withdrawal of the guidewire back into the lead.

Threshold testing

The initial biventricular (BiV) systems incorporated 'dual unipolar pacing'. In this configuration, unipolar leads were placed either endocardially or epicardially. Using a Y-adapter, one lead was connected to the anode and the other to the cathode. The bipolar Y-adapter was then connected to a bipolar device with a single ventricular port. This system has also been called split bipolar pacing. These systems have been abandoned because of high-threshold problems. Dual site cathodal stimulation is now commonly used. This arrangement stimulates LV and RV cathodes simultaneously through an internal or external Y-adapter with a connection between the two cathodes and anodes, respectively. Dual cathodal ventricular stimulation can have several configurations.

1 Two unipolar leads with a Y-adapter are connected to the negative pole of a unipolar pacemaker and the positive pole of the pacemaker can.

2 The 'shared common-ring bipolar' or 'extended bipolar' system is presently the most commonly used system. The RV lead is bipolar and the LV lead is unipolar. The LV lead shares the ring or anode of the RV lead. This configuration allows for extended bipolar pacing of the LV lead and limits sensing to the heart, thereby avoiding myopotential oversensing or muscle stimulation seen with configuration 1.

3 The 'dual ventricular bipolar' is the most desirable configuration of the future, in which both the RV and LV leads are bipolar, and independently programmable to enable easy and precise determinations of acute and chronic BiV, RV and LV thresholds and sensing (Figure 1.16).

In presently available dual cathodal systems where the outputs to both chambers and sensing are common and simultaneous, the absence of independent outputs for separate pacing of each ventricle makes determination of the individual RV and LV threshold problematic at the time of follow-up. There is no problem during implantation in testing the RV and LV independently using standard threshold testing techniques. Yet, when testing is performed in a biventricular system through a Y-adapter configuration, defining biventricular, RV, and LV thresholds can be difficult and frustrating as it is during follow-up testing of the chronic thresholds. Occasionally, the RV and LV thresholds are nearly identical, and determining loss of capture in a given ventricle can be challenging. Usually,

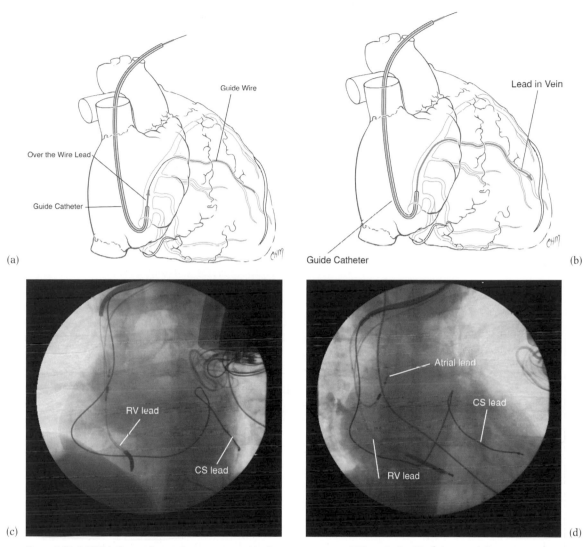

Figure 1.15 (a) With the guiding catheter supported in the coronary sinus (CS) os, the lead for left ventricular pacing is advanced over the guidewire. (b) Over-the-wire left ventricular lead placed in the distal part of the posterolateral branch of the CS. (c) Radiograph of the CS lead in the right anterior oblique projection and (d) left anterior oblique projection.

the threshold is determined by reducing the pulse amplitude or pulse duration until there is loss of capture in the chamber with the highest threshold.

Threshold testing is a two-step process. First the LV threshold is determined. If this is unacceptable or complicated by diaphragmatic stimulation, the lead requires adjusting or repositioning. If the unipolar LV threshold is acceptable, the biventricular threshold is then determined. Present LV leads with only one electrode at the tip are tested in the unipolar mode for threshold measurement so that the cath-

ode is connected to the lead tip. Threshold testing requires identification of loss of capture in one ventricle, then both (Figure 1.17a,b). This requires monitoring surface ECG, markers, and the ventricular electrogram to establish the template or morphology of LV, RV and BiV capture. Capture threshold is usually determined by decrementing the pulse amplitude in volts with the pulse width maintained at 0.5 ms. The measured pacing impedance reflects the combination of the two ventricular leads in parallel and is therefore less than the individual

Ventricular Lead Polarity

Shared Common Ring Bipolar Sensing/Pacing

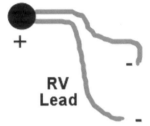 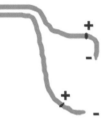 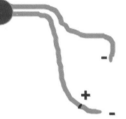

(a) Dual Ventricular Unipolar   **(b) Dual Ventricular Bipolar**   **(c) Shared Common Ring Bipolar**

Figure 1.16 Diagrammatic representation of the various ventricular lead configurations: (a) dual unipolar (split bipolar); (b) dual bipolar; and (c) shared common ring 'bipolar'.

impedances. The sensing threshold is a combination of sensing from both ventricles. It is important to monitor the biventricular electrogram for:

1. far-field sensing of the atrial electrogram to avoid inhibition of biventricular pacing. This form of oversensing is usually associated with basilar LV electrode positions and is less common with the more posterolateral LV positions achieved by the over-the-wire leads. Far-field atrial sensing on the ventricular channel is best determined using the marker channels through the device. Furthermore, as far-field atrial sensing may occur with later lead displacement, ventricular sensitivity is best programmed at about 5 mV to prevent this form of oversensing; and

2. prevention of double counting and inappropriate shocks in biventricular ICDs. Sufficient separation of the RV and LV electrograms is important if a biventricular ICD with common RV and LV sensing is being implanted. Double counting may also occur with far-field atrial sensing.

The biventricular threshold should be < 3.0 V (3.0 V is borderline) at 0.5 ms pulse duration. The endocardial R-wave signal should be = 5 mV. Pacing impedance should range between 300 and 1000 Ω (Table 1.5). Lead repositioning in another branch is necessary with unacceptable thresholds,

Table 1.5 Acceptable biventricular pacing and sensing thresholds.

1 Voltage threshold = 3.0 V at 0.5 ms pulse duration
2 R-wave amplitude = 5.0 mV
3 Pacing impedance 300–1000 Ω

or extracardiac and diaphragmatic stimulation. Phrenic nerve or diaphragmatic stimulation can be problematic and is usually associated with the more posterior branches of the coronary sinus. To exclude the possibility of extracardiac stimulation, LV pacing should be tested in the unipolar or extended bipolar configurations at outputs of 10 V or greater. Although extracardiac stimulation may sometimes be avoided by decreasing voltage output and increasing pulse duration to maintain capture, most cases of extracardiac stimulation require repositioning of the coronary sinus electrode into another vein.

Removing the guiding catheter

After successful positioning of the coronary sinus lead, the delivery system sheath and guiding catheter should be left in place if the right-sided leads have not been placed. In this situation, the guiding

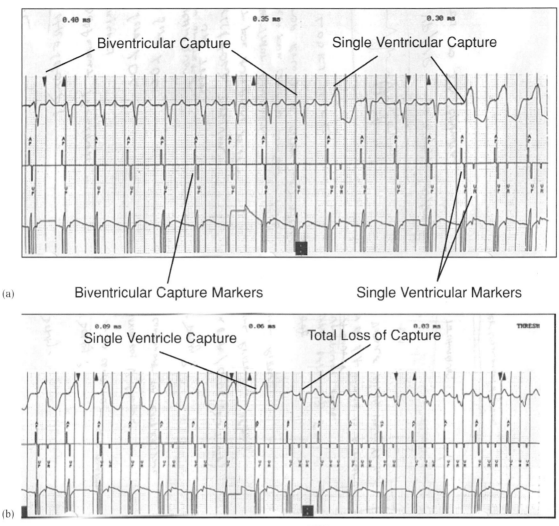

Figure 1.17 (a) Biventricular threshold testing. The left side of the strip shows biventricular capture. As the output of the pacemaker is decreased, there is intermittent capture of either the right or left ventricle as indicated by a change in QRS configuration. (b) Further decrease in the output causes total loss of ventricular capture.

catheter and sheath offer stability to prevent dislodgement of the coronary sinus lead. With previous implantation of the right-sided system, it is necessary to remove the delivery system, lead, stylet, guidewire, guiding sheath and the initial entry hemostatic sheath. This part of the procedure is critical because removal of guidewires and sheaths can easily dislodge the coronary sinus lead. The guiding catheter and introducer sheaths must be peeled or slid away without dislodging the lead. This procedure requires lead stabilization while guiding catheters and sheaths are removed. Guiding catheters can be removed by two techniques. One technique involves sliding the guiding sheath while stabilizing the lead in a simultaneous maneuver. A second technique utilizes careful retraction of the guiding catheter over the coronary sinus lead, stabilizing the lead with a stylet. Both techniques require an acquired skill, operator experience, extreme patience and care. If an outer peel-away sheath is used, its prior removal requires skill in maintaining lead and guiding catheter stability. Once the guiding catheter has been removed and stable lead position confirmed, all supporting guidewires or stylets may finally be removed. The lead is then secured, and tied down by use of the suture sleeve.

Table 1.6 Complications.

1 Air embolization
2 Minor coronary sinus dissection
3 Major coronary sinus dissection
4 Coronary sinus perforation
5 Cardiac tamponade
6 Diaphragmatic stimulation
7 Arrhythmias such as far-field atrial sensing

Complications

Although safe, transvenous LV lead placement via the coronary sinus is associated with some potentially life-threatening complications. The major complications are listed in Table 1.6.

The procedure with conscious sedation carries the risk of aspirating large quantities of air causing air embolization, which can be obviated by adequate patient preparation and utilization of sheaths incorporating hemostatic valves and guiding catheters equipped with hemostatic mechanisms.

Major coronary sinus dissection may occur during introduction of the guiding catheter or EP catheter, or during balloon angiography, either from trauma or from overexpansion of the balloon catheter (Figure 1.18). A major dissection requires termination of the procedure, careful monitoring, and a repeat attempt postponed for several weeks.

Occasionally the guiding catheter, guiding catheter, EP electrode or lead may cause coronary sinus perforation, which is easily diagnosed with contrast venography. This complication is a medical emergency, and the patient should be evaluated with echocardiography and hemodynamic monitoring, and managed in a critical care unit.

Extracardiac stimulation is not life-threatening but very bothersome. Diaphragmatic stimulation is more common with posterolateral coronary sinus branch placement. At the time of implantation, this problem should always be ruled out by LV and biventricular pacing at 10 V in the unipolar or extended bipolar configurations. Extracardiac stimulation mandates lead repositioning in a new tributary or a completely new branch.

Upgrading

When a patient with a pre-existing pacemaker

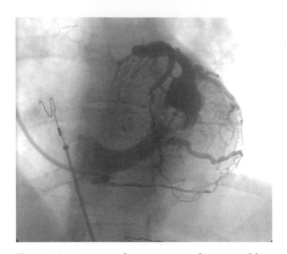

Figure 1.18 Angiogram demonstrating a dissection of the coronary sinus. Courtesy of Guidant Corporation.

system requires ventricular resynchronization, the procedure can be simply performed by the addition of a coronary sinus lead adapted to a dedicated biventricular pacemaker. Despite concerns about venous access, it can usually be easily accomplished. If the patient requires a biventricular ICD, two new leads are needed: a ventricular lead for pacing and shocking capability, and a coronary sinus lead for LV pacing. Consequently, extraction of the inactive leads must be considered. Clinical experience has shown that extraction is not absolutely necessary because the addition of an ICD and coronary sinus leads to a pre-existing dual-chamber system is usually accommodated without complications. In terms of venous access, the question arises as to whether to reaccess the venous circulation with a single or multiple punctures. Using the principle of the retained guidewire has proven to be extremely successful in this operator's experience. In extreme instances, the contralateral subclavian or axillary vein may be used, and tunneling techniques to advance the additional leads back to the original pocket [33]. Upgrade approaches are shown in Table 1.7.

Epicardial approach

Recently, thoracoscopic approaches, less risky than thoracotomy, have been developed for the placement of left ventricular leads [22,34–36]. The issues of lead instability and unreliable sensing/pacing characteristics remain problematic. On the

Table 1.7 Upgrading techniques for biventricular pacing and ICD systems.

---

1 Add coronary sinus lead ipsilaterally
2 Add coronary sinus lead contralaterally with tunneling
3 Add coronary sinus lead plus endocardial pacing and shocking electrode ipsilaterally
4 Add coronary sinus lead ipsilaterally plus contralateral endocardial pacing and shocking electrode placement
5 Add coronary sinus lead, extract chronic ventricular electrode, add endocardial pacing and shocking electrode ipsilaterally
6 Add coronary sinus lead and endocardial pacing and shocking electrode contralaterally with extraction of chronic lead system ipsilaterally

---

horizon is a percutaneous epicardial technique utilizing robotics for left-sided lead placement.

Conclusions

LV lead implantation for cardiac resynchronization therapy calls upon the skills of device implantation techniques, electrophysiologic monitoring and interventional/angioplasty techniques. A thorough knowledge of both the gross and radiologic anatomy is essential for success of the procedure. The tools for cardiac resynchronization are still quite inadequate at this juncture for swift LV lead placement but they continue to undergo rapid evolution [37]. With the development of tools for rapid access of the coronary sinus os and precise sites in the coronary venous system, the procedure will most probably become shorter and safer in the future. In addition, it is quite possible that the development of an improved epicardial approach using modern robotics may ultimately pave the way for reliable implantation of LV leads. At present, given the current development tools and techniques, the operator requires extreme patience and persistence.

References

1 Abraham WT, Fisher WG, Smith AL et al. Cardiac resynchronization in chronic heart failure. *N Engl J Med* 2002; **346**: 1845–53.
2 Saxon LA, DeMarco T. Cardiac resynchronization: a cornerstone in the foundation of device therapy for heart failure. *Am J Cardiol* 2001; **38**: 1971–3.

3 Stellbrink C, Breithardt AO, Franke A et al. Impact of cardiac resynchronization therapy using hemodynamically optimized pacing of left ventricular remodeling in patients with congestive heart failure and ventricular conduction disturbances. *J Am Coll Cardiol* 2002; **38**: 1957–65.
4 Grass D, Leclercq C, Tang AS et al. Cardiac resynchronization therapy in advanced heart failure, the Multicenter Insync clinical study. *Eur J Heart Fail* 2002; **4**: 311–20.
5 Auricchio A, Stellbrink C, Sack S. Long-term clinical effect of hemodynamically optimized cardiac resynchronization therapy in patients with heart failure and ventricular conduction delay. *J Am Coll Cardiol* 2002; **39** (12): 2026–33.
6 Auricchio H, Kloss M, Trautmann SL et al. Exercise performance following cardiac resynchronization therapy in patients with heart failure and ventricular conduction delay. *Am J Cardiol* 2002; **89**: 198–203.
7 Linde C, Leclercq C, Rex S et al. Long-term benefits of biventricular pacing in congestive heart failure, results from the multisite stimulation in cardiomyopathy (MUSTIC) study. *J Am Coll Cardiol* 2002; **40**: 111–18.
8 Leporte V, Pizzarelli G, Dernevik L. Inadvertent trans-atrial pacemaker insertion: an unusual complication. *Pacing Clin Electrophysiol* 1987; **10**: 951–4.
9 Daubert JC, Ritter P, Le Breton H et al. Permanent left ventricular pacing with transvenous leads inserted into the coronary veins. *Pacing Clin Electrophysiol* 1998; **21**: 239–45.
10 Greenberg P, Castellanett M, Messenger J et al. Coronary sinus pacing. *Circulation* 1978; **57**: 98–103.
11 Hunt D, Sloman G. Long-term electrode catheter placement from coronary sinus. *Br Med J* 1968; **4**: 495–6.
12 Spitzberg JW, Milstoc M, Wertheim AR. An unusual site for ventricular pacing occurring during the use of the transvenous catheter pacemaker. *Am Heart J* 1969; **77**: 529–33.
13 Kemp A, Johansen JK, Kjaergaard E. Malplacement of endocardial pacemaker electrodes in the middle cardiac vein. *Acta Med Scand* 1976; **199**: 7–11.
14 Shattigar UR, Loungani RR, Smith CA. Inadvertent permanent ventricular pacing from the cardiac vein: an electrocardiographic roentgenographic and echocardiographic assessment. *Clin Cardiol* 1989; **12**: 267–269.
15 Bai Y, Strathmore N, Mond H et al. Permanent ventricular pacing via the great cardiac vein. *Pacing Clin Electrophysiol* 1994; **17**: 678–83.
16 Bakker PF, Meijburg H, de Jonge N et al. Beneficial effects of biventricular pacing in congestive heart failure [abstract]. *Pacing Clin Electrophysiol* 1994; **17**: 820.

17 Cazeau S, Ritter P, Bakdach S *et al.* Four-chamber pacing in dilated cardiomyopathy. *Pacing Clin Electrophysiol* 1994; **17**: 1974–9.

18 Netter FH. In: Yonkman FF, ed. *Ciba Collection of Medical Illustrations*, Vol. V. *Heart*. New Jersey: Summit, 1969: 8.

19 Yen Ho S, Anderson RH, Sanchez-Quintana D. Rose structure of the atriums: more than an anatomical curiosity. *Pacing Clin Electrophysiol* 2002; **25**: 342–50.

20 Ho S. Understanding atrial anatomy: implications for atrial fibrillation ablation. In: *Cardiology International for a Global Perspective on Cardiac Care*. London: Graycoat Publishing Ltd, 2002: S17–S20.

21 Cabrera JA, Sanchez-Quintana D, Ho SY *et al.* Angiographic anatomy of the inferior right atrial isthmus in patients with and without history of common atrial flutter. *Circulation* 1999; **99**: 3017–23.

22 Jansens JL, Jottrand M, Preumont N *et al.* Cardiac resynchronization therapy with robotic thoracoscopy [abstract]. *Europace* 2002; **3**: 92.

23 Gilard M, Mansourati J, Etienne Y *et al.* Angiographic anatomy of the coronary sinus and its tributaries. *Pacing Clin Electrophysiol* 1998; **21**: 2280–4.

24 Niazi I. Power point presentation on cardiac anatomy. St Paul, MN: Guidant, 2002.

25 Belott PH, Reynolds DW. Permanent pacemaker and implantable cardioverter defibrillator implantation. In: Ellenbogen KA, Kay GN, Wilkoff BL, eds. *Clinical Cardiac Pacing and Defibrillation*, 2nd edn. Philadelphia: W.B. Saunders Company, 2000: 578–9.

26 Belott PH, Reynolds DW. Permanent pacemaker and implantable cardioverter defibrillator implantation. In: Ellenbogen KA, Kay GN, Wilkoff BL, eds. *Clinical Cardiac Pacing and Defibrillation*, 2nd edn. Philadelphia: W.B. Saunders Company, 2000: 576–7.

27 Blanc JJ, Benditt D, Gilard M *et al.* A method for permanent transvenous left ventricular pacing. *Pacing Clin Electrophysiol* 1998; **21**: 2021–4.

28 Auricchio A, Klein H, Tockman B *et al.* Transvenous biventricular pacing for heart failure: can the obstacles be overcome? *Am J Cardiol* 1999; **83**: 136–42.

29 Belott PH. Retained-guidewire-introducer technique for unlimited access to the central circulation: a review. *Clin Progr Electrophysiol Pacing* 1983; **1**: 59–63.

30 Belott PH. A variation on the introducer technique for unlimited access to the subclavian vein. *Pacing Clin Electrophysiol* 1981; **4**: 43–8.

31 Moss AJ, Zareba W, Hall WJ *et al.* Prophylactic implantation of a defibrillator in patients with myocardial infarction and reduced ejection fraction. *N Engl J Med* 2002; **346**: 877–83.

32 Meisel E, Pfeiffer D, Engelmann L *et al.* Investigation of coronary venous anatomy by retrograde venography in patients with malignant ventricular tachycardia. *Circulation* 2001; **104**: 442–7.

33 Belott PH. Use of the contralateral subclavian vein for placement of atrial electrodes in chronically VVI paced patients. *Pacing Clin Electrophysiol* 1983; **6**: 781–3.

34 Kleine P, Grönefeld G, Dogan S *et al.* Robotically enhanced placement of left ventricular epicardial electrodes during implantation of a biventricular implantable cardioverter defibrillator system. *Pacing Clin Electrophysiol* 2002; **25**: 989–91.

35 McVenes R. The future of left ventricular stimulation: transvenous, endocardial or epicardial? [abstract]. *Europace* 2002; **3**: A13.

36 SantAnna J, Prates P, Kalil R. Robotically assisted implantation for biventricular stimulation [abstract]. *Europace* 2002; **3**: A92.

37 Daoud E, Kalbfleisch S, Hummel J *et al.* Implantation techniques and chronic lead parameters of biventricular pacing dual-chamber defibrillators. *J Cardiovasc Electrophysiol* 2002; **13**: 971–9.

CHAPTER 2

Pacing in Vasovagal Syncope: Are Too Many or Too Few Pacemakers Implanted?

David G. Benditt and Mary E. McGrory-Usset

Introduction

Published recommendations from the American College of Cardiology/American Heart Association (ACC/AHA) [1], the British Pacing and Electrophysiology Group (BPEG) [2] and the European Society of Cardiology guidelines task force on the management of syncope [3] endorse cardiac pacing therapy for selected patients with recurrent vasovagal syncope. It is likely that, given the body of evidence available, the current deliberations by the pacemaker indications guidelines committee of the European Society of Cardiology will follow suit. Thus, the most important agencies governing appropriate use of cardiac pacing therapy concur on the potential value of pacing for prevention of recurrent vasovagal faints.

Despite this favorable institutional attitude, cardiac pacemakers remain infrequently used in the treatment of vasovagal syncope. This chapter examines the evidence addressing pacemaker treatment strategy in vasovagal syncope, and attempts to quantitate the current status of pacing for this indication.

Considerations in treatment selection

Current strategies for treatment to prevent recurrent vasovagal syncope comprise: (i) education and reassurance; (ii) salt and volume management usually in conjunction with physical maneuvers; (iii) pharmacologic therapies; and (iv) cardiac pacing. The first three of these approaches, although continually evolving, have been the subject of several recent reviews [3–5] and lie outside the scope of this chapter.

In the vast majority of individuals who experience vasovagal faints, the events are solitary (or exceedingly infrequent), and without long-term consequences. These individuals, if they seek medical advice at all, require primarily education and reassurance. Not infrequently, however, patients may experience numerous syncopal or near-syncopal episodes over an extended period of time. In such cases, the addition of salt and volume counseling, and perhaps physical maneuvers (e.g. tilt-training, leg crossing [6–8]), may be sufficient. Occasionally, drugs are also needed (e.g. beta-adrenergic blockers, midodrine [9–12]) although their efficacy (with perhaps the exception of midodrine [11,12]) remains the subject of considerable uncertainty.

Notwithstanding the fact that most vasovagal syncope patients can be managed with the treatment strategies noted above, there is nevertheless a subset of afflicted individuals in whom prevention of vasovagal symptom recurrences requires more aggressive medical intervention. For example, some patients may be extremely alarmed at the prospect of a recurrence. Others may have suffered economic loss (e.g. job loss, insurance issues, driving restrictions) due to their susceptibility to recurrent faints. In yet others, syncope may have occurred without warning leading to an unacceptable risk of accident and physical injury. The latter scenario (i.e. absence of usual premonitory symptoms) is particularly prevalent in older patients with vasovagal spells [13]; these individuals are especially susceptible to fractures or other musculoskeletal injuries. Finally, even infrequent vasovagal recurrences may be unacceptable in certain occupational or avocation settings (e.g. pilots, machinery operators, commercial vehicle operators, window-washers, sky-divers, scuba-divers, etc.). It is in these scenarios that consideration of pacemaker implantation may be reasonable.

Selecting pacemaker candidates

Tilt-table testing has provided important insights into understanding of the electrophysiologic and hemodynamic features associated with vasovagal syncope. Findings suggest that the relative importance of bradycardia and vasodilatation varies among patients being evaluated for vasovagal syncope. Further, it seems that few patients exhibit either a 'pure' cardioinhibitory (i.e. bradycardia being the principal cause of the faint) or a 'pure' vasodilatation (i.e. vascular dilatation is the crucial factor causing systemic hypotension) syndrome. The vast majority of fainters appear to exhibit a combination of both features (i.e. 'mixed') [14–17]. However, subsequent clinical observations suggest that tilt-table findings may have underestimated the frequency with which marked bradycardia is crucial to symptom development in spontaneous vasovagal faints.

Initial studies examining the potential value of cardiac pacing in vasovagal syncope focused on symptomatic individuals in whom there was some evidence of a bradycardic component to the faint. In this regard, the VPS1 study utilized a relatively complex system to identify bradycardia [18]. The VASIS trial used a more intuitive classification scheme [16,19,20]. In both cases (see later), randomized controlled trials vs. conventional medical treatment at the time showed pacing to be highly effective in a subset of relatively symptomatic individuals with recurrent vasovagal faints. Conversely, absence of demonstrable bradycardia was used to exclude pacemaker candidacy. The recently reported ISSUE trial results now shed doubt on whether it is reasonable to exclude such individuals [21]. In fact, it appears that tilt-table testing (for reasons as yet unknown) may overestimate the importance of the vasodilatation component in vasovagal fainters.

Current status of evidence supporting pacing for vasovagal syncope

Initial studies of cardiac pacing efficacy undertaken in the tilt-testing laboratory found that pacing did not prevent induced vasovagal syncope; however, pacing did tend to prolong the presyncope warning period [3]. As a result, for many years the prevailing opinion was that cardiac pacing had either no role, or at best only a minor role, to play in treatment of patients with vasovagal faints. Nevertheless, pacing remained the subject of a number of small clinical studies, and the reader is referred to these non-randomized uncontrolled observational reports for the important background information they provide [22–28].

The validity of cardiac pacing as a treatment candidate for very symptomatic vasovagal fainters has been markedly altered following publication of the results of three randomized controlled trials [18,19,29]. Each of these demonstrated pacemakers to be effective for reducing syncope recurrence rates in patient populations characterized by multiple recurrent faints and some evidence of bradycardia. As noted earlier, the focus of the multicenter trials was treatment of individuals who appeared to demonstrate predominantly cardioinhibitory faints. In the case of the North American study, syncope recurrence rate was substantially less in the pacemaker group than in control patients. The result was an actuarial 1-year rate of recurrent syncope of 18% for pacemaker patients and 60% for controls [18]. The results of the VASIS trial [19] were similar to those of the North American study. However, VASIS comprised a longer follow-up in less severely affected patients than was the case in the VPS1 study. In VASIS, 5% of patients in the pacemaker arm experienced recurrence of syncope compared with 61% in the no-pacemaker arm during a mean follow-up of 3.7 years ($P = 0.0006$). More recently, Ammirati *et al.* [29] reported results in 93 patients (> 55 years of age) who had experienced > 3 syncopal events over a 2-year period of time, and who had positive tilt tests with evidence of bradycardia. Patients were randomized to either pacing (DDD mode with rate-drop algorithm, $n = 46$) or beta-adrenergic blocker therapy ($n = 47$). Paced patients had 2 syncope recurrences during a mean follow-up of 390 days, compared to 12 syncopal recurrences over a mean follow-up of 135 days in beta-blocker-treated patients.

In summary, several well-designed clinical studies support the validity of cardiac pacing therapy for patients with recurrent vasovagal syncope. Despite these observations, cardiac pacing appears to be only infrequently prescribed for this indication. In part this reluctance relates to the fact that many affected patients are young, whereas the trials examined primarily older individuals. Further, there remain uncertainties regarding the potential placebo effect associated with implantation of a medical device [5,30]. The latter concern was addressed retrospectively in the VPS1 study [18] by noting the absence of pacemaker impact on presyncopal symptoms. This same issue has also been assessed directly in VPS2 (in which all patients had devices implanted) [31]. The VPS2 study results did not show a statistically significant pacing benefit at 6 months follow-up, despite an apparent divergence in the curves suggesting a pacing benefit.

Pacemaker implantation rates for syncope: registry observations

The frequency with which pacemakers are currently implanted for vasovagal syncope is not precisely known. Even less well established is any quantitative estimate of the appropriate number of vasovagal syncope patients who warrant this form of therapy. We have, however, attempted to derive an estimate of implant frequency and trends for this indication from both a database maintained by a major pacemaker manufacturer (Medtronic, Inc., Minneapolis, MN) and a recent survey of pacemaker-implanting physicians regarding their thoughts on this issue.

The database was queried with regard to the monthly number of US pacemaker implantations designated for a primary indication of 'syncope', and more specifically for the 'primary' indication 'vasovagal syncope/carotid sinus syndrome' (VVS/CSS). Data are provided for the months September 2000 through March 2002. Over this time frame the method of device registration remained relatively constant with respect to syncope classification with the exception that VVS/CSS was separated out as a specific subgroup beginning February 2001 (Figures 2.1 & 2.2). Other indications, such as atrioventricular (AV) block or sinus node dysfunction,

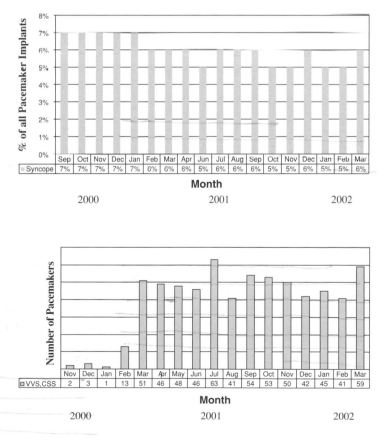

Figure 2.1 Graph depicting monthly pacemaker implantation rates for a 'primary' diagnosis of syncope from one major device manufacturer. Findings show a relatively stable rate of approximately 7% up to February 2001 at which time vasovagal syncope/carotid sinus syndrome (VVS/CSS) began to be classified separately. After February 2001, implants for a diagnosis of 'syncope' stabilized at 5–6% (see Figure 2.2 and text).

Figure 2.2 Graph illustrating the month-by-month frequency of pacemaker implantation for a 'primary' diagnosis of vasovagal syncope (VVS) or carotid sinus syndrome (CSS). After February 2001, the VVS/CSS implant rate ranges from 0.4 to 0.6% of all implants The apparent increment in VVS/CSS implant frequency in February 2001 relates to the registration card listing these conditions separately from the primary diagnosis of 'syncope' (see text for explanation).

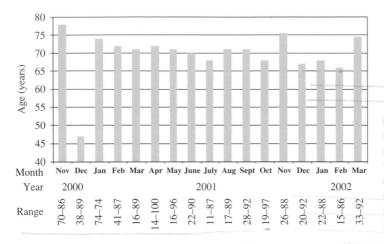

Month   Nov Dec Jan Feb Mar Apr May June July Aug Sept Oct Nov Dec Jan Feb Mar

Year   2000   2001   2002

Range   70–86 38–89 74–74 41–87 16–89 14–100 16–96 22–90 11–87 17–89 28–92 19–97 26–88 20–92 22–88 15–86 33–92

Figure 2.3 Graph indicating the trend in median patient age for individuals receiving pacemakers for a primary vasovagal syncope/carotid sinus syndrome (VVS/CSS) indication (see text). The apparent reduction in median patient age suggests that more VVS patients are being included.

in which 'syncope' may have been a secondary indication, were excluded.

Findings in Figure 2.1 suggest that 'syncope' (as a primary diagnosis) consistently accounted for approximately 5–6% of all pacemaker indications on a monthly basis for at least 13 months (i.e. after February 2001), but was about 7% prior to that time. For the purposes of this registry, 'syncope' can reasonably be assumed to encompass many conditions, but since VVS/CSS was identified as a separate diagnosis code beginning February 2001, we assume only a minor overlap with this group. In fact, prior to February 2001 (Figure 2.1), the 'syncope' category accounted for about 7% of pacemaker implants. Thus, assuming the difference between pre-February 2001 data and post-February 2001 data is due to separate classification of VVS/CSS, we conclude that VVS/CSS made up approximately 1% of all pacemaker implants. In support of this 1% estimate, Figure 2.2 depicts the monthly pacemaker implantation rates when either of these were considered the 'primary' diagnosis (i.e. when this code was separated out beginning February 2001). Again, the implantation rate has been relatively stable, comprising approximately 0.4–0.6% of all pacemaker implants each month. Although speculative, the difference between the 0.4–0.6% values, and the 1% noted above, may represent failure of some physicians to use the newly identified VVS/CSS category.

Whether there has been an overall trend towards greater use of pacemakers in VVS is the key issue of interest here. Unfortunately, a direct answer to this question is not available. However, as depicted in Figure 2.3, there appears to be a downward trend in

the age of patients receiving pacemakers in the VVS/CSS group. Albeit a tenuous interpretation, this latter observation could be taken to suggest that a greater number of VVS patients are entering the combined VVS/CSS pool. In any case, it is too early to tell whether the positive clinical trial results have had an impact on the use of pacemakers in VVS patients.

Physician inclination

The impact of published clinical trials on physician decision-making and subsequent clinical care patterns is often delayed. This careful attitude is likely to be exaggerated in instances such as vasovagal syncope in which the condition itself is considered to be relatively benign. However, ultimately lifestyle and morbidity concerns [32] can be expected to enter into the equation if the therapy itself is considered safe, effective and acceptable to most patients.

In order to assess the potential impact of clinical data on physician treatment inclination, a survey of 191 US physicians who implanted 25 or more pacemakers per year was undertaken. The venues were two large cardiology meetings in the US in the first half of 2001. Table 2.1 summarizes the estimated diagnosis breakdown of device implants by these physicians. Note that VVS (3%) and CSS (2%) accounted for approximately 5% of all indications. This number is consistent with the registration for 'syncope' summarized above, but significantly greater than device registration results for the newly added VVS/CSS primary diagnosis code. One conclusion from these results is that patients coded

Table 2.1 Physician survey: estimates of pacemaker implants for each diagnostic category.

Primary pacing condition	Total no. IPGs	% of total IPGs
Sinus node dysfunction, not drug-induced	4109	38
Atrioventricular block, not drug-induced	3569	33
Sinus node dysfunction or atrioventricular block, drug-induced	1190	11
Ablate and pace	649	6
Atrial tachyarrhythmia	324	3
Vasovagal syncope	324	3
Hypersensitive carotid sinus syndrome	216	2
Hypertrophic cardiomyopathy	216	2
DCM w/prolonged PR	216	2
Other	54	< 1
Total	10 867	100

IPG, implanted pulse generator; DCM, dilated cardiomyopathy.

Figure 2.4 Bar graphs illustrating percentage of physicians surveyed in the first half of 2001 who estimated that they had increased the number of pacemakers implanted for each of the diagnostic categories during the previous 2 years (light bars), or expected to increase the number during the following 2 years (dark bars). See text for discussion. Abbreviations: SND, sinus node dysfunction; Ab&P, ablate and pace; AVB, atrioventricular block; VVS, vasovagal syncope; CCS, carotid sinus syndrome; HOCM, hypertrophic cardiomyopathy.

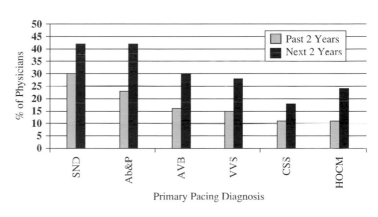

with the 'primary' diagnosis of 'syncope' in the registry may represent primarily VVS/CSS patients. Other conditions which cause syncope (e.g. AV block) presumably were listed appropriately in the specific registry categories which had been historically assigned to them.

Figure 2.4 summarizes the percentage of physicians surveyed who experienced an increase in pacemaker implantations for each diagnostic category over the previous 2 years, and the percentage who expected to increase implants for each diagnostic category over the following 2 years. In essence, about 25% of physicians surveyed expected to use pacing more frequently for VVS/CSS indications in the near future. Considering the robustness and consistency of the clinical trial data (i.e. following VPS1 [18] and VASIS [19], but prior to ISSUE [21], Rome [29] and SAFE PACE [31]), this finding

reflects the conservative stance present in the medical community at the time of the survey.

Conclusion

At the present time several randomized clinical studies support the view that cardiac pacing is of considerable value in selected symptomatic vasovagal syncope patients. The findings provided by VPS1 [18], VASIS [19] and the Rome trial [29] are very supportive while VPS2 [31] is less positive. Further, given findings from both the ISSUE study [21] and the RAST study [33], suggesting that bradycardia is more frequent in spontaneous vasovagal faints than had previously been expected (independent of findings in the tilt-table laboratory), pacing therapy may be applicable to a far larger vasovagal syncope population than has been previously acknowledged.

The size of the VVS population which might be better treated with cardiac pacing is currently unknown. Further, maximum benefit from this therapeutic avenue will not be attained until we achieve greater understanding of the spectrum of manifestations of vasovagal syncope and devise techniques to recognize onset of an episode at an early stage. Diagnostic features in current pacing systems for recognizing vasovagal syncope are limited; significant abrupt bradycardia must develop before a vasovagal event can be recognized, and pacing is triggered. In the future, more sophisticated sensor systems may prove helpful [34]. Nonetheless, even if pacing is restricted to the most severely affected individuals, it appears that this treatment option is markedly underutilized. Perhaps as the findings of the studies examining spontaneous arrhythmia in vasovagal syncope (i.e. ISSUE, RAST, ISSUE2) become more widely appreciated, the positive outcomes of the pacing clinical trials (VPS1, VASIS, Rome, and perhaps VPS2) will begin to have a greater impact on the overall fabric of clinical care in vasovagal fainters.

Acknowledgment

The authors would like to thank Barry L. S. Detloff for technical assistance, and Wendy Markuson for preparation of the manuscript.

References

1 Gregoratos G, Cheitlin MD, Conill A et al. ACC/AHA guidelines for implantation of cardiac pacemakers and antiarrhythmia devices: Executive Summary. A report of the American College of Cardiology/American Heart Association Task Force on Practice Guidelines (Committee on Pacemaker Implantation). *Circulation* 1998; **97**: 1325–35.

2 Clarke M, Sutton R, Ward D et al. Recommendations for pacemaker prescriptions for symptomatic bradycardia. British Pacing and Electrophysiology Group Working Party Report. *Br Heart J* 1991; **66**: 185–91.

3 Brignole M, Alboni P, Benditt DG et al. Guidelines on management (diagnosis and treatment) of syncope. *Eur Heart J* 2001; **22**: 1256–1306.

4 Benditt DG, Sakaguchi S, Lurie KG et al. Pathophysiology of neurally mediated syncope. In: Saksena S, Luderitz B, eds. *Interventional Electrophysiology: A Textbook*, 2nd edn. Armonk, NY: Futura Publishing Company, Inc., 1996: 133–43.

5 Sutton R. Therapy of vasovagal syncope: is there a role for drugs today? In: Raviele R, ed. *Arrhythmias*. Milan: Springer, 2001: 75–82.

6 Ector H, Reybrouck T, Heidbuchel H, Gewillig M, Van de Werf F. Tilt training: a new treatment for recurrent neurocardiogenic syncope or severe orthostatic intolerance. *Pacing Clin Electrophysiol* 1998; **21**: 193–6.

7 Di Girolamo E, Di Iorio C, Leonzio L, Sabatini P, Barsotti A. Usefulness of a tilt training program for prevention of refractory neurocardiogenic syncope in adolescents. A controlled study. *Circulation* 1999; **100**: 1798–1801.

8 Wieling W, Van Lieshout JJ, Van Leeuwen AM. Physical maneuvers that reduce postural hypotension in autonomic failure. *Clin Autonom Res* 1993; **3**: 57–65.

9 Milstein S, Buetikofer J, Dunnigan A, Benditt DG, Gornick C, Reyes WJ. Usefulness of disopyramide for prevention of upright tilt-induced hypotensionbradycardia. *Am J Cardiol* 1990; **65**: 1339–44.

10 Brignole M, Menozzi C, Gianfranchi L, Lolli G, Bottoni N, Oddone D. A controlled trial of acute and long-term medical therapy in tilt-induced neurally mediated syncope. *Am J Cardiol* 1992; **70**: 339–42.

11 Samniah N, Sakaguchi S, Lurie KG, Iskos D, Benditt DG. Efficacy and safety of midodrine hydrochloride in patients with refractory vasovagal syncope. *Am J Cardiol* 2001; **88** (1): 80–3.

12 Perez-Lugones A, Schweikert R, Pavia S et al. Usefulness of midodrine in patients with severely symptomatic neurocardiogenic syncope: a randomized control study. *J Cardiovasc Electrophysiol* 2001; **12**: 935–8.

13 Fitzpatrick A, Theodorakis G, Vardas P et al. The incidence of malignant vasovagal syndrome in patients with recurrent syncope. *Eur Heart J* 1991; **12**: 389–94.

14 Almquist A, Goldenberg IF, Milstein S et al. Provocation of bradycardia and hypotension by isoproterenol and upright posture in patients with unexplained syncope. *N Engl J Med* 1989; **320**: 346–51.

15 Fish FA, Strasburger JF, Benson DW Jr. Reproducibility of a symptomatic response to upright tilt in young patients with unexplained syncope. *Am J Cardiol* 1992; **70**: 605–9.

16 Sutton R, Petersen M, Brignole M et al. Proposed classification for tilt induced vasovagal syncope. *Eur J Cardiac Pacing Electrophysiol* 1992; **2**: 180–3.

17 Benditt DG, Goldstein MA, Adler S, Sakaguchi S, Lurie KG. Neurally mediated syncopal syndromes: pathophysiology and clinical evaluation. In: Mandel WJ, ed. *Cardiac Arrhythmias*, 3rd edn. Philadelphia: J. B. Lippincott Co, 1995: 879–906.

18 Connolly SJ, Sheldon R, Roberts RS, Gent M. Vasovagal pacemaker study investigators. Cardiac pacing for the prevention of vasovagal syncope. *J Am Coll Cardiol* 1999; **33**: 16–20.

19 Sutton R, Brignole M, Menozzi C *et al.* Dual-chamber pacing is efficacious in treatment of neurally mediated tilt-positive cardioinhibitory syncope. Pacemaker versus no therapy: a multicentre randomized study. *Circulation* 2000; **102**: 294–9.

20 Brignole M, Menozzi C, Del Rosso A *et al.* New classification of hemodynamics of vasovagal syncope: beyond the VASIS classification, analysis of the presyncopal phase of the tilt test without and with nitroglycerin challenge. Vasovagal Syncope International Study. *Europace* 2000; **2**: 66–76.

21 Moya A, Brignole M, Menozzi C *et al.* Mechanism of syncope in patients with isolated syncope and in patients with tilt-positive syncope. *Circulation* 2001; **104**: 1261–7.

22 McLeod KA, Wilson N, Hewitt J *et al.* Cardiac pacing for severe childhood neurally mediated syncope with reflex anoxic seizures. *Heart* 1999; **82**: 721–5.

23 Fitzpatrick AP, Travill CM, Vardas PE *et al.* Recurrent symptoms after ventricular pacing in unexplained syncope. *Pacing Clin Electrophysiol* 1990; **13**: 619–24.

24 Fitzpatrick A, Theodorakis G, Ahmed R, Williams T, Sutton R. Dual chamber pacing aborts vasovagal syncope induced by head-up 60 degree tilt. *Pacing Clin Electrophysiol* 1991; **14**: 13–19.

25 Samoil D, Grubb BP, Brewster P, Moore J, Temesy-Armos P. Comparison of single and dual chamber pacing techniques in prevention of upright tilt induced vasovagal syncope. *Eur J Cardiac Pacing Electrophysiol* 1993; **1**: 36–41.

26 Sra J, Jazayeri MR, Avitall B *et al.* Comparison of cardiac pacing with drug therapy in the treatment of neurocardiogenic (vasovagal) syncope with bradycardia or asystole. *N Engl J Med* 1993; **328**: 1085–90.

27 Petersen MEV, Chamberlain-Webber R, Fizpatrick AP, Ingram A, Williams T, Sutton R. Permanent pacing for cardio-inhibitory malignant vasovagal syndrome. *Br Heart J* 1994; **71**: 274–81.

28 Benditt DG, Sutton R, Gammage M *et al.* Clinical experience with Thera DR rate drop response pacing algorithm in carotid sinus syndrome and vasovagal syncope. *Pacing Clin Electrophysiol* 1997; **20**: 832–9.

29 Ammirati F, Colivicchi F, Santini M *et al.* Permanent cardiac pacing versus medical treatment for the prevention of recurrent vasovagal syncope. A multicenter, randomized, controlled trial. *Circulation* 2001; **104**: 52–6.

30 Benditt DG. Cardiac pacing for prevention of vasovagal syncope [editorial]. *J Am Coll Cardiol* 1999; **33**: 21–3.

31 Connolly SJ, Sheldon R, Thorpe KE *et al.* Pacemaker therapy for prevention of syncope in patients with recurrent severe vasovagal syncope. Second vasovagal pacemaker study (VPSII): a randomised trial. *JAMA* 2003; **289**: 2224–9.

32 Kenny RAM, Richardson DA, Steen N *et al.* Carotid sinus syndrome: a modifiable risk factor for nonaccidental falls in older adults (SAFE PACE). *J Am Coll Cardiol* 2001; **38**: 1491–6.

33 Krahn A, Klein GJ, Yee R, Skanes AC. Randomized assessment of syncope trial. Conventional diagnostic testing versus a prolonged monitoring strategy. *Circulation* 2001; **104**: 46–51.

34 Benditt DG. Hemodynamic sensors: clinical value in vasovagal syncope. In: Raviele A, ed. *Cardiac Arrhythmias*. Milan: Springer, 2001: 602–7.

CHAPTER 3

Unusual Indications for Cardiac Pacing

Chu-Pak Lau, Hung-Fat Tse, Kathy Lai-Fun Lee and S. Serge Barold

Introduction

Originally a primary therapy for patients with symptomatic bradyarrhythmias, cardiac pacing is now increasingly used for non-traditional indications without bradycardia or conduction system disease [1–5]. This chapter reviews some of the unusual indications for permanent pacing with emphasis on recent and controversial developments. The role of pacing for atrial fibrillation, congestive heart failure and neurocardiogenic syncope is covered in other chapters of this book.

Unusual conditions in atrioventricular block

First-degree atrioventricular block
The hemodynamic disturbance produced by marked first-degree atrioventricular (AV) block (> 0.30 s) has been called the 'pacemaker syndrome without a pacemaker' [6] because inadequate timing of atrial and ventricular systole forms the basis of the pacemaker syndrome. Both sinus rhythm with a very long PR interval and VVI pacing with retrograde ventriculoatrial conduction are associated with a P wave too close to the preceding ventricular complex and share the same abnormal physiology [7–9] (Figures 3.1 & 3.2). Hence symptomatic patients with marked first-degree AV block are sometimes described as having the 'pseudopacemaker syndrome' [10]. The 1998 joint American College of Cardiology and American Heart Association (ACC/AHA) guidelines for pacemaker implantation state that 'first-degree AV block with symptoms suggestive of pacemaker syndrome and documented alleviation of symptoms with temporary pacing' constitutes a class II indication [11]. This recommendation for a dual-chamber pacemaker with a more physiologic AV interval applies primarily to patients with basically well-preserved left ventricular (LV) function. (Patients with a poor LV fraction < 35% should be considered for biventricular pacing especially in the setting of congestive heart failure.) Invasive hemodynamic measurements may be helpful in questionable cases but need not be routine [3]. During a resting study it may not be possible to demonstrate symptomatic improvement, and the execution of exercise studies with a temporary dual-chamber pacemaker in place is difficult. An invasive hemodynamic study (that entails risk and cost) is not mandatory in patients with preserved LV function if the diagnosis is obvious and the PR interval does not shorten during an exercise test in association with effort intolerance.

A DDD pacemaker can restore a relatively normal AV interval, but it necessarily induces a paced sequence from the right ventricle that can adversely affect cardiac hemodynamics and LV myocardial perfusion and function [12–16]. Thus, in the individual patient with a long PR interval (LPRI) as an isolated abnormality, the clinician must decide whether there will be a net benefit provided by two opposing factors: a positive effect from AV delay optimization with a shorter AV delay, and a negative inotropic effect produced by pacing-induced aberrant ventricular depolarization. This determination can sometimes be made clinically and non-invasively, but a hemodynamic study with temporary pacing may be required in selected cases (Figure 3.3). In this respect, Iliev et al. [17] recently compared the AAI and DDD modes in patients with sick sinus syndrome (DDD pacemakers) and native but long AV conduction in otherwise normal hearts. At a pacing rate of 70 p.p.m. at rest, there

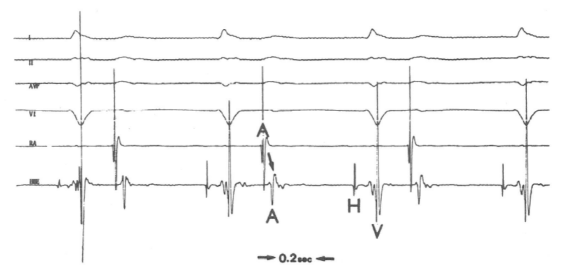

Figure 3.1 Surface ECG and intracardiac recording from a patient with symptomatic marked first-degree atrioventricular block. RA, high right atrial electrogram; HBE, electrogram at site of His bundle recording. Note the sequence of atrial activation (RA to HBE) is consistent with sinus rhythm and rules out retrograde atrial activation. The AH interval is markedly prolonged.

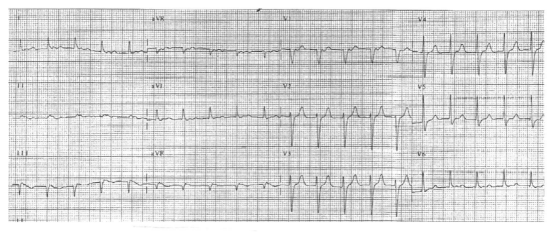

Figure 3.2 Twelve-lead ECG in the same patient as in Figure 3.1. During sinus tachycardia the sinus P wave is close to the preceding QRS complex on the initial portion of the T segment. This pattern mimics a reentrant supraventricular tachycardia.

was no overall difference in the aortic flow time velocity integral (which reflects cardiac output) during AAI and DDD pacing. However, when the patients were divided according to the AV interval (AVI), those with AVI < 270 ms showed a higher aortic flow velocity integral during AAI pacing. When the AVI was > 270 ms, the aortic flow velocity integral was higher during DDD pacing. These workers established that during DDD pacing the resultant increments in cardiac output were greater with longer native AV intervals. Conversely, with a normal or near-normal PR interval, a higher cardiac output was found during AAI pacing with a conducted QRS complex and spontaneous ventricular depolarization. Knowing the physiology of the LPRI syndrome, it is not surprising these workers found that at a pacing rate of 90 p.p.m., DDD was superior to AAI pacing. These data provide an important guideline in the management of patients with LPRI in that the improvement with pacing outweighs the negative impact on LV function when the PR interval is > 0.28 s.

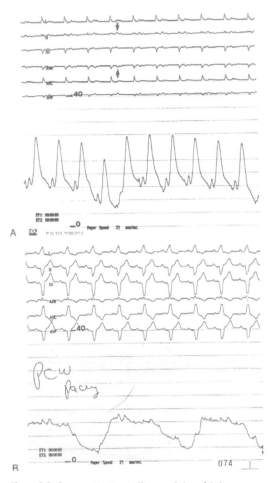

Figure 3.3 Same patient as in Figures 3.1 and 3.2.
(a) Pulmonary capillary wedge pressure shows large
cannon waves during sinus rhythm with a very long
PR interval (scale 0–40 mmHg). (b) Note the normal
pulmonary capillary wedge pressure after temporary
dual-chamber pacing with a physiologic atrioventricular
delay (scale 0–40 mmHg).

Pacing in patients with first-degree AV block may
be associated with functional atrial undersensing
sustained by circumstances that direct the P wave
toward the postventricular atrial refractory period
(PVARP) and the preceding ventricular complex
(Figures 3.4 & 3.5) [7,18]. The combination of a relatively fast sinus rate and prolonged AV conduction
provides a favorable setting for the development of
functional atrial undersensing [19–21]. During
functional atrial undersensing the electrocardiogram (ECG) shows sinus rhythm, a long PR interval
(exceeding the programmed AV delay) and con-

ducted QRS complexes but no pacemaker stimuli.
The P waves remain trapped in the PVARP and the
conducted QRS complexes activate the ventricle.
Functional atrial undersensing can be initiated and
terminated by appropriately timed atrial and ventricular extrasystoles [18].

Optimal pacing. During functional atrial undersensing patients may be symptomatic, with complaints
suggestive of the pacemaker syndrome [19].
Pacemaker syndrome secondary to functional atrial
undersensing differs from the other conditions associated with pacemaker syndrome in that the pacemaker remains inhibited and the hemodynamic
abnormality stems from the disturbed relationship
of spontaneous atrial and ventricular activity. In
effect the pacemaker functions as a bystander to the
hemodynamic situation. Functional atrial undersensing can also occur with a short programmed
PVARP whenever a ventricular extrasystole activates an automatic PVARP extension [18]. In this
situation an unsensed P wave within the extended
PVARP gives rise to a conducted QRS complex
which the pacemaker interprets as a ventricular
extrasystole whereupon it generates another
PVARP extension. The extended PVARP is perpetu-
ated from cycle to cycle as long as the pacemaker
interprets the conducted QRS as a ventricular
extrasystole.

Functional atrial undersensing can often be corrected or reduced by shortening the PVARP and AV
delay [19]. A relatively short PVARP can often be
used to prevent functional atrial undersensing
because retrograde VA block is common in patients
with first-degree AV block. Automatic mode switching may have to be turned off in devices where
the algorithm controls the PVARP duration as
a function of the tachycardia detection rate.
Other programming maneuvers may be useful, but
symptomatic refractory cases of functional atrial
undersensing should undergo ablation of the AV
junction [22,23].

Provocable AV block
Exercise
Permanent pacing is recommended as a class I indication in symptomatic or asymptomatic patients with
exercise-induced AV block (absent at rest) because
most cases are due to tachycardia-dependent block
in the His–Purkinje system and carry a poor prog-

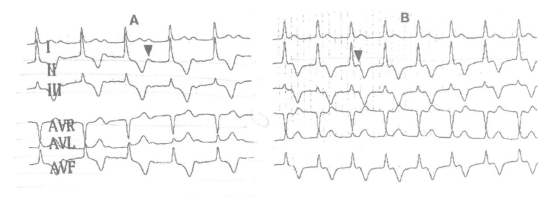

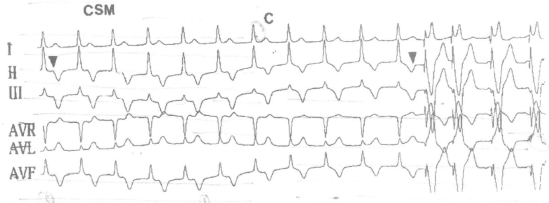

Figure 3.4 Six-lead ECG showing marked first-degree atrioventricular (AV) block and sinus tachycardia in a patient with a DDD pacemaker. The postventricular atrial refractory period (PVARP) was 360 ms. The arrowheads point to sinus P waves. (a) Sinus rhythm at a rate of 88 b.p.m. with an RP interval of approximately 360 ms. Note the positive P wave near the end of the T wave in leads I, II, III and aVF. (b) Sinus tachycardia at a rate of 112 b.p.m. and a longer PR interval than in panel (a). The RP interval now measures only 150 ms. At that time the PVARP was shortened to 200 ms, but the tachycardia continued. (c) Carotid sinus massage (CSM) caused a gradual slowing of the sinus rate with eventual restoration of AV synchrony. The arrowhead points to a P wave beyond the 200 ms PVARP. The succeeding two ventricular stimuli occur after completion of the upper rate interval. The basic AV delay was 120 ms and, the rate-adaptive function was programmed on (from [21] with permission).

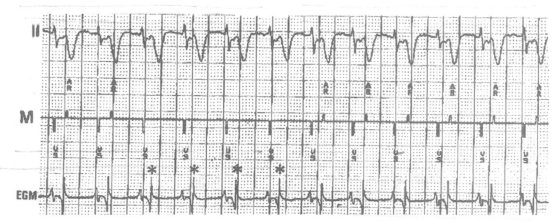

Figure 3.5 Same patient as in Figure 3.4. PVARP = 360 ms. There is sinus tachycardia at a rate of 110 b.p.m. and a long PR interval. The RP interval was about 150 ms. The pacemaker detects P waves in the 360 ms PVARP but not when the RP interval becomes shorter than the 150 ms postventricular atrial blanking period (no AR representation—asterisks). AR, atrial event sensed in the PVARP; AS, atrial sensed event; EGM, electrogram; M, markers; VS, ventricular sensed event. Paper speed = 25 mm/s (from [21] with permission).

nosis in terms of the development of complete AV block [3,24–27]. This form of AV block is often reproducible in the electrophysiologic laboratory by rapid atrial pacing (provided the atrial rate is increased gradually to avoid functional infra-Hisian block) because it is tachycardia dependent and rarely due to AV nodal disease. AV block secondary to myocardial ischemia occurring during exercise (or spontaneously) is rare and does not require pacing unless ischemia cannot be alleviated [28].

During electrophysiologic study
Barring a markedly prolonged HV interval [11], when an electrophysiologic study is performed for the evaluation of syncope, many workers believe that AV block or delay in the following circumstances constitutes an indication for permanent pacing.

1 Second- or third-degree His–Purkinje block induced by a 'stress test' of the conduction system that involves rapid atrial pacing performed in stages with a gradual increase in the rate. It is widely believed that His–Purkinje block induced by gradually increasing rates of atrial pacing, although an insensitive sign of conduction system disease, should be listed as a class I indication for permanent pacing (provided functional infranodal block is ruled out) because it correlates with a high incidence of third-degree AV block or sudden death [24, 29].

2 The fatigue phenomenon in the His–Purkinje system is a rare manifestation of conduction disease in which anterograde infranodal AV block, sometimes not inducible by rapid atrial pacing, occurs following cessation of ventricular burst pacing generally performed from the right ventricular (RV) apex. In this respect it is not always appreciated that a substantial number of the reported cases of the His–Purkinje fatigue phenomenon also demonstrated previous anterograde AV block in situations other than RV pacing [30–35]. When investigating the fatigue phenomenon in a patient with bundle branch block, a negative response to burst pacing of the RV apex and outflow tract should be followed by rapid ventricular pacing and programmed premature stimulation (same protocol as for ventricular tachycardia) from the RV apex and the outflow tract because such a protocol may be the only way to unmask AV block [35]. If negative, the stimulation protocol should be repeated after a pharmacologic challenge with a type IA antiarrhythmic agent because the fatigue phenomenon may occasionally become manifest only after such a challenge [36,37].

3 Bradycardia-dependent (phase 4) block (not bradycardia associated as in vagally induced AV block) is rare and always infranodal and should be evaluated by carotid sinus pressure and with His bundle recordings by producing bradycardia and pauses by the electrical induction of atrial or ventricular premature beats.

4 Diagnostic challenge with drugs such as procainamide that depress His–Purkinje conduction to provoke HV prolongation or actual His–Purkinje block in susceptible patients are underutilized in the US [36,37]. A positive response consists of doubling the HV interval or the induction of second- or third-degree AV block.

Neuromuscular disease
Conduction system disease may be an important cause of mortality in patients with neuromuscular disease (e.g. myotonic muscular dystrophy, Kearns–Sayre syndrome, Emery Dreifuss muscular dystrophy, etc.). Pacing should be considered early in the course of the disease in asymptomatic patients whenever there is bifascicular block, a long PR interval or progression of any conduction abnormality (PR interval, left anterior hemiblock, increased QRS duration) without waiting for the development of second- or third-degree AV block [3,38–41]. A PR interval > 275 ms presumably due to infra-Hisian conduction delay may be predictive of sudden death. Invasive electrophysiologic studies should be performed in questionable cases to determine the need for pacing. In the setting of spontaneous or inducible ventricular tachyarrhythmias, an implantable defibrillator should be considered.

Rare causes of AV block
Syncope with paroxysmal AV block may be precipitated by a variety of unusual triggering stimuli. Whether pacing is indicated depends on the clinical severity and whether the trigger can be controlled or avoided. These situations are almost never related to carotid hypersensitivity and cannot usually be reproduced by vagal maneuvers. Rarely vasovagal syncope may be associated with a head-up tilt-table test producing AV block without significant sinus bradycardia [42–44].

Deglutition (swallowing) syncope occurs in patients with organic or functional abnormalities of the esophagus and rarely without demonstrable esophageal disease [24]. The mechanism seems related to an esophagocardiac vagal reflex from activation of receptors in the esophageal wall secondary to distention of the esophagus. This form of AV block occurs almost always with swallowing food or hot or cold liquids and permanent pacing provides long-term benefit. This form of syncope may rarely be associated with carotid sinus hypersensitivity or vasovagal syncope [45,46]. Also related to a reflex involving the gastrointestinal tract, AV block from defecation syncope can also be treated with a permanent pacemaker [47].

Cough syncope is associated with loss of consciousness after prolonged bouts of violent coughing. Syncope often occurs because of lower cerebral perfusion consequent to increase in intrathoracic pressure that lowers the cardiac output and impairs venous return from the brain. In some cases AV block may play a complicating role and a permanent pacemaker can produce symptomatic relief [48–50].

Paroxysmal AV block in the absence of orthostatic hypotension can be triggered by modest changes in posture such as sitting up from the supine position. This type of AV block is not due to decreased vagal tone, but to an increase in the atrial rate in the form of a tachycardia-dependent block. In the case of AV nodal block, an increase in the standing heart rate may override the decrease in vagal tone and precipitate AV block. Postural AV block can also occur in the His–Purkinje system [51–54].

Orthostatic hypotension

Orthostatic hypotension, whether primary or secondary to autonomic dysfunction, remains a medical challenge. In 1980, Moss et al. [55] reported the use of atrial tachypacing at 100 p.p.m. to treat a case of primary orthostatic hypotension. However, this was soon followed by a negative report using temporary atrial pacing [56]. Nevertheless, infrequent case reports from several centers have suggested that pacing may be effective in selected patients [55–62] (Table 3.1). Most case reports are of relatively short follow-up and suggest that tachypacing should not be used as sole therapy. Adjunctive therapy with fludrocortisone is important and should be supplemented by midodrine, beta-blockers, added salt intake and other measures. The proposed mechanism of tachypacing is to treat the concomitant 'chronotropic incompetence' of patients with orthostatic hypotension with pacing [59]. By shortening diastole, tachypacing may reduce the rapid run-off associated with low peripheral resistance present in these patients. Some residual adrenergic tone is necessary, and it seems that patients with total autonomic failure do not benefit from tachypacing.

An ordinary activity sensor-driven DDDR pacemaker can be programmed to increase its rate rapidly upon standing, a response that can be supplemented by having the patient or a family member tap on the device. This allows an acceptable pacing rate (75–80 p.p.m.) when pacing for orthostatic hypotension is not required. Ideally the pacemaker should automatically set a lower pacing rate at night. However, it is preferable to use more refined

Table 3.1 Clinical efficacy of pacing for orthostatic hypotension.

Study	No. of patients	Pacemaker	Rate (p.p.m.)	Follow-up	Benefit
Moss et al. (1980)	1	AAI	100	10 months	Yes
Goldberg et al. (1980)	1	Temporary atrial	90–100	No	No
Kristinsson et al. (1983)	2	AAI	95 (day) 55 (night)	2 years	Yes
Cunha et al. (1990)	1	AAI	96 (day) 60 (night)	9 months	Yes
Weissman et al. (1992)	5	3 AAI, DDD, DDDR	90–100	1 year	4 improved
Grubb et al. (1993)	1	DDDR	*	4 months	Yes
Abe et al. (2000)	2	DDD	100	5 and 6 months	Yes

* Rate driven by detecting the change in pre-injection period.

pacing technology to activate tachypacing automatically only when the device detects the upright posture because persistent tachypacing is likely to be poorly tolerated.

Grubb *et al.* [60] reported the use of the right ventricular pre-ejection interval sensor in a patient with orthostatic hypotension (Figure 3.3). In the upright posture, venous return decreases and the fall in blood pressure led to an increase in sympathetic tone and shortening of the pre-ejection interval. Alternatively, the fall in the pulmonary systolic pressure might have reduced the afterload of right ventricular ejection with resultant shortening of the pre-ejection interval. The device detected the change and delivered tachypacing at 110–120 p.p.m. effectively suppressing orthostatic hypotension, thereby avoiding continuous tachypacing and its potential harmful effects on the heart. This experience suggested that developments in sensor technology may allow earlier and more appropriate response to alterations in blood pressure and posture and greater applicability of this form of therapy.

Hemodynamic sensors such as the first derivative of right ventricular pressure and the peak endocardial acceleration sensors may also provide effective detection of orthostatic pressure changes. Sensing of posture could also be achieved with an activity sensor such as a triaxial accelerometer which defines the body position by the relative input of the three dimensional acceleration detected [64,65]. Refinement of sensor-derived algorithms should eventually provide a way to rapidly control the pacing rate automatically with orthostatic changes in the waking state.

All patients considered for atrial pacing should undergo repeated testing in the supine and upright positions with or without pacing (90–100 p.p.m.) by a temporary atrial or AV sequential pacing system. The procedure is best done on a tilt-table so the patient is always supported. If rapid atrial pacing blunts the degree of hypotension, pacing therapy is probably going to be helpful but the test has poor predictive value.

Hypertrophic cardiomyopathy

Many observational studies have suggested that dual-chamber pacing can be effective therapy for symptomatic relief in patients with obstructive hypertrophic cardiomyopathy (OHCM) [4,65–67]. Pacing reduces the left ventricular outflow tract (LVOT) gradient by about 50%. However data from controlled crossover randomized trials (that involved only three relatively small studies discussed below) are far less impressive and even controversial [68–70]. In the European Pacing in Hypertrophic Cardiomyopathy study (PIC study), 83 patients with OHCM (refractory or intolerant to drug therapy) and a resting LVOT gradient > 30 mmHg underwent a randomized, crossover study between AAI (at 30 p.p.m.) and DDD pacing with short AV interval, each for a 12-week period [68]. Patients in the DDD pacing period had a significantly lower LVOT gradient improved NYHA class and improved walking time than those with the inactive pacemaker. Seventeen of 83 patients (20%) required early reprogramming from AAI to DDD because of persistent symptoms or deterioration. Seventy-nine of the 83 patients (95%) preferred DDD pacing. Subsequent follow-up of patients for 1 year showed that pacing was beneficial for pressure gradient and symptoms in 72 patients [87%]. Subgroup analysis of the PIC data showed that improvement depended upon age, with a marked improvement between the ages of 60 and 70 which was statistically significant compared to other decades [71].

On the other hand, the M-PATHY study, which randomized 48 patients with resting LVOT ≥ 50 mmHg to receive 3 months of DDD and 3 months of AAI pacing, showed that the symptoms were not improved despite a significant reduction of LVOT by DDD pacing [69]. However, when the patients were unblinded and were followed for an additional 6 months, patients in the DDD phase were symptomatically improved. This response suggests a strong placebo effect of pacing. In a subgroup of 6 elderly patients (> 65 years), more striking clinical improvement was noted. In a smaller study with a similar double-blind randomized crossover design (21 patients with 19 completing the study) Nishimura *et al.* showed that pacing produced no symptomatic response despite significant reduction of LVOT gradient when DDD pacing was compared to AAI back-up pacing (30/min), an observation consistent with a placebo effect [70].

Some observations suggest that improvement with pacing is based on more than a placebo effect.

Linde *et al.* [72] demonstrated that during inactive pacing, there was a significant improvement in perceived chest pain, dyspnea and palpitations associated with a statistically significant decrease of the LVOT gradient from 71± 32 to 52± 34 mmHg. During active pacing the perceived symptoms were similar but there was improvement in alertness and 'strenuous' exercise associated with a decrease of the LVOT gradient from 70± 24 to 33± 27 mmHg. The difference in gradient reduction between the two groups was statistically highly significant. Gadler *et al.* [73] analysed the quality of life in patients from the PIC study during 1 year of follow-up. Patients were randomized to two arms: active and inactive. After 3 months the pacemaker was reprogrammed to the alternate mode and a further 3 months followed. After this period subsequent pacemaker programming corresponded to the mode preferred by the patient. A last assessment was made 1 year after baseline examinations. Eighty patients completed the first crossover period and 75 completed the full 1-year follow-up. Active pacing induced a significant improvement in the quality of life, in the order of 9–44%, regardless of programming sequence. Discontinuation of pacing after the first active period resulted in return of symptoms. Fourteen patients requested early reprogramming after having been programmed to inactive pacing after a first period of active pacing. Seventy-six patients preferred active pacing after the crossover period. A further 6 months of pacing induced progressive improvement in symptoms already favorably influenced.

The mixed findings in the three randomized trials are difficult to explain. OHCM is a complex heterogeneous disease with variable symptoms and gradients so that an intervention such as pacing is liable to produce variable results. Furthermore, changes in exercise capacity and NYHA class are not necessarily associated with a reduction in LVOT gradient.

The implantation of dual-chamber pacing is not primary therapy and should not be considered as replacement for drug therapy [69]. Pacing should be weighed against the risk and efficacy of surgical left ventricular myectomy and percutaneous transcoronary septal myocardial ablation with ethanol injection into the first septal artery (chemical myectomy) [74]. The latter procedure may require pacing because AV block occurs in 15–20% of patients

[75]. There are no prospective randomized studies comparing pacing with other therapeutic strategies. The 1998 ACC/AHA guidelines for implantation of pacemakers list medically refractory symptomatic HOCM with significant resting or provoked LV outflow obstruction as a class IIb indication based on data from observational reports [11]. These guidelines are probably based on favorable data derived mostly from retrospective uncontrolled studies. The guidelines are vague on what constitutes a 'significant resting or provoked gradient' in HOCM patients. As a rule, pacing should only be considered with a resting gradient > 30 mmHg or a provoked LVOT gradient > 50 mmHg [2]. We believe that pacing for HOCM should be considered only in drug-refractory patients (especially the elderly) in whom surgical myectomy (superior to pacing in symptom relief and gradient reduction according to a recent comparison study [74]) is either contraindicated or rejected (or where the patients are not optimal candidates), or where there is lack of access to experienced surgical treatment for this disease [76]. Patients receiving a pacemaker should be warned of the uncertainty of this form of therapy. Pacing is also indicated in patients who develop bradycardia secondary to successful pharmacologic therapy.

Indications for a dual-chamber defibrillator

Pacing does not reduce mortality or sudden cardiac death. Now that the implantation procedure for a dual-chamber defibrillator is similar to that for a dual-chamber pacemaker, the question arises as to whether it would be preferable to implant a dual-chamber defibrillator (with DDDR pacing capability) because OHCM patients are at risk of malignant ventricular tachyarrhythmias and sudden death. At this juncture a prophylactic implantable cardioverter defibrillator (ICD) should at least be considered in high-risk patients (family history of sudden death, recurrent syncope, abnormal blood pressure response to exercise, septal or LV thickness > 30 mm and Holter-documented non-sustained ventricular tachycardia) [77,78]. Atrial tachyarrhythmias often result in serious hemodynamic consequences and an ICD with atrial defibrillation capability would also be a consideration. Unfortunately, financial restrictions will limit the application of an attractive universal mode of therapy.

Pacing for sleep apnea

Sleep apnea is a common medical problem, and affects 2–4% of the middle-aged population of the United States [79–81]. It increases the risk of hypertension and cardiovascular disease, and causes daytime somnolence with a resultant higher risk of traffic accident. Approximately 90% of sleep apnea is due to obstruction of the upper airways, and 10% is of central origin. Drug treatment is ineffective. While continuous airway pressure devices are the gold standard of treatment, these are poorly tolerated and long-term compliance is limited.

During apneic episodes there is a high incidence of cardiac arrhythmias amenable to treatment. As the patients are asleep, these arrhythmias are asymptomatic. In a study of eight patients referred for permanent pacing for bradyarrhythmias occurring during the sleeping hours (sinus pauses in eight, AV block in four), seven out of eight of them were found to have symptoms of sleep apnea. Sleep apnea was subsequently confirmed, bradyarrhythmias were corrected with mechanical treatment and pacing was not required. Thus in patients presenting with asymptomatic bradyarrhythmias during the sleeping period in the absence of causes such as bradyarrhythmias due to athletic training, sleep apnea should be considered as an underlying cause.

In a recent publication, Garrigue *et al.* [82] reported that pacing may reduce the incidence of apnea/hyponea episodes. Of 152 patients with sinus node disease in their pacemaker population, 31% were found to have symptoms of sleep disorder. Fifteen of the 26 consenting patients (58%) had documented sleep apnea with an apnea/hyponea index ≥ 5/h. Half of them were suffering from central apnea. The patients were randomized to AAI pacing at > 15 b.p.m. over the nocturnal rate, or to VVI pacing at 40 b.p.m., each for 1 day. There was a significant reduction from 9 to 3 episodes/h after pacing without changing the sleeping duration or the overall pacing rate. Interestingly, not only was central sleep apnea improved, but patients with obstructive sleep apnea improved as well.

These observations are interesting but raise a number of issues. The authors postulated that pacing by preventing bradyarrhythmias could counteract the sustained increases in vagal tone by maintaining sympathetic activity. Hemodynamic changes by pacing may affect barorespiratory reflexes and reduce parasympathetic outflow. A reduction in parasympathetic outflow may relax genioglossus muscles and improve the obstructive form of sleep apnea. However, the current acute study only examined a pacing population with relatively mild apnea of the central types. Whether the results in terms of rate control or pacing are applicable on a long-term basis to the general population of sleep apnea patients remains to be investigated [83,84].

References

1 Glikson M, Hayes DL, Nishimura RA. Newer clinical applications of pacing. *J Cardiovasc Electrophysiol* 1997; **8**: 1190–1203.
2 Hayes DL, Barold SS, Camm AJ *et al.* Evolving indications for permanent cardiac pacing. An appraisal of the 1998 ACC/AHA guidelines. *Am J Cardiol* 1998; **82**: 1082–6.
3 Hayes DL. Evolving indications for permanent pacing. *Am J Cardiol* 1999; **83** (5B): 161D–165D.
4 Barold SS. New and evolving indications for cardiac pacing. In: Singer I, ed. *Interventional Electrophysiology*. Lippincott, Baltimore: Williams & Wilkins, 2001: 781.
5 Wolbrette DL, Naccarelli GV. Emerging indications for permanent pacing. *Curr Cardiol Rep* 2000; **2**: 353–60.
6 Chirife R, Ortega DF, Salazar AI. 'Pacemaker syndrome' without a pacemaker. Deleterious effects of first-degree AV block [abstract]. *RBM* 1990; **12**: 22.
7 Barold SS. Optimal pacing in first-degree AV block. *Pacing Clin Electrophysiol* 1999; **22**: 1423–4.
8 Mabo P, Cazeau S, Forrer A *et al.* Isolated long PR interval as only indication of permanent DDD pacing [abstract]. *J Am Coll Cardiol* 1992; **19**: 66A.
9 Kim YH, O'Nunain S, Trouton T *et al.* Pseudopacemaker syndrome following inadvertent fast pathway ablation for atrioventricular nodal reentrant tachycardia. *J Cardiovasc Electrophysiol* 1993; **4**: 178–82.
10 Zornosa JP, Crossley GH, Haisty WK Jr *et al.* Pseudo pacemaker syndrome: a complication of radiofrequency ablation of the AV junction. *Pacing Clin Electrophysiol* 1992; **15**: 590.
11 Gregoratos G, Cheitlin MD, Freedman RA *et al.* ACC/AHA guidelines for implantation of cardiac pacemakers and antiarrhythmia devices; a report of the American College of Cardiology/American Heart Association task force on practice guidelines (Committee on pacemaker implantation). *J Am Coll Cardiol* 1998; **31**: 1175–209.

12 Tse HF, Lau CP. Long-term effect of right ventricular pacing on myocardial perfusion and function. *J Am Coll Cardiol* 1997; **29**: 744–9.

13 Leclercq C, Gras D, Le Helloco A *et al.* Hemodynamic importance of preserving the normal sequence of ventricular activation in permanent cardiac pacing. *Am Heart J* 1995; **129**: 1133–41.

14 Rosenqvist M, Isaaz K, Botvinick EH *et al.* Relative importance of activation sequence compared to atrioventricular synchrony in left ventricular function. *Am J Cardiol* 1991; **67**: 148–56.

15 Rosenqvist M, Bergfeldt L, Haga Y *et al.* The effect of ventricular activation sequence on cardiac performance during pacing. *Pacing Clin Electrophysiol* 1996: **19**: 1279–86.

16 Prinzen FW, Van Oosterhout MF, Vanagt WY *et al.* Optimization of ventricular function by improving the activation sequence during ventricular pacing. *Pacing Clin Electrophysiol* 1998; **21**: 2256–60.

17 Iliev II, Yamachika S, Muta K *et al.* Preserving normal ventricular activation versus atrioventricular delay optimization during pacing: the role of intrinsic atrioventricular conduction and pacing rate. *Pacing Clin Electrophysiol* 2000; **23**: 74–80.

18 Barold SS. Timing cycles and operational characteristics of pacemakers. In: Ellenbogen K, Kay N, Wilkoff B, eds. *Clinical Cardiac Pacing and Defibrillation*, 2nd edn. Philadelphia: W. B. Saunders, 2000: 727–825.

19 Bode F, Wiegand U, Katus HA *et al.* Pacemaker inhibition due to prolonged native AV interval in dual-chamber devices. *Pacing Clin Electrophysiol* 1999; **22**: 1425–31.

20 Wilson JH, Lattner S. Undersensing of P waves in the presence of adequate P wave due to automatic postventricular atrial refractory period extension. *Pacing Clin Electrophysiol* 1989; **10**: 1729–32.

21 Jaïs P, Barold SS, Shah DC *et al.* Pacemaker syndrome induced by the mode switching algorithm of a DDDR pacemaker. *Pacing Clin Electrophysiol* 1999; **22**: 682–5.

22 Kuniyashi R, Sosa E, Scanavacca M *et al.* Pseudo-sindrome de marcapasso. *Arq Bras Cardiol* 1994; **62**: 111–15.

23 Pitney M, Davis M. Catheter ablation of ventriculoatrial conduction in the treatment of pacemaker mediated tachycardia. *Pacing Clin Electrophysiol* 1991; **14**: 1013–17.

24 Barold SS, Falkoff MD, Ong LS *et al.* Atrioventricular block. In: Barold SS, Mugica J, eds. *New Perspectives in Cardiac Pacing 2*. Mount Kisco, NY: Futura Publishing Company, 1991: 23–52.

25 Sumiyoshi M, Nakata Y, Yasuda M *et al.* Clinical and electrophysiologic features of exercise-induced atrioventricular block. *Am Heart J* 1996; **132** (6): 1277–81.

26 Luscure M, Dechandol AM, Lagorge P *et al.* Blocs auriculo-ventriculaires d'effort. *Ann Cardiol Angeiol* 1995; **44**: 486–92.

27 Barold SS, Jaïs P, Shah DC *et al.* Exercise-induced second-degree AV block: is it type I or type II? *J Cardiovasc Electrophysiol* 1997; **8** (9): 1084–6.

28 Deaner A, Fluck D, Timmis AD. Exertional atrioventricular block presenting with recurrent syncope: successful treatment by coronary angioplasty. *Heart* 1996; **75** (6): 640–1.

29 Petrac D, Radic B, Birtic K *et al.* Prospective evaluation of infrahisal second-degree AV block induced by atrial pacing in the presence of chronic bundle branch block and syncope. *Pacing Clin Electrophysiol* 1996; **19**: 784–92.

30 Runge M, Narula OS. 'Fatigue' phenomenon in the human His–Purkinje system (HPS). *Circulation* 1973; **48** (Suppl. IV): 103.

31 Narula OS, Runge M. Accommodation of AV nodal conduction and 'fatigue' phenomenon in the His–Purkinje system. In: Wellens HJJ, Lie KI, Janse M, eds. *The Conduction System of the Heart*. Leiden: Stenfert Kroese, 1976: 529–44.

32 Wald RW, Waxman MB. Depression of AV conduction following ventricular pacing. *Pacing Clin Electrophysiol* 1981; **4**: 84–91.

33 DiLorenzo DR, Sellers D. Fatigue of the His–Purkinje system during routine electrophysiologic studies. *Pacing Clin Electrophysiol* 1988; **11**: 263–70.

34 Sasano T, Okishige K, Azegami K *et al.* Transient complete atrioventricular block provoked by ventricular pacing in a patient with nonsustained ventricular tachycardia. *J Electrocardiol* 1999; **32**: 185–90.

35 Barold SS, Barold HS. Demonstration of the fatigue phenomenon of the His–Purkinje system by right ventricular outflow tract stimulation. *J Interv Card Electrophysiol* 2000; **4**: 489–91.

36 Englund A, Bergfeldt L, Rosenqvist M. Disopyramide stress test. A sensitive and specific tool for predicting impending high-degree AV block in patients with bifascicular block. *Br Heart J* 1995; **74**: 650–5.

37 Englund A, Bergfeldt L, Rosenqvist M. Pharmacological stress testing of the His–Purkinje system in patients with bifascicular block. *Pacing Clin Electrophysiol* 1998; **21**: 1979–87.

38 Mammarella A, Paradiso M, Antonini G *et al.* Natural history of cardiac involvement in myotonic dystrophy (Steinert's disease): a 13-year follow-up study. *Adv Ther* 2000; **17**: 238–51.

39 Fragola PV, Autore C, Magni G *et al.* The natural course of cardiac conduction disturbances in myotonic dystrophy. *Cardiology* 1991; **79**: 93–8.

40 Himmrich E, Popov S, Liebrich A *et al.* Hidden intracardiac conduction disturbances and their spontan-

eous course in patients with progressive muscular dystrophy. *Z Kardiol* 2000; **89**: 592–8.

41 Polak PE, Zijlstra F, Roelandt JR. Indications for pacemaker implantation in the Kearns–Sayre syndrome. *Eur Heart J* 1989; **10**: 281–2.

42 de Meester A, Chaudron JM. Paroxysmal atrioventricular block induced during head-up tilt test. *Acta Cardiol* 1999; **54**: 101–3.

43 Abe H, Hanada H, Kohshi K *et al.* Treatment of advanced atrioventricular block with beta-adrenergic blockade therapy. *Pacing Clin Electrophysiol* 1999; **22**: 1097–9.

44 Sumiyoshi M, Nakata Y, Mineda Y. Paroxysmal atrioventricular block induced during head-up tilt testing in an apparently healthy man. *J Cardiovasc Electrophysiol* 1997; **8**: 561–4.

45 Antonelli D, Rosenfeld T. Deglutition syncope associated with carotid sinus hypersensitivity. *Pacing Clin Electrophysiol* 1997; **20**: 2282–3.

46 Kakuchi H, Sato N, Kawamura Y. Swallow syncope associated with complete atrioventricular block and vasovagal syncope. *Heart* 2000; **83**: 702–4.

47 Newton JL, Allan L, Baptist M *et al.* Defecation syncope associated with splanchnic sympathetic dysfunction and cured by permanent pacemaker insertion. *Am J Gastroenterol* 2002; **96**: 2276–8.

48 Baron SB, Huang SK. Cough syncope presenting as Mobitz type II atrioventricular block—an electrophysiologic correlation. *Pacing Clin Electrophysiol* 1987; **10**: 65–9.

49 Nakagawa S. Vagally mediated paroxysmal atrioventricular block presenting as 'Mobitz type II' block. *Pacing Clin Electrophysiol* 1988; **11**: 471–2.

50 Lee D, Beldner S, Pollaro F *et al.* Cough-induced heart block. *Pacing Clin Electrophysiol* 1999; **22**: 1270–1.

51 Seda PE, McAnulty JH, Anderson CJ. Postural heart block. *Br Heart J* 1980; **44**: 221–3.

52 Belhassen B, Danon L, Shoshani D *et al.* Paroxysmal atrioventricular block triggered by orthostatic hypotension. *Am Heart J* 1986; **112**: 1107–9.

53 Klein HO, DiSegni E, Kaplinsky E. Paroxysmal heart block triggered by sitting up. A usually undetected cause of cerebral ischemia. *Heart Lung* 1988; **17**: 648–50.

54 Schwela H, Oltmanns G. Postural-induced complete heart block. *Am Heart J* 1987; **114**: 1532–4.

55 Moss AJ, Glaser W, Topol E. Atrial tachypacing in the treatment of a patient with primary orthostatic hypotension. *N Engl J Med* 1980; **302**: 1456–7.

56 Goldberg MR, Robertson RM, Robertson D. Atrial tachypacing for primary orthostatic hypotension. *N Engl J Med* 1980; **303**: 885–6.

57 Cunha UG, Machado EL, Santana LA. Programmed atrial pacing in the treatment of neurogenic orthostatic hypotension in the elderly. *Arq Brasil Cardiol* 1990; **55**: 47–9.

58 Kristinsson A. Programmed atrial pacing for orthostatic hypotension. *Acta Med Scand* 1983; **214**: 79–83.

59 Weissmann P, Chin MT, Moss AJ. Cardiac tachypacing for severe refractory idiopathic orthostatic hypotension. *Ann Intern Med* 1992; **116**: 650–1.

60 Grubb BP, Wolfe DA, Samoil D *et al.* Adaptive rate pacing controlled by right ventricular preejection interval for severe refractory orthostatic hypotension. *Pacing Clin Electrophysiol* 1993; **16**: 801–5.

61 Abe H, Numata T, Hanada H *et al.* Successful treatment of severe orthostatic hypotension with cardiac tachypacing in dual chamber pacemakers. *Pacing Clin Electrophysiol* 2000; **23**: 137–9.

62 Clémenty J, Gencel L, Garrigue S *et al.* Permanent cardiac pacing in the treatment of orthostatic hypotension: literature update and five additional cases. In: Blanc JJ, Benditt D, Sutton R, eds. *Neurally Mediated Syncope.* Armonk, NY: Futura Publishing Co., 1996: 127–36.

63 Mai J, Park E, Bornzin GA *et al.* Enhanced rate response algorithm for orthostatic compensation pacing. *Pacing Clin Electrophysiol* 2000; **23**: 1809–11.

64 Duru F, Bloch KE, Weilenmann D *et al.* Clinical evaluation of a pacemaker algorithm that adjusts the pacing rate during sleep using activity variance. *Pacing Clin Electrophysiol* 2000; **23**: 1509–15.

65 Fananapazir L, Epstein ND., Curiel RV *et al.* Long-term results of dual-chamber (DDD) pacing in obstructive hypertrophic cardiomyopathy. Evidence for progressive symptomatic and hemodynamic improvement and reduction of left ventricular hypertrophy. *Circulation* 1994; **90**: 2731–42.

66 Fananapazir L, Atiga W, Tripodi D *et al.* Therapy in obstructive hypertrophic cardiomyopathy. The role of dual chamber (DDD) pacing. In: Barold SS, Mugica J, eds. *Recent Advances in Cardiac Pacing. Goals for the 21st Century.* Armonk, NY: Futura Publishing Co., 1998; 35–50.

67 Fananapazir L, McAreavey D. Therapeutic options in patients with obstructive hypertrophic cardiomyopathy and severe drug-refractory symptoms. *J Am Coll Cardiol* 1998; **31**: 259–64.

68 Kappenberger L, Linde C, Daubert C *et al.* Pacing in hypertrophic obstructive cardiomyopathy. A randomized crossover study. PIC Study Group. *Eur Heart J* 1997; **18**: 1249–56.

69 Maron BJ, Nishimura RA, McKenna WJ *et al.* Assessment of permanent dual-chamber pacing as a treatment for drug-refractory symptomatic patients with obstructive hypertrophic cardiomyopathy. A

randomized, double-blind, crossover study (M-PATHY). *Circulation* 1999; **99**: 2927–33.

70 Nishimura RA, Trusty JM, Hayes DL *et al.* Dual-chamber pacing for hypertrophic cardiomyopathy: a randomized, double-blind, crossover trial. *J Am Coll Cardiol* 1997; **29**: 435–41.

71 Meisel E, Rauwolf TP, Burkhard M *et al.* Older patients with obstructive hypertrophic cardiomyopathy benefit most from pacemaker therapy. Results from the PIC Study. *Circulation* 1999; **100** (Suppl I): I–78.

72 Linde C, Gadler F, Kappenberger L. Placebo effect of pacemaker implantation in obstructive hypertrophic cardiomyopathy. PIC Study Group. Pacing in Cardiomyopathy. *Am J Cardiol* 1999; **83**: 903–7.

73 Gadler F, Linde C, Daubert C *et al.* Significant improvement of quality of life following atrioventricular synchronous pacing in patients with hypertrophic obstructive cardiomyopathy. Data from 1 year of follow-up. PIC study group. Pacing in Cardiomyopathy. *Eur Heart J* 1999; **20**: 1044–50.

74 Ommen SR, Nishimura RA, Squires RW *et al.* Comparison of dual chamber pacing versus septal myectomy for the treatment of patients with hypertrophic obstructive cardiomyopathy: a comparison of objective hemodynamic and exercise end points. *J Am Coll Cardiol* 1999; **34**: 191–6.

75 Gietzen FH, Leuner CJ, Hegselmann J *et al.* Hemodynamic effects of adjunct DDD pacing in patients with total AV block after transcoronary ablation of septum hypertrophy for hypertrophic obstructive cardiomyopathy. *Circulation* 1999; **100** (Suppl I): I-464.

76 Erwin JP III, Nishimura RA, Lloyd MA *et al.* Dual chamber pacing for patients with hypertrophic obstructive cardiomyopathy: a clinical perspective in 2000. *Mayo Clin Proc* 2000; **75**: 173–80.

77 Maron BJ, Shen WK, Link MS *et al.* Efficacy of implantable cardioverter-defibrillators for the prevention of sudden death in patients with hypertrophic cardiomyopathy. *N Engl J Med* 2000; **342**: 365–73.

78 Watkins H. Sudden death in hypertrophic cardiomyopathy. *N Engl J Med* 2000; **342**: 42–3.

79 Mooe T, Rabben T, Wiklund U *et al.* Sleep-disordered breathing in men with coronary artery disease. *Chest* 1996; **109**: 659–63.

80 Harbison J, O'Reilly P, McNicholas WT. Cardiac rhythm disturbances in the obstructive sleep apnea syndrome: effects of nasal continuous positive airway pressure therapy. *Chest* 2000; **118**: 591–5.

81 Stegman SS, Burroughs JM, Henthorn RW. Asymptomatic bradyarrhythmias as a marker for sleep apnea: appropriate recognition and treatment may reduce the need for pacemaker therapy. *Pacing Clin Electrophysiol* 1996; **19**: 899–904.

82 Garrigue S, Bordier P, Jais P *et al.* Benefit of atrial pacing in sleep apnea syndrome. *N Engl J Med* 2002; **346**: 404–12.

83 Gottlieb DJ. Cardiac pacing—a novel therapy for sleep apnea? *N Engl J Med* 2002; **346**: 444–5.

84 Kato I, Shiomi T, Sasanabe R *et al.* Effects of physiological cardiac pacing on sleep-disordered breathing in patients with chronic bradydysrhythmias. *Psychiatry Clin Neurosci* 2002; **55**: 257–8.

CHAPTER 4

Pacing for Prevention of Atrial Fibrillation: Fact or Fancy?

Panos E. Vardas and Emmanuel M. Kanoupakis

Introduction

Prevention of recurrences of atrial fibrillation (AF) is an issue that has attracted ever-increasing interest in recent years. The limitations of antiarrhythmic drugs, as regards their efficacy and potential side-effects [1–3], have stimulated the development of non-pharmacologic approaches over the last decade. Thorough research into the pathophysiologic mechanisms of AF has led to the development of preventive pacing strategies, targeted at modifying the electrophysiologic properties of the arrhythmogenic atrial substrate and inhibiting AF initiation.

Conventionally, AF is established when various conditions serving as triggers, initiators or perpetuators coincide [4]. It has been suggested that AF is developed on an electrically unstable atrial substrate that is usually triggered by early atrial extrasystoles. Unstable atrial tissue is characterized by regional conduction delays, resulting from organic or functional conduction blocks, and an increased dispersion of refractoriness [5–8]. Furthermore, the interaction with the autonomic nervous system [9], atrial stretch [10] and cellular non-uniform anisotropy due to fibrosis may also influence such an arrhythmogenic substrate. Atrial premature beats coupled early beyond the refractory period may further accentuate these conduction delays.

Atrial pacing may intervene at different targets in this pathophysiologic concept to prevent atrial tachyarrhythmias. Overdrive suppression of ectopic atrial activity and prevention of bradycardia and excessive rate decays may abolish the triggers. Pacing algorithms can also eliminate potential initiators such as spatial electrical heterogeneity due to pauses and short–long cycles. Finally, pacing from different atrial sites may change the conduction sequence and compensate the intra-atrial or inter-atrial conduction delay, modifying the perpetuators.

Evidence to date that atrial pacing may prevent atrial arrhythmias comes from those paced principally for a bradyarrhythmic indication, those paced for paroxysmal AF in the absence of a bradyarrhythmic indication and those with postoperative AF. Atrial pacing modalities evaluated include conventional single-site right atrial appendage pacing, alternative-site and multisite pacing, and the use of special algorithms.

Atrial-based vs. single-chamber ventricular pacing

First evidence that atrial pacing may prevent atrial arrhythmias in clinical practice comes from a broad group of patients: those paced principally for a bradyarrhythmic indication, especially sinus node disease.

Beneficial effects of permanent antibradycardia pacing for the prevention of AF were primarily recognized in several retrospective studies. In a review of 10 of these trials Connolly et al. [11] estimated that in patients with sick sinus syndrome the incidence of AF is lower in those receiving atrial or dual chamber pacemakers compared with those with ventricular pacing alone (relative risk reduction 62%). The possibility that selection bias in uncontrolled retrospective studies could be responsible for the apparent clinical superiority of physiologic pacing modes raised the need for prospective clinical trials of pacemaker mode selection.

In the first prospective, randomized trial Andersen et al. [12] compared AAI with VVI pacing in 225 patients with sick sinus syndrome. At the first analysis after a mean follow-up of 3.3 ± 1.5 years there was a non-significant trend towards reduction of AF in patients receiving AAI pacemakers compared with the VVI group, but after extended follow-up at 5.5 ± 2.4 years, up to 8 years, the reduction in chronic AF became significant [13].

Lamas et al. [14] in the Pacemaker Selection in the Elderly trial (PASE) enrolled 407 consecutive patients paced for sinus node disease (175), atrio-ventricular block (201) and other indications (31). All patients received a dual-chamber rate adaptive (DDDR) system that was randomly programmed to VVIR or DDDR mode. After a mean follow-up of 30 months, intention-to-treat analysis revealed no significant mode-related difference in the incidence of AF in the overall group, although a non-significant trend favored atrial-based pacing in the sinus node disease group.

The Canadian Trial of Physiologic Pacing (CTOPP) [15] was a multicenter, prospective, randomized trial comparing clinical outcomes including AF in 2568 patients randomized to atrial-based or ventricular pacing with mean follow-up of 3.5 years. Physiologic pacing was associated with an 18% relative risk reduction of development of chronic AF.

The Pacemaker Atrial Tachycardia (Pac-A-Tach) Study [16] compared the efficacy of VVIR and DDDR pacing for the prevention of atrial tachyarrhythmias in patients with the bradycardia–tachycardia syndrome. One hundred patients were randomized to DDDR mode and 98 to VVIR mode. The intention-to-treat analysis did not reveal a significant difference in atrial tachyarrhythmia recurrence between the two groups, neither did the addition of antiarrhythmic drugs alter arrhythmia recurrence.

Thus there is some evidence that in paced patients, particularly for sick sinus syndrome, atrial-based pacing may prevent AF compared with single ventricular pacing. However, atrial pacing offers no clear improvement in the incidence of AF, strokes and cardiovascular mortality in other groups of paced bradyarrhythmic patients [14,15].

Use of special algorithms

It is a fact that the onset of AF shows a large inter- and intrapatient variation but the majority of episodes start after events which pacing therapy can potentially influence. The most common onset mechanisms were premature atrial captures (PAC) related (30%), early reinitiation (26%) and preceding bradycardia (17%). Several ongoing trials investigate the onset mechanisms of AF, the preventative effects of conventional atrial pacing and the effects of specific pacing algorithms [17]. These specific pacing algorithms include minimal increment overdrive pacing, rate smoothing to prevent abrupt changes in rate, and algorithms specifically to suppress atrial ectopic triggers for AF and to eliminate the short–long cycles of those that occur. The separate and combined effects of four algorithms are under evaluation: pace conditioning, postexercise rate control, PAC suppression and post-PAC pause elimination.

Alternative pacing sites

Small clinical studies further suggest that alternative atrial pacing sites may assist in preventing AF. Yu et al. [18] showed that premature stimulation in the high right atrium causes a greater delay in conduction to the His bundle area, right posterior septum and distal coronary sinus than does premature atrial stimulation in the distal coronary sinus. By pre-exciting the area where conduction typically is slow, recovery of atrial excitability is advanced uniformly and atrial premature beats are less likely to encounter conduction delay so that conduction block and re-entry do not occur and AF is prevented. Padeletti et al. [19] have reported the elimination of episodes of AF in patients with sinus bradycardia and paroxysmal AF following single-site pacing in the posterior triangle of Koch. Others [20] have demonstrated a trend towards a lower rate of development of chronic AF in a group with paroxysmal AF and an indication for pacing with the pacing site randomized to the anterior superior interatrial septum (in the region of Bachmann's bundle), compared to a group randomized to right atrial appendage pacing.

Multisite atrial pacing has been suggested as another alternative pacing treatment to prevent recurrences of atrial tachyarrhythmias. However, not only are the underlying electrophysiologic mechanisms of these preventive effects largely speculative, there are also a number of controversies regarding the selection of patients, the pacing sites and the proven clinical benefit.

Multisite pacing to prevent AF

Electrophysiologic basis for multisite atrial pacing

Interatrial conduction delay may represent another important factor facilitating the induction of AF or serving as a perpetuator. When the high right atrium and distal coronary sinus were driven simultaneously, the conduction delay caused by premature stimulation in the high right atrium was significantly reduced. Prakash *et al.* [21] have shown that dual site right atrial pacing and biatrial pacing were equally effective in reducing P-wave duration, a measure of global atrial conduction delay, and homogenizing local activation times in the atrial septum, crista terminalis, the His bundle area and coronary sinus ostium region, in comparison with spontaneous sinus rhythm and single-site atrial pacing.

The inducibility of AF under conditions of multisite pacing was first examined acutely using programmed atrial stimulation. Despite a number of weak points in these studies, mainly regarding the method of arrhythmia induction and the type and number of patients who were studied, they found that either biatrial pacing or dual-site right atrial pacing can reduce the inducibility of AF [22–24].

Clinical benefit of multisite pacing to prevent AF

The clinical benefit of multisite pacing for the prevention of AF relapses has been investigated in an increasing number of patients who have already completed quite a long follow-up period. At the same time, more properly designed prospective, randomized studies have been aimed at an assessment of the therapeutic effect of multisite pacing in patients with a chronic history of atrial tachyarrhythmias.

Early clinical results suggested a high efficacy in AF prevention by multisite pacing in patients with interatrial conduction delay with P wave > 120 ms and an interatrial conduction time ≥ 100 ms [25]. Similarly a long-term experience in 86 patients showed that biatrial pacing was able to maintain sinus rhythm in 64% of patients with previously drug-refractory AF [26]. Recently, results of the latest randomized, prospective, crossover SYNBIA-PACE study were presented [27]. This trial compared 'synchronous' biatrial pacing, single-site atrial pacing and support pacing at a low rate, in patients with a long-lasting history of recurrent and drug-refractory atrial tachyarrhythmias associated with interatrial conduction delay, most of whom did not have a conventional bradycardiac indication for pacing [25]. Biatrial pacing was achieved via two atrial electrodes positioned at the right atrial appendage and within the coronary sinus. The primary endpoint was to compare the time to first atrial arrhythmia recurrence, as monitored by the Holter functions of the pacemaker. This study showed a trend towards a reduction in the incidence of atrial arrhythmias during biatrial pacing, but no real benefit of this pacing mode was demonstrated in this selected population.

One of the first prospective, randomized, single-blinded studies [28] comparing either biatrial or right atrial pacing with no pacing in patients with drug-refractory, persistent or paroxysmal AF showed that there was a significant reduction in the overall duration of AF with either right atrial or biatrial pacing, when compared with the unpaced control period. However, there was no effect on the number of AF episodes. Furthermore, when right atrial pacing was compared with biatrial pacing no difference could be demonstrated in either the frequency or the duration of AF episodes. An advantage of this study was that AF recurrence was based on data derived from long-term pacemaker Holter analysis and not only on symptomatic episodes. In this study the indication for biatrial pacing was solely arrhythmia prevention in all cases and we cannot be certain whether these results obtained with unselected patients would be comparable to those from selected patients with interatrial conduction disturbances or structural heart disease, or who require a pacemaker for conventional indications.

Another method proposed for compensation of mainly intra-atrial conduction delay has been implantation of two leads in the right atrium. AF prevention by dual-site right atrial pacing has been attributed to a reduction of the dispersion of right atrial refractoriness rather than right–left resynchronization, because a decrease in P-wave duration did not correlate with arrhythmia suppression by dual-site right atrial pacing. Delfaut *et al.* in a prospective, crossover study [29] compared the efficacy of dual-site right atrial pacing and single-site right atrial pacing in the prevention of AF in patients with drug-refractory AF or flutter who had, in contrast to two previously mentioned studies, a documented primary or drug-induced bradycardia. Two atrial leads were positioned at the high right atrium and at the ostium of the coronary sinus. They were connected to the atrial output of a standard DDDR pacemaker programmed to a lower rate between 80 and 90 b.p.m., to obtain continuous overdrive atrial pacing. Also, in this study patients were without marked interatrial conduction delay. Both pacing strategies resulted in a significant increase in the duration of arrhythmia-free intervals when compared with no pacing, while dual-site pacing was superior to single atrial pacing. However, recurrence of atrial tachyarrhythmias in this study was based mainly on the patients' symptoms and no data were available from long-term pacemaker Holter monitoring to establish a truly depressant effect of pacing. Furthermore, all patients had sinus bradycardia and in the majority this appears to have been induced by antiarrhythmic drugs, rather than intrinsic sinus node disease. Thus, the observed antiarrhythmic effect of pacing could have been because of improved tolerance and/or higher doses of antiarrhythmic drugs and might possibly have been due to an enhanced antiarrhythmic drug efficacy at higher rates or to a reduction in bradycardia-related AF onset.

This study also leads us to speculate that atrial overdrive pacing may continue to play a significant role in the reduction of AF recurrence. It is perhaps for this reason that the results of Delfaut et al. [29], who included bradycardic patients, are so encouraging. Indeed, continuous pacing inhibits the mechanisms that trigger arrhythmia and thus protects the atrium from the process of remodeling, which is one of the main determinants for AF initiation and perpetuation. This may be why the study of Levy et al. [28] detected no difference between biatrial and right atrial pacing.

The DAPPAF study [30] compared high right atrial, dual-site right atrial and support pacing in 121 patients with recurrent symptomatic AF and bradycardia in the presence or absence of antiarrhythmic drugs in a crossover study design. Patient tolerance and adherence was superior with dual-site right atrial pacing as compared with support or high right atrial pacing. Freedom from any symptomatic AF recurrence tended to be greater with dual RA but not with high RA pacing compared to support pacing. When dual RA pacing was compared to high RA pacing there was a reduced relative risk of recurrent AF but this did not achieve significance. Combined symptomatic and asymptomatic AF frequency in patients measured by device datalogs was significantly reduced during dual RA pacing as compared to high RA pacing. However, in antiarrhythmic drug-treated patients, dual RA pacing increased symptomatic AF-free survival compared to support pacing and high RA pacing. Analysis of this study shows that dual-site right atrial pacing is safe and effective for the long-term prevention of AF and maintenance of rhythm control and proposed that adjuvant antiarrhythmic therapy is required for optimal results.

The New Indication for Pacing Prevention of Atrial Fibrillation (NIPP-AF) study [31] compared dual-site pacing with high right atrial pacing in 15 patients with paroxysmal AF and maintained on sotalol, for prevention of AF. Compared to pacing in the high right atrium the combination of dual site pacing with a consistent pacing algorithm was associated with prolonged intervals between AF episodes and a shorter time in AF. Preliminary results of the Dual Site Atrial Pacing for Prevention of Atrial Fibrillation (DRAPPAF) study have been reported by Ramdat-Misier et al. [32]. In a prospective, randomized crossover study in patients with no recurrent drug-refractory AF patients were randomized to either single-site or dual-site pacing after implantation of a DDD device, combined with antiarrhythmic drug therapy. In the first 26 patients reported after completion of the study protocol the arrhythmia-free interval was not significantly different in either group, although the need for electrical cardioversion because of recurrent AF lasting more than 24 h was less during dual-site pacing.

Despite some promise, the role of multisite pacing for the prevention of AF remains investigational. We are hopeful that with the suitable selection of patients and following the improvement of pacing technology, multisite atrial pacing will prove efficacious.

Another aspect that has to be resolved from the experience with multisite pacing for AF prevention is the method for evaluating clinical effectiveness. The most common method has been the measurement of the 'time to first recurrence' of the symptomatic AF episode, but it is not certain that this is the best approach. Studies relying solely on symptom endpoints before or without ECG verification in persistent AF are more likely to underestimate AF events, or the burden and measurement of asymptomatic AF may be particularly important in this patient group.

Epicardial multisite atrial pacing in postoperative patients

During the immediate postoperative period in patients who undergo cardiac surgery, a high incidence of atrial tachyarrhythmias has been observed (40–60%), with a concomitant increase in morbidity and in hospitalization costs [33,34]. In spite of the reduction in postoperative AF resulting from prophylactic treatment with beta-blockers, sotalol or amiodarone, the incidence of arrhythmia is still about 25%, and concerns about potential side-effects or contraindications in many patients exist [35–38]. Temporary pacing with the use of epicardial wires has been tried as a non-pharmacologic therapy. The findings are again conflicting. In a very recent study, and in their effort to achieve continuous modification of the electrical substrate, Bloomaert et al. [39] evaluated the efficacy of a specific algorithm with continuous atrial dynamic overdrive pacing to prevent AF after coronary artery bypass grafting (CABG). Ninety-six patients in sinus rhythm without antiarrhythmic therapy on the second postoperative day were randomized to AAI pacing or no pacing for 24 h, and Holter ECGs used to detect AF occurrence. The incidence of AF was significantly lower in the paced group (10%) compared with control subjects (27%), particularly in patients with preserved left ventricular function.

Daoud et al. [40] and Orr et al. [41] reported that simultaneous right and left atrial pacing significantly reduced the incidence of AF following open heart surgery, to 17.9% and 10%, respectively. In contrast, Gerstenfeld et al. [42] in a first report from a study of 61 patients, found no significant difference in the proportion of patients developing AF after CABG, whether atrial pacing alone, biatrial pacing or no atrial pacing was applied. Another prospective randomized investigation by Kurz et al. [43] examined the effect of biatrial pacing in postoperative cardiac patients, assessing the incidence and the possible proarrhythmic effects of pacing. This study was terminated very early because its pacing protocol was observed to promote AF, possibly as a consequence of undersensing of atrial signals by the epicardial leads that resulted in asynchronous atrial

pacing. Of course, it is true that postoperative AF may be influenced by other factors, such as high catecholamine state, postoperative pericarditis, fluid and electrolyte shifts and respiratory compromise, that alter the arrhythmiogenic substrate and that might lessen the effectiveness of pacing. On the other hand, if agents such as alpha-blockers are needed, the combination of these with pacing may be more promising, as shown by the trend in the study of Gerstenfeld et al. [42] that was confirmed at a level of statistical significance by the study of Greenberg et al. [44]. However, even this latter study does not appear to attribute any advantage to multisite pacing, since the best results were achieved with right atrial pacing.

Conclusions

The use of atrial pacing to prevent atrial arrhythmias is best explained when examined in the context of patients with symptomatic bradycardia receiving physiologic pacing for sick sinus syndrome. Additionally, recent evidence allows some optimism that atrial pacing may have a role in the prevention of drug-resistant paroxysmal AF. It is likely that the maximum therapeutic effect of pacing will be realized when combined with antiarrhythmic drug prescription. Pacing with dedicated algorithms and optimal pacing sites may reduce the number of atrial tachy-arrhythmia episodes in a subgroup of patients. Nevertheless, the evidence base for the value of pacing to prevent AF remains remarkably conflicting, as does the evidence for the use of alternative single-site and multisite atrial pacing.

However, there are sufficient encouraging data to justify a continuation of our investigative efforts, focusing on clinical efficacy and optimal patient selection.

References

1 Crijns HJ, Van Gekder IC, Van Gilst WH et al. Serial antiarrhythmic drug treatment to maintain sinus rhythm after electrical cardioversion of chronic atrial fibrillation or atrial flutter. Am J Cardiol 1991; **68**: 335–41.
2 Gosselink AT, Grijns HJ, Van Gelder IC et al. Low-dose amiodarone for maintenance of sinus rhythm after cardioversion of atrial fibrillation or flutter. JAMA 1992; **267**: 3289–93.

3 Falk RH. Proarrhythmia in patients treated for atrial fibrillation or flutter. *Ann Intern Med* 1992; **117**: 141–50.

4 Allessie MA, Konings K, Kirchoff CJHJ, Wijffels M. Electrophysiologic mechanisms of perpetuation of atrial fibrillation. *Am J Cardiol* 1996; **77**: 10A–23A.

5 Cosio FG, Palacios J, Vidal JM *et al.* Electrophysiologic studies in atrial fibrillation. Slow conduction of premature impulses: a possible manifestation of the background for reentry. *Am J Cardiol* 1983; **51**: 122–30.

6 Brachmann J, Karolyi L, Kubler W. Atrial dispersion of refractoriness. *J Cardiovasc Electrophysiol* 1998; **9**: S35–9.

7 Buxton AE, Waxman HL, Marchlinski FE *et al.* Atrial conduction: effects of extrastimuli with and without atrial dysrhythmias. *Am J Cardiol* 1984; **54**: 755–61.

8 Simpson R, Foster JR, Gettes LS. Atrial excitability and conduction in patients with interatrial conduction defects. *Am J Cardiol* 1982; **50**: 1331–7.

9 Liu L, Nattel S. Differing sympathetic and vagal effects on atrial fibrillation in dogs: role of refractoriness heterogeneity. *Am J Physiol* 1997; **273** (2 Pt 2): H805–16.

10 Satoh T, Zipes DP. Unequal atrial stretch in dogs increases dispersion of refractoriness conducive to developing atrial fibrillation. *J Cardiovasc Electrophysiol* 1996; **7**: 833–42.

11 Connolly SJ, Kerr C, Gent M, Yusuf S. Dual chamber pacing versus ventricular pacing: critical appraisal of the literature. *Circulation* 1996; **94**: 578–83.

12 Andersen HR, Thuesen L, Bagger JP, Vesterlund T, Thomsen PE. Prospective randomised trial of atrial versus ventricular pacing in sick sinus syndrome. *Lancet* 1994; **344**: 1523–8.

13 Andersen HR, Nielsen JC, Thomsen PE *et al.* Long-term follow-up of patients from a randomised trial of atrial versus ventricular pacing for sick-sinus syndrome. *Lancet* 1997; **350**: 1210–16.

14 Lamas GA, Orav EJ, Stambler BS *et al.* Quality of life and clinical outcomes in elderly patients treated with ventricular pacing as compared with dual chamber pacing: Pacemaker Selection in the Elderly Investigators. *N Engl J Med* 1998; **338**: 1097–1104.

15 Connolly SJ, Kerr CR, Gent M *et al.* Effects of physiologic pacing versus ventricular pacing on the risk of stroke and death due to cardiovascular casues. *N Engl J Med* 2000; **342**: 1385–91.

16 Wharton JM, Sorrentino RA, Campbell P and the PAC-A-TACH Investigators. Effect of pacing modality on atrial tachyarrhythmia recurrence in the tachycardia–bradycardia syndome: Preliminary results of the Pacemaker Atrial Tachycardia Trial. *Circulation* 1998; **98**: 1–494.

17 Jacob MJ, Markert T, Dokumaci B *et al.* Atrial arrhythmia prevalence in paced patients: the first results of the AIDA II study. *Eur Heart J* 2000; **21**: 195.

18 Yu WC, Chen SA, Tai CT *et al.* Effects of different atrial pacing modes on atrial electrophysiology: implicating the mechanism of biatrial pacing in prevention of atrial fibrillation. *Circulation* 1997; **96**: 2992–6.

19 Padeletti L, Porciani C, Michelucci A *et al.* Interatrial septum pacing: a new approach to prevent recurrent atrial fibrillation. *J Interv Card Electrophysiol* 1999; **3**: 35–43.

20 Bailin S, Adler SW, Giudici MC *et al.* Bachmann's bundle pacing for the prevention of atrial fibrillation: initial trends in a multicenter randomized prospective study. *Pacing Clin Electrophysiol* 1999; **22**: 727 [abstract].

21 Prakash A, Delfaut P, Krol RB *et al.* Regional right and left atrial activation patterns during single- and dual-site atrial pacing in patients with atrial fibrillation. *Am J Cardiol* 1998; **15**: 1197–1204.

22 Prakash A, Saksena S, Hill M *et al.* Acute effects of dual-site right atrial pacing in patients with spontaneous and inducible atrial flutter and fibrillation. *J Am Coll Cardiol* 1997; **29**: 1007–14.

23 Papageorgiou P, Anselme F, Kirchhof CJ *et al.* Coronary sinus pacing prevents induction of atrial fibrillation. *Circulation* 1997; **96**: 1893–8.

24 Manios EG, Igoumenidis NE, Kochiadakis GE *et al.* Inducibility of atrial tachyarrhythmia in patients with lone atrial fibrillation. *Pacing Clin Electrophysiol* 1999; **22**: 843.

25 Daubert C, Mabo P, Berder V. Arrhythmia prevention by permanent atrial resynchronization in advanced interatrial blocks. *Eur J Cardiac Pacing Electrophysiol* 1994; **1**: 35–44.

26 Revault d'Allones, Pavin D, Leclerq C *et al.* Long-term effects of biatrial synchronous pacing to prevent drug-refractory atrial tachyarrhythmia: a nine year experience. *J Cardiovasc Electrophysiol* 2000; **11**: 1081–91.

27 Mabo P, Daubert JC, Bohour A. Biatrial synchronous pacing for atrial arrhythmia prevention: The SYNBIAPACE study. *Pacing Clin Electrophysiol* 1999; **22**: 755.

28 Levy T, Walker S, Rochelle J *et al.* Evaluation of biatrial pacing, right atrial pacing, and no pacing in patients with drug refractory atrial fibrillation. *Am J Cardiol* 1999; **8**: 426–9.

29 Delfaut P, Saksena S, Prakesh A, Krol RB. Long-term outcome of patients with drug-refractory atrial flutter and fibrillation after single- and dual-site right atrial pacing for arrhythmia prevention. *J Am Coll Cardiol* 1998; **32**: 1900–8.

30 Saksena S, Prakash A, Ziegler P *et al. The Dual Site Atrial Pacing for Permanent Atrial Fibrillation Trial: improved suppression of drug refractory AF with dual site*

atrial pacing and antiarrhythmic drugs. Presented at the 22nd Annual NASPE meeting, Boston, Massachusetts, May 5, 2001.

31 Lau CP, Tse HF, Yu CM *et al.* Dual site right atrial pacing in paroxysmal atrial fibrillation without bradycardia (NIPP-AF study). *Pacing Clin Electrophysiol* 1999; **22**: 804.

32 Ramdat Misier AR, Beukema WP, Oude Luttikhuis HA, Willems R. Multisite atrial pacing: An option for atrial fibrillation prevention. Preliminary results of the Dutch Dual-Site Right Atrial Pacing for Prevention of Atrial Fibrillation Study. *Am J Cardiol* 2000; **86** (Suppl): 20K–24K.

33 Aranki SF, Shaw DP, Adams DH *et al.* Predictors of atrial fibrillation after coronary artery surgery. Current trends and impact on hospital resources. *Circulation* 1996; **94**: 390–7.

34 Mathew JP, Parks R, Savino JS *et al.* Atrial fibrillation following coronary artery bypass graft surgery: predictors, outcomes, and resource utilization. Multicenter Study of Perioperative Ischemia Research Group. *JAMA* 1996; **276**: 300–6.

35 Kowey PR, Taylor JE, Rials SJ *et al.* Meta-analysis of the effectiveness of prophylactic drug therapy in preventing supraventricular arrhythmia early after coronary artery bypass grafting. *Am J Cardiol* 1992; **69**: 963–5.

36 Daoud EG, Strickberger SA, Man KC *et al.* Preoperative amiodarone as prophylaxis against atrial fibrillation after heart surgery. *N Engl J Med* 1997; **337**: 1785–91.

37 Guarnieri T, Nolan S, Gottlieb SO *et al.* Intravenous amiodarone for the prevention of atrial fibrillation after open heart surgery: the Amiodarone Reduction in Coronary Heart (ARCH) trial. *J Am Coll Cardiol* 1999; **34**: 343–7.

38 Gomes JA, Ip J, Santoni-Rugiu F *et al.* Oral d,l sotalol reduces the incidence of postoperative atrial fibrillation in coronary artery bypass surgery patients: a randomized, double-blind, placebo-controlled study. *J Am Coll Cardiol* 1999; **34**: 334–9.

39 Blommaert D, Gonzalez M, Mucumbitsi J *et al.* Effective prevention of atrial fibrillation by continuous atrial overdrive pacing after coronary artery bypass surgery. *J Am Coll Cardiol* 2000; **35**: 1411–15.

40 Daoud EG, Riba A, Strickberger A *et al.* Simultaneous right and left atrial epicardial pacing for prevention of post open-heart surgery atrial fibrillation. *Pacing Clin Electrophysiol* 1999; **22**: 707 [abstract].

41 Orr WP Tsui S, Stafford PJ *et al.* Synchronized bi-atrial pacing for the prevention of atrial fibrillation after coronary artery bypass surgery. *Pacing Clin Electrophysiol* 1999; **22**: 755 [abstract].

42 Gerstenfeld EP, Hill MR, French SN *et al.* Evaluation of right atrial and biatrial temporary pacing for the prevention of atrial fibrillation after coronary artery bypass surgery. *J Am Coll Cardiol* 1999; **33**: 1981–8.

43 Kurz DJ, Naegeli B, Kunz M *et al.* Epicardial, biatrial synchronous pacing for prevention of atrial fibrillation after cardiac surgery. *Pacing Clin Electrophysiol* 1999; **22**: 721–6.

44 Greenberg MD, Katz NM, Iuliano S *et al.* Atrial pacing for the prevention of atrial fibrillation after cardiovascular surgery. *J Am Coll Cardiol* 2000; **35**: 1416–22.

CHAPTER 5

Extraction of Pacing and Defibrillator Leads: Current Concepts and Methods

Charles J. Love

Needs and definitions

Extraction of chronic pacing and implantable cardioverter defibrillator (ICD) leads is a procedure that has been growing in volume at a rapid rate [1–3]. This increase is likely attributable to patients living longer, the introduction of new technologies, and the failure of established technologies. Pacing leads have a finite longevity, although unlike the devices to which they are attached, no 'recommended replacement time' or 'end of life' indicator is present. Lead longevity varies widely depending on lead model, construction, composition and implant technique. It is not infrequent that the lead fails to outlive the pacemaker. Patients are living longer (relative to the 1950s when pacing was introduced) and often require one or more lead replacements. This is especially true of pediatric and young adult patients. As new technologies are introduced that require additional or specialized leads, older leads may become superfluous. Many leads have been placed on 'alert' or have been recalled due to design or material problems discovered years after the products were implanted. For some designs (such as the Telectronics Accufix), abandoning the lead does not prevent the possibility of injury from lead failure.

The growing number of pacemaker and ICD implants combined with the shift to dual-chamber devices has resulted in many more leads being implanted. Newer devices may not have connectors compatible with the older large unipolar and bipolar leads. This makes abandonment or use of bulky adapters necessary during device replacement or upgrade to dual-chamber bipolar devices. We are now seeing a rise in cardiac resynchronization therapy with addition of another lead being placed into a coronary vein. All of these factors have resulted in a need for a procedure that can safely, quickly and efficiently remove superfluous leads while maintaining or recreating venous access. Based on these needs, a small group of physicians in partnership with industry created the techniques of transvenous lead extraction. Lead extraction is a specific term that is now defined as the removal of a transvenous lead that is more than a year old, or any time that specialized equipment (locking stylets, sheaths, snares) is required. Otherwise, the procedure is simply referred to as a lead removal. Success in lead extraction is defined in two ways: radiographic and clinical. Radiographic success is complete if the entire lead is removed, partial if the tip and/or a small piece of conductor coil (< 4 cm) remains, and there is failure if more than the latter remains. A clinical success is when the goal of the procedure has been attained (e.g. creation of venous access, resolution of infection, etc.). Clinical failure is when the goal has not been attained or a significant complication occurs [4]. Note that clinical success may be achieved in the setting of a radiographic failure.

Indications

Until the conference of 1998 held at the North American Society of Pacing and Electrophysiology (NASPE) annual scientific sessions, the Byrd clinical indication scheme was widely accepted [5–7]. This scheme described the indications as 'mandatory, necessary and discretionary'. Though this scheme evolved and served us well for many years, a new

Table 5.1 Indications for lead extraction.

Class I *(conditions for which there is general agreement that leads should be removed). When a lead or lead fragment causes:*
Sepsis (including endocarditis).
Life-threatening arrhythmias.
An immediate or imminent physical threat to the patient (including retained extraction hardware).
Clinically significant thromboembolic events.
Obliteration or occlusion of all useable veins, with the need to implant a new transvenous pacing system.
Interference with the operation of another implanted device.

Class 2 *(conditions for which leads are often removed, but there is some divergence of opinion with respect to the benefit vs. risk of removal). When a lead or lead fragment causes or is thought to cause:*
A localized pocket infection, erosion or chronic draining sinus that does not involve the transvenous portion of the lead
    system, when the lead can be cut through a clean incision that is totally separate from the infected area.*
An occult infection for which no source can be found.
Chronic pain at the pocket or lead insertion site that causes significant discomfort for the patient, is not manageable by
    medical or surgical technique without lead removal, and for which there is no acceptable alternative.
A threat to the patient due to its design or its failure, though not immediate or imminent if left in place.
Interference with the treatment of a malignancy.
Interference with reconstruction at the site of a traumatic injury to the entry site of the lead.
Prevention of access to the venous circulation for newly required implantable devices.
No immediate problem but is non-functional in a young patient.

Class 3 *(conditions for which there is general agreement that removal of leads is unnecessary)*
Any situation where the risk posed by removal of the lead is significantly higher than the benefit of removing the lead.
A single non-functional transvenous lead in an older patient.
Any normally functioning lead that may be reused at the time of pulse generator replacement, provided the lead has a
    reliable performance history.

---

* The lead can be cut and the clean incision closed; then the infected area can be opened, the clean distal portion of the lead pulled into the infected area, and that portion removed. This allows a total separation of the retained lead fragment from the infected area.

description of indications based on the familiar 'class 1, 2, 3' categories widely used for other procedures has now been accepted. A panel of experts consisting of surgeons, cardiologists and industry representatives were assembled in a public forum to discuss the available data and share their expertise. A document was published in the June 2000 issue of *Pacing and Clinical Electrophysiology* (PACE) [4]. A summary of the indications by class is listed in Table 5.1.

Of these indications, the one that generated (and continues to generate) significant controversy is the removal of superfluous leads. These are leads that are abandoned for a variety of reasons, including recalls, alerts, insulation failures, conductor coil failures, poor reliability records, exit block, undersensing, incompatible connectors and other issues.

Some experts feel that any old lead that is non-functional or abandoned should be routinely removed to prevent future problems in the vasculat-

ure. This would also allow access to the circulation via the extraction sheath, and prevent a more difficult extraction procedure when the leads are older. Other experts feel that leads which are not infected and do not pose a threat to the patient at the present time should be left in place [8]. The latter feel that it may be safer and easier to abandon old leads, unless they are causing a current problem or are infected. Recently Bohm and colleagues published a paper on a series of patients who had superfluous, non-infected leads abandoned rather than extracted [9]. They followed 60 patients and found that complications due to the retained leads occurred in 20% of the patients. Complications included lead migration, skin erosion, venous thrombosis and muscle stimulation. The series did not deal with the more complex issue of ICD leads in which current shunting and chatter between the leads can lead to ineffective shocks and inappropriate shocks, respectively. Overall, it is up to the physician and the patient to weigh the risks and benefits of and alternatives to a lead extraction in each situation. Factors such as the physician's experience or local access to a center with extraction expertise may play a significant role in the decision to extract a lead.

Historical perspective

In the past, very few tools were available to extract pacing and ICD leads. Usually direct manual traction was (and still is) applied to the lead for some period of time, and to a degree that was felt to be safe by the physician. When direct traction over a short term was not effective, longer-term traction was applied. This was done by tying a string to the exposed end of the lead, then placing a small weight (e.g. 0.25 kg) on the other end of the string. The string was placed over a pulley and the patient was placed in a monitored setting. When the weight was heard hitting the floor, the lead was extracted. Unfortunately, both of these direct traction methods are unreliable, time-consuming and potentially dangerous. Placing excessive direct traction on a lead may invaginate the myocardium and increase the risk of creating a serious avulsion. In addition, leaving the incision open for any period of time outside of the operating room would likely prohibit reimplant at the same site due to the possibility of infection.

In some cases, abandoning a lead in place is appropriate and the safest alternative for the patient. If this is done, the lead should be capped or cut and tied off, with some portion of the lead remaining in the pocket. No exposed conductor coil should be left in the pocket. One procedure that experts strongly discourage is that of cutting the lead and allowing the free end to retract into the vein. This makes a future lead extraction attempt very difficult. Allowing the lead to retract should never be done if the pocket and/or lead are colonized with bacteria, or if the pocket is infected. Doing so may allow the lead to be a constant source of bacterial seeding.

If traction or abandonment were not options, a primary thoracotomy was required. This is a much more invasive approach, and in many cases requires a median sternotomy and use of cardiopulmonary bypass. More recently, Byrd described a limited thoracotomy procedure that allows access to the right atrium and the ability to extract the leads

[10]. Though effective, thoracotomy has significant morbidity and recovery issues. Thoracotomy may still be the most appropriate approach for certain clinical situations (see below).

Preparation

In preparation for performing a lead extraction, the patient must be fully informed of what the procedure is, how it will be done, and what results are expected. The patient must also understand that there are significant risks, including the possibility of extensive surgical intervention and death. The degree to which these risks exist depends on a number of factors (see 'Complications', p. 58). Once informed consent has been obtained, the patient should be physically prepared for the procedure. This includes placement of good intravenous access, typing and screening for red blood cells, and obtaining some basic laboratory values (CBC, differential, electrolytes, BUN, creatinine, PT, PTT and platelets). If the patient has been on anticoagulation, this should be discontinued in advance of the operation if possible. For patients who have a mechanical valve prosthesis, hospitalization and heparinization while the INR returns to baseline have been used. It should be noted that when heparin is restarted after the operation, pocket bleeding and hematoma formation is not uncommon. Therefore, the risk of embolic events from stopping the anticoagulation needs to be balanced against the risk of bleeding from the operation. A preoperative chest X-ray may be useful, though examination by fluoroscopy may be sufficient. A lateral view of the lead system may alert the physician to the possibility of an anomalous course of the lead. Placement of the lead in the left ventricle or cardiac veins may change the approach used to remove the lead.

The operation may be performed in an operating room (OR) or an electrophysiology (EP) laboratory. Modern EP laboratories are now equipped as operating rooms. In our hospital the EP laboratory must meet the same epidemiology requirements as the ORs. One advantage of the EP laboratory over a standard OR is the quality of the fluoroscopy and monitoring equipment. Constant observation of the lead during the extraction procedure and sheath advancement is mandatory. Being able to see the sheath at all times is a great advantage. The small monitors and limited capability of most portable

C-arm fluoroscopy units in the ORs is often less than optimal. In addition, the monitoring systems in the EP laboratory used for display of intracardiac signals are often very useful during the implant portion of the operation.

Another controversy that continues is the type of anesthesia that should be used during lead extraction. Some feel that general anesthesia with endotrachial intubation is the best way to assure patient comfort. General anesthesia allows for extensive debridement of infected tissues in the device pocket when necessary. It also minimizes the time required to open the chest should this be required. The ability to easily pass a transesophageal echocardiography probe to monitor the ventricle and pericardial space is another advantage of general anesthesia. Others prefer using local anesthesia with conscious sedation. This is fast and safe and allows the patient to communicate unusual pain to the operator. I have found that the patient often lets me know verbally that a problem has occurred before the blood pressure, pulse rate or oxygenation change. Both approaches are acceptable, and the choice should be left to the operator based on experience and the particular clinical situation.

A similar controversy exists regarding the use of an arterial monitoring line. The ability to have instantaneous access to the patient's blood pressure is a very valuable tool. However, newer non-invasive blood pressure monitoring devices give rapid and accurate readouts. Pulse oximetry probes can give a pressure waveform that is proportional to the blood pressure, giving information similar to the arterial line. One advantage of an arterial line placed via the femoral artery is that it can be used to access the circulation for the purpose of placing the patient on percutaneous extracorporeal membrane oxygenation (ECMO). Having a femoral arterial and venous line in place may allow the rapid use of ECMO to sustain a patient until a definitive operation to correct the vascular accident or myocardial tear can be completed.

On other topics, there is no controversy among the experts. If the operator is not a cardiothoracic surgeon, the latter should be on site and readily available. Having access to a peripheral vascular surgeon is also helpful, as some of the vascular complications require a team approach to resolve successfully. Open-heart procedures must be available at the hospital where the extraction is being performed. Should a problem occur, there is no time to transfer a patient to another institution. A pericardiocentesis tray needs to be immediately accessible, as should be a thoracotomy tray. The team assisting the operator should be experienced with, or well instructed on the procedure. These people must know the equipment being used and how to monitor the patient properly. I have repeatedly stated that the best safety factor in our laboratory is the staff that assist me.

Though it should go without saying, the operator should also be well trained. The viewing of an instructional videotape or watching someone else do several extractions is insufficient as a means of obtaining competency. One should perform a minimum of 20 'hands-on' lead extractions under the instruction of an operator well experienced in all of the techniques and tools available. Even this level of training is unlikely to cover all situations and complications that are likely to occur during extraction procedures. As with all procedures, simply achieving a minimum number does not by itself imply that an operator is competent.

Before beginning an extraction procedure, one should have available a wide array of tools to assist in the performance of the operation. This includes sheaths of different sizes and compositions, locking stylets, tools for superior and femoral approaches, and miscellaneous snares and catheters. Powered sheaths such as the Spectranetics Laser Sheath (SLS™) or the Cook Vascular Electrosurgical Dissection Sheath (EDS™) may increase the success rate and reduce the time required to perform the extraction. To date, there is no evidence that use of powered sheaths decrease the complication rate of the procedure. In summary, the more experienced the operator and the wider the array of tools available, the more likely a successful and safe procedure.

Procedure description

The approach to the extraction will depend on the condition and location of the leads, as well as any evidence of vascular anomalies that might be present. Typically, an extraction is performed from the site of venous access (i.e. superior approach). If the lead has been cut or fractured and has retracted into the vascular space, the femoral approach is most often used. If any portion of the lead is present in the pocket, the lead must be exposed and dissected free

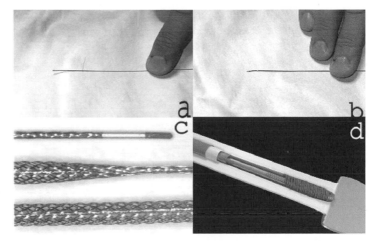

Figure 5.1 Locking stylets. (a) Original Cook Locking Stylet uses a small piece of fine wire that 'bunches up' when the stylet is rotated. (b) Second-generation Cook Wilkoff™ Locking Stylet has a 'barb' that protrudes. (c) Spectranetics LLD™ Lead Locking Device uses a wire mesh stretched over a stylet that expands when released. (d) Third-generation Cook Liberator™ Locking Stylet uses a spring at the end of the stylet that is compressed by an outer hollow stylet.

from the adherent tissues. All suture and suturing sleeve material must be removed. The latter is critical if an infection is present in the pocket, as retained foreign material will prevent the infection from being eradicated.

Leads that have been in place for less than 1 year, as well as other leads that are isodiametric and active fixation in design, are often removed using direct traction and rotation of the lead. If the lead will not release from the myocardium with minimal to moderated traction (up to 1 kg of force), then use of a locking stylet and extraction sheaths is recommended. Until recently, the use of a locking stylet required precise sizing of the internal lumen of the central conductor coil. The development of the Spectranetics Lead Locking Device (LLD™) and the Cook Vascular Liberator™ locking stylet has not only made the precise measurements unnecessary, but has resulted in an improved and more secure 'lock' in the lead. The LLD reduced the number of sizes to 3, and the Liberator is a 'one size fits all' design. The original Cook locking stylets in iterations of 0.001 inch are no longer in production (Figure 5.1).

Once the lead has been dissected free, the end is clipped cleanly, and the inner coil is exposed and dilated if necessary. A standard stylet is placed into the central coil lumen to assure that it is patent, and to clear any debris that may be present. In some cases a stylet may not pass due to debris in, or kinking of, the central coil. A locking stylet is then passed to the tip of the lead (or as far as it will go if a kink or obstruction is present). The stylet is then locked, and a suture is placed tightly around the proximal end

of the lead with the free end of the suture then attached to the locking stylet. The ligature compresses the insulation and outer coil (if present) onto the inner coil, preventing both the insulation from 'bunching' in front of the extraction sheath, and the conductor coils from unraveling. If a locking stylet cannot be placed, the amount of traction that can be placed on the lead before the lead breaks is limited. This makes the extraction more difficult, and may require the use of a powered sheath system or a femoral approach.

Once the lead is prepared, an appropriate sheath is applied to the lead. Sheath choices include non-powered types made of Teflon, polypropylene or stainless steel (Figure 5.2). The latter are used only to enter the central circulation when significant scar tissue or calcification prevents insertion of the more flexible sheaths. Optionally, a powered sheath may be used. These utilize either ultraviolet laser energy delivered through the Spectranetics SLS™

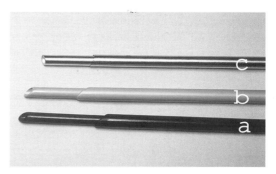

Figure 5.2 Non-powered telescoping extraction sheaths: (a) Teflon; (b) polypropylene; (c) stainless steel.

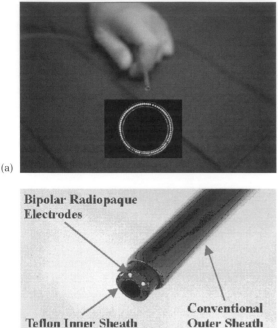

(a)

(b)

Bipolar Radiopaque Electrodes

Conventional Outer Sheath

Teflon Inner Sheath with Beveled Tip

Figure 5.3 Powered sheaths: (a) Spectranetics SLS™ Laser Sheath; (b) Cook Vascular EDS™ Electrosurgical Dissection Sheath.

sheath, or electrosurgical radiofrequency energy via the Cook EDS™ sheath (Figure 5.3). The characteristics, advantages and disadvantages of the different sheath types are summarized in Table 5.2. The sheath system is advanced over the lead under constant fluoroscopic observation, staying in line (coaxial) with the lead and using 'counterpressure'. Counterpressure is the process of advancing the sheath system using forward pressure, while applying an equal and opposite amount of force to the lead. As binding sites are encountered, the sheaths are manipulated or energized to move forward. There are two sites that are critical during the advancement of the sheaths. The first is the junction of the inominate vein with the superior vena cava. The acute bend in the venous anatomy is prone to tearing as the sheath makes the bend. If the tear is above the pericardial reflection, bleeding will enter the right pleural space with resultant hemothorax. If the right-sided (venous) pressures are high, rapid exsanguination may occur. The second critical site is the junction of the superior vena cava with the right atrium. Fibrosis frequently occurs at this site, and there appears to be some relative structural weakness of the tissues predisposing to tears. A tear in this area will usually result in pericardial tamponade.

Once the sheaths are advanced to approximately 1 cm from the tip of the lead, the lead is pulled up against the sheath using 'countertraction'. The traction force applied to the lead is countered by the end of the sheath (Figure 5.4). This has the effect of localizing the force on the myocardium to prevent a large avulsion of the tissue where the lead is attached to the heart. The lead is then pulled into the sheath, and the myocardium is allowed to fall back to its normal position. If an infection is not present and a new lead is to be placed from the same site, a guidewire may be passed through the extraction sheath before the sheath is removed.

A variation on the superior approach utilizing the jugular vein has been advocated by some as possibly being more safe and effective than the traditional approach [11]. After the lead is dissected free from the tissues in the pocket, venous entry is made via the right internal jugular vein. A snare is then used to grasp the lead, the free end of which is then pulled through the jugular vein. The lead is then extracted using the methods noted above. It is felt that since this provides a more linear approach to the lead (eliminating sharp bends), a reduction in shearing force as the sheaths make acute bends will be reduced or eliminated. The downside to this approach is an

Table 5.2 Advantages and disadvantages of sheath types.

Sheath type	Cost per sheath	Accessory cost	Time reduction	Safety	Efficacy
Teflon sheaths	$	0	0	+	+
Polypropylene sheaths	$	0	0	+	++
Stainless steel sheaths	$	0	+	+	N/A
Laser sheath	$$$$	$$$$	+++	+	++++
Electrosurgical sheath	$$	$$	+++	+	++++

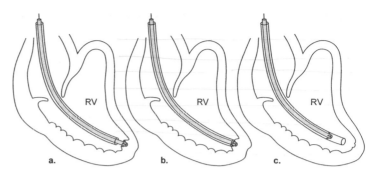

Figure 5.4 Countertraction. (a) Sheath is advanced to about 1 cm from the myocardium. (b) The lead and myocardium are drawn up to the sheath. (c) Traction is applied until the lead releases and the myocardium falls safely away.

additional venous entry site, additional time required to perform the operation, and not retaining venous access from the subclavian insertion site.

In some cases, the lead may not be accessible from the superior approach. Given this scenario, or as a primary approach at the desire of the operator, the femoral approach may be used to snare the lead and extract it via the femoral vein. As the proximal portion of the lead is not available, locking stylets are not used when a femoral extraction approach is performed. In performing a femoral extraction, if any portion of the lead remains attached in the pocket, it must be dissected free. If the connector is present, it is cut off. The femoral vein is accessed using a 16F femoral workstation. This is a long Teflon sheath with a hemostatic valve. A number of different types of snares are available to entangle the lead and pull it into the sheath. A snare is placed into the sheath, and the lead is grasped and pulled into the sheath. The sheath is advanced over the lead to near the electrode tip and countertraction is used to remove the lead.

Occasionally, a lead cannot be removed using a transvenous approach, or a situation may be present that precludes the use of intravascular sheaths. This may be due to the presence of calcification around the lead, large vegetations on the lead, or the presence of a known vascular anomaly. In addition, in some cases a transvenous approach may have failed, resulting in retention of the lead and/or extraction tools. In such situations, a thoracotomy may be required to remove the lead and/or retained extraction tools. Thus, thoracotomy may serve as a primary or secondary procedure for the extraction. The approach may be a median sternotomy, lateral thoracotomy or the Byrd transthoracic approach. The latter uses a small incision over the right parasternal region with removal of a piece of the 4th

or 5th costochondral cartilage. The right atrium is then accessible to enter and remove the lead [10].

Some situations require extreme caution and special consideration of the planned approach. These include inadvertent placement of the lead on the left side of the heart, coronary sinus leads, and leads placed into a descending cardiac vein. Historically, leads were placed into the coronary sinus to pace the atrium or were placed there inadvertently. Similarly, leads placed into a descending cardiac vein were typically thought to have been put into the right ventricle. With the advent of ICD therapy, coronary sinus leads were placed intentionally. More recently, lead placement into the descending coronary veins for biventricular pacing is becoming routine. These venous structures make extraction difficult due to their small size and tortuosity. In addition, should a tear of one of these posterior structures occur, surgical repair may be quite challenging. For leads that have been placed inadvertently into the left ventricle or left atrium via a septal defect or patent foramen ovale, the risk of causing a cerebral or systemic embolic event is present. Most lead extraction experts prefer to approach these cases by primary thoracotomy. This allows the lead to be removed directly, and any extraneous fibrotic tissue, fibrous sheath material and thrombus to be removed.

Results

In the early years of lead extraction, complete success was achieved in 88% of cases (as defined by removal of all intravascular lead material) [2]. This included the need to resort to a femoral approach in a significant number of cases. Over more than a decade of experience and tool development the complete success rate has risen to 93% with a reduction in the time required to perform the procedure. Currently, in skilled hands, when combined with partial success rates of 5%, the overall success rate is in the range of 98% [12]. This increase in efficacy has been accomplished without an increase in complications. The major contributing factors to the increased success have been the development of the newer type of locking stylets, and the laser and EDS-powered sheath systems.

Complications

Unfortunately, extraction of chronically implanted pacing and ICD leads has inherent risks. These are related to the fibrous attachment of the leads to the vein and the myocardium, to unforeseen vascular anomalies, and to the inability of the operator to maintain a coaxial alignment to the lead. As noted above, the sharp bend from the inominate vein into the superior vena cava represents an area of common vascular tear, as does the junction of the superior vena cava with the right atrium. Avulsions of atrial or ventricular myocardium are also possible. The latter often occur while traction is being applied to a lead while attempting to advance an extraction sheath. In attempting to safely advance the sheath system around a bend, the traction applied to the lead may be in excess of that needed to avulse the lead from the myocardium. If the fibrous tissue–myocardium attachment is strong, a transmural avulsion will occur with subsequent pericardial tamponade. Other complications that have been reported are listed in Table 5.3.

As with any invasive procedure, complications will occur even when appropriate precautions, techniques and experienced hands are used. Preparation for this eventuality is critical if the patient is going to be rescued. The immediate availability of

Table 5.3 Complications of lead extraction.

Major complications
Death
Cardiac avulsion or tear requiring intervention
Vascular avulsion or tear requiring intervention
Hemothorax or severe bleeding from any source requiring transfusion
Pneumothorax requiring chest tube drainage
Pulmonary embolism requiring surgical intervention
Respiratory arrest
Septic shock
Stroke

Minor complications
Pericardial effusion not requiring pericardiocentesis or surgical intervention
Hemodynamically significant air embolism
Pulmonary embolism not requiring intervention
Vascular repair near the implant site or venous entry site
Arrhythmia requiring cardioversion
Hematoma at the pocket requiring drainage
Arm swelling or thrombosis of implant veins resulting in medical intervention
Sepsis in a previously non-septic patient with infection
Pacing system-related infection of a previously non-infected site

Observations
Transient hypotension that responds to fluids or minor pharmacologic
   intervention
Non-significant air embolism
Small pneumothorax not requiring intervention
Ectopy not requiring cardioversion
Arm swelling or thrombosis of implant veins without need for medical
   intervention
Pain at cut-down site
Myocardial avulsion without sequelae
Migrated lead fragment without sequelae

pericardiocentesis and thoracotomy instruments is critical. Blood should be screened ahead of time, and both cardiac and peripheral vascular surgeons should be available on site to deal with a cardiac or vascular tear. Having access to diagnostic and interventional radiology services is also very helpful to determine the exact site and nature of a vascular tear or anomaly. Rapid response to a complication will nearly always result in a good outcome. However, some situations such as a slow blood leak into the pleural space may not be recognized until the patient can no longer be resuscitated. Hypotension is very frequent during lead extraction as a result of vagal stimulation from visceral traction. Differentiating this benign atropine- and fluid-responsive problem from a life-threatening tear or avulsion can be a challenge. For this reason, having echocardiography immediately available is also important. Physicians who perform lead extraction under general anesthesia should consider the use of transesophageal echo to monitor the pericardial space during the critical phases of the extraction. Some physicians have also reported on the use of intravenous ultrasound to observe the progress of the sheath system, and to evaluate the structure of the fibrous encapsulation surrounding the lead [13]. In the future, this may assist in finding arteriovenous fistulae and leads that have eroded into the extravascular space.

Summary

Lead extraction has become a true procedure, with an organized and logical set of steps. These have evolved to allow the safe and effective removal of pacing and ICD leads by a transvenous approach. The pioneering efforts of a core group of physicians dedicated to lead extraction, as well as the efforts of industry to provide the tools needed, have been instrumental in bringing us the current state of the art. In well-trained hands, lead extraction can be performed quickly and safely. There remain challenges to be overcome as pacing continues to evolve. Coronary sinus and cardiac venous leads will continue to present us with a higher level of risk and complexity. Hopefully, newer technologies and techniques will be developed to assist in these special situations. Finally, the pacing industry is developing new lead systems that will have 'extractability' built into the basic design of pacing and ICD leads. This may reduce or eliminate the need for specialized extraction techniques in the future.

References

1 Wilkoff BL, Smith HJ, Fearnot NE et al. Intravascular lead extraction: multicenter update for 523 patients [abstract]. *Pacing Clin Electrophysiol* 1992; **15**: 513.

2 Smith HJ, Fearnot NE, Byrd CL et al. Five-years experience with intravascular lead extraction. *Pacing Clin Electrophysiol* 1994; **17**: 2016–20.

3 Byrd CL, Wilkoff BL, Love CJ, Sellers TD, Reiser C. Clinical Study of the Laser Sheath for Lead Extraction: the total expenerice in the United States. *PACE* 2002; **25**: 804–8.

4 Love CJ, Wilkoff BL, Byrd CL et al. Recommendations for extraction of chronically implanted transvenous pacing and defibrillator leads: indications, facilities, training. North American Society of Pacing and Electrophysiology Lead Extraction Conference Faculty. *Pacing Clin Electrophysiol* 2000; **23** (4–1): 544–51.

5 Byrd CL, Schwartz SJ, Hedin N. Lead extraction: indications and techniques. *Cardiol Clin* 1992; **10**: 735–48.

6 Byrd CL, Schwartz SJ, Hedin NB. Lead extraction: techniques and indications. In: Barold SS, Mugica J, eds. *New Perspectives in Cardiac Pacing*, 3. Mt. Kisco, NY: Futura, 1993: 29–55.

7 Byrd CL. Management of implant complications. In: Ellenbogen KA, Kay GN, Wilkoff BL, eds. *Clinical Cardiac Pacing*. Philadelphia: W.B. Saunders, 2000; 669–709.

8 Levine PA. Should lead explantation be the practice standard when a lead needs to be replaced? *Pacing Clin Electrophysiol* 2000; **23** (4–1): 421–2.

9 Bohm A, Pinter A, Duiray G et al. Complications due to abandoned noninfected pacemaker leads. *Pacing Clin Electrophysiol* 2001; **24**: 1721–4.

10 Byrd CL, Schwartz SJ. Transatrial implantation of transvenous pacing leads as an alternative to implantation of epicardial leads. *Pacing Clin Electrophysiol* 1990; **13** (12–2): 1856–9.

11 Soldati E, Bongiorni MG, Arena G et al. A ten-year single-center experience in transvenous removal of pacing and defibrillating leads: results and complications in more than 1000 leads. *Pacing Clin Electrophysiol* 2002; **25** (4–2): 562.

12 Wilkoff BL, Byrd CL, Love CJ et al. Pacemaker lead extraction with the laser sheath: results of the pacing lead extraction with the excimer sheath (PLEXES) trial. *J Am Coll Cardiol* 1999; **33** (6): 1671–6.

13 Arena G, Bongiorni MG, Soldati E et al. Usefulness of intracardiac echography for transvenous leads extraction. *Pacing Clin Electrophysiol* 2002; **25** (4–2): 545.

PART II
Multisite Pacing in Heart Failure

CHAPTER 6

Multisite Pacing for Heart Failure: From Electrophysiology to Hemodynamics

Luigi Padeletti, Alessandra Sabini, Cristina Tosti Guerra, Andrea Colella, Gabriele Demarchi, Paolo Pieragnoli, Antonio Michelucci and Maria Cristina Porciani

Effects of left bundle branch block on ventricular function: experimental and clinical studies

The effects of artificial stimuli on the mammalian ventricle were first studied in 1925 by Wiggers [1] who demonstrated in the canine heart that 'when artificial stimuli are given to the inhibited ventricles at rates corresponding to the normal for any heart, the initial slower rise of intraventricular pressure is prolonged, the isometric contraction phase is lengthened, the gradient is not so steep, the pressure maximum is lower and the duration of systole is increased . . . When a local artificial stimulus is applied to any portion of the ventricular surface the impulse spreads somewhat radically from the point of stimulation and induces a series of local fractionate contractions responsible for the initial slow rise of intraventricular pressure . . . Consequently, two different contraction processes almost imperceptibly merge: the first one is a localized fractionate contraction occasioned by a relatively slow fiber to fiber excitation and the second one is a more generalized contraction of the remaining ventricular muscle excited via bundle branches in more rapid sequence'.

Since this original observation, many other animal and human studies have suggested that left bundle branch block (LBBB) induced by ventricular pacing results in an abnormal activation pattern with depressed ventricular function, alterations in regional myocardial perfusion, and myocardial structural changes.

Park et al. [2] demonstrated in closed-chest dogs that ventricular pacing produces a rightward shift of the left ventricular (LV) end-systolic pressure–volume relation. The extent of this shift was related to the degree of LV dyssynchrony as estimated by QRS duration. In contrast, this shift did not occur during atrial pacing.

Burkhoff et al. [3] investigated the influence of the pacing site in an isolated heart preparation and observed an inverse linear correlation between QRS duration and peak LV pressure. These workers suggested that the loss of ventricular pump function during ventricular pacing was caused by a decrease in effective or functional muscle mass. It was postulated that the epicardial regions activated early did not contribute to the function of the entire ventricle because they underwent a relatively unloaded contraction.

Prinzen et al. [4] confirmed these finding in a study involving opened-chest dogs paced from the right atrium, right ventricular outflow tract (RVOT) and LV apex. Ventricular pacing was associated with a significant non-uniform LV distribution of epicardial fiber strain and blood flow. Asynchronous ventricular electrical activation secondary to ventricular pacing decreased contractile force in regions activated early, and increased it in epicardial regions activated late. In both RVOT and LV apical pacing, similar non-uniformities in epicardial electrical activation time, fiber strain and blood flow were observed, albeit in the opposite direction.

A subsequent study by the same group [5] quantified by magnetic resonance the degree and extent of local myofiber shortening and work during asynchronous electrical activation, evoked by ventricular pacing from the LV base and right ventricular apex (RVA). Both pacing modes caused pronounced redistribution of midwall fiber shortening and work, with work values ranging from 50% of normal at the pacing site to about 150% in sites farthest from the pacing sites. The reduction in systolic shortening and external work as well as the size of the hypofunctioning zone around the pacing site were significantly larger during RVA pacing than during basal LV pacing. These local changes may be responsible for the depression in ventricular function during RVA pacing.

The same workers also demonstrated that the propagation velocity of mechanical activation during ventricular pacing is similar to the velocity of electrical propagation in the myocardium. The propagation of mechanical activation for an LV wall pacing site produced homogeneous LV activation, whereas propagation for the right ventricular pacing sites generated dishomogeneous mechanical responses [6].

Two different echocardiographic investigations in dogs during epicardial LV pacing documented that regions activated early became thinner but the septum became thickened (the late activated region) after 6 months [7,8]. Postmortem examinations showed that myocytes were significantly thicker in the septum than in the LV free wall [8].

In humans the impact of LBBB on LV performance remains controversial. Bourassa and Takeshita studied the effects of intermittent LBBB on LV performance and demonstrated that, in abnormal hearts, intermittent LBBB causes significant deterioration of LV performance manifested by a decrease in systolic pressure, cardiac output (CO) and LV contractility [9,10]. In contrast, Wong [11] found no change in the timing of left heart events, hemodynamic pressures and indices of LV function during normal intraventricular conduction and during intermittent LBBB in a subject with a normal heart.

Different results were obtained by Grines et al. [12] who compared 18 patients with isolated LBBB with 10 normal subjects by performing apex cardigrams, phonocardiograms, electrocardiograms (ECGs), two-dimensional dual M-mode echocardiograms and radionuclide ventriculograms. There was no evidence of heart disease in the group with LBBB and the etiology was considered primary conduction disease in all patients. The results suggested that altered electrical activation in patients with isolated LBBB caused global ventricular abnormalities manifested by abnormal findings in diastolic filling times, abnormal heart sounds, interventricular septal motion and LV ejection fraction.

In a retrospective echocardiographic study of patients with LBBB, Prinzen et al. [7] found that the septal site activated early was significantly thinner than the posterior wall activated late, but there was no difference in regional wall thickness in a control group.

Xiao et al. [13] compared the effect of right ventricular pacing and classic LBBB on LV function in a retrospective and prospective study of 48 patients, 24 with a VVI pacemaker and 24 with LBBB. They investigated the two functional situations with electrocardiography, and M-mode, cross-sectional and Doppler echocardiography. The LV was activated much more rapidly with RV pacing than with LBBB. This occurred even when LBBB was present before pacing. The two situations produced different electromechanical delays, contraction and relaxation times and extent of uncoordinated ventricular wall motion. These workers concluded that in humans, the influence of right ventricular pacing and LBBB on LV function is not identical and questioned the use of right ventricular pacing as an experimental model for LBBB.

Right ventricular pacing, even in the presence of atrioventricular (AV) synchrony and rate adaptation, is associated with reduced local myocardium perfusion at the site of pacing as detected by thallium-201 exercise myocardial scintigraphy. These perfusion abnormalities with RVA pacing may result from alterations in myocardial activation and contraction. Furthermore, the incidence of impaired perfusion increases with time. In the long term, these perfusion abnormalities may produce regional wall motion abnormalities, resulting in impaired global LV function [14].

In 1998 Murkofsky et al. [15] correlated QRS duration with LV ejection fraction (EF) and observed that non-specific prolonged QRS duration (> 0.10 s) on a standard resting 12-lead ECG in the absence of typical bundle branch block is indicative of decreased resting LV systolic function.

Recently, Das et al. [16] evaluated ejection fraction (EF) and QRS duration and concluded that in LBBB, the QRS duration has a significant inverse relationship with EF and that a value ≥ 170 ms is a marker of significant LV systolic dysfunction.

Effects of left bundle branch block on prognosis in dilated cardiomyopathy

In 1944 White wrote: 'There seem to be two general clinical groups of cases with bundle branch block: (1) with a rapidly bad prognosis based largely on the presence of evidence of extensive heart disease, usually considerable enlargement and some degree of myocardial or coronary insufficiency: (2) with a fairly good prognosis of years of life and activity in which the bundle branch block is the only abnormal finding; despite this general trend accurate prognosis in an individual case is usually impossible' [17].

In 1951 Johnsons *et al.* reported on survival in a series of 555 consecutive patients with LBBB [18]. Heart size was definitely related to survival time. Patients with hearts of normal size survived approximately 1 year longer than the average patient, whereas those with marked enlargement of the heart had a shorter survival period by about 1 year.

Patients with dilated cardiomyopathy and ventricular activation disturbances characterized by ECG criteria for LBBB are at greater risk of clinical deterioration and mortality. Xiao *et al.* [19], in a retrospective study on 56 patients with dilated cardiomyopathy, observed that changes in ventricular conduction, readily quantifiable from the standard ECG, may carry significant prognostic information. In the patients who died, there was a striking acceleration in the rate of increase in QRS duration (to 4–5 times—in terms of the rate of increase, and not to the absolute value—in the months before death compared to that of clinically stable patients). The ventricular cavity size, PR interval and QRS duration increased progressively with time in all patients. These findings were confirmed by Venkateshawar *et al.* [20] who observed that the 6-year mortality rate in patients with chronic heart failure (CHF) and altered LV function was significantly higher, regardless of the degree of LV impairment, in patients with a QRS duration > 110 ms. An important contribution was provided by the data from the Italian Network on Congestive Heart Failure Patients Registry [21]. The study population included 5517 patients with CHF, and complete LBBB in 1391 (25.2%). LBBB was associated with a significantly higher prevalence of NYHA classification III to IV CHF, reduced systolic blood pressure, third heart sound, abnormally increased cardiothoracic ratio, and severely reduced EF measured by echocardiography. All-cause mortality and sudden death mortality rates were significantly greater in patients with LBBB.

Cardiac pacing for heart failure patients

Initial clinical studies of pacing in patients with heart failure focused on the effects of shortening the atrioventricular (AV) delay [22–24] but the results were disappointing [25–28]. The lack of benefit may be due to the potential detrimental effect of pacing-induced widening of the QRS complex, outweighing the beneficial effect of increased ventricular filling time. Consequently, interest has now shifted to LV-based pacing, mainly biventricular pacing (BVP). The valuable lessons learned from optimization of the AV delay from these early studies should not be ignored because they form part of the total resynchronization strategy in the CHF patient. After the first report in 1983 involving four patients [29], nearly 13 years elapsed before the first reported systematic analysis of multisite pacing in CHF. In 1996 Cazeau *et al.* [30] evaluated eight patients with a wide QRS and end-stage CHF by performing invasive hemodynamic studies with different pacing configurations (RVA/RVOT pacing and two configurations of BVP: RVOT/LV and RVA/LV). BVP configurations increased the mean cardiac index, decreased the mean V wave and decreased pulmonary capillary wedge pressure (PCWP). Several subsequent studies compared the hemodynamic effect of right ventricular, LV and biventricular temporary pacing (Table 6.1) [31–34]. In 1997 Blanc *et al.* [31] performed an acute hemodynamic evaluation in 27 patients with CHF and either first-degree AV block and/or intraventricular conduction disturbances. Pacing of LV either alone or in combination with right ventricular pacing resulted in a significant increase of systolic blood pressure and a decrease in both PCWP and mean V-wave amplitude. These findings were confirmed in 1998 by Leclercq *et al.* [32] who studied the acute hemodynamic response to BVP in patients with severely symptomatic CHF with intraventricular conduction delay. Cardiac index improved and PCWP decreased significantly with BVP configuration. Several others'

Table 6.1 Studies comparing the effect of multisite pacing on hemodynamics.

Authors	n	Pacing site	PCWP	CO	LV dP/dt
Cazeau et al. [30]	8	RV	=	=	
		LV	=	=	N/A
		LV + RVA	=	↑	
		LV + RVOT	=	↑	
Blanc et al. [31]	23	RVA	=		
		LV	↓	N/A	N/A
		LV + RVA	↓		
Leclercq et al. [32]	18	RV	↑	↑	
		BV	↑	↑	N/A
Kass et al. [34]	18	RV	=		=
		LV	=	N/A	↓
		BV	=		↓
Auricchio et al. [33]	27	RV	=		=
		LV	↑	N/A	↑
		LV + RVA	↓		↑

CO, cardiac output; PCWP, pulmonary capillary wedge pressure; RV, right ventricular (various sites); BV, biventricular; LV, left ventricular; RVA, RV apex; RVOT, RV outflow tract; N/A, not applicable.

hemodynamic studies have now confirmed these observations and have also demonstrated that BVP enhances ventricular systolic function as assessed by maximal rate of pressure rise [33,34] and pressure–volume loops [34], and improves the magnitude and synchrony of wall contraction [35,36].

Recent clinical trials [37,38] suggest that cardiac resynchronization therapy (CRT) may be of clinical benefit (Table 6.2) in terms of improvement in NYHA functional class status, ability to cover a greater distance during a 6-min walking test, higher peak oxygen consumption during exercise testing, and a reduced score on the Minnesota Living with Heart Failure Questionnaire.

Nelson et al. [39] recently performed cardiac catheterization in 10 patients with dilated cardiomyopathy and LBBB during LV or BVP, and compared the results to intravenous dobutamine. They demonstrated that both BVP and LV-only pacing can generate systolic improvement while concomitantly reducing myocardial energy or oxygen consumption. By contrast the inotropic agents improve dP/dt but at the cost of an increased oxygen consumption.

Hamdan et al. [40] reported that short-term BVP increases arterial blood pressure and reduces sympathetic nerve activity. Saxon et al. [41] reported a decrease in serum norepinephrine levels after 12 weeks of BV pacing in patients with CHF and conduction delay. Inflammatory cytokines are known to contribute to the progression of heart failure, and are related to patient prognosis [42]. Insulin-like growth factor I (IGF-I) is a cell survival factor that inhibits tumor necrosis factor alpha (TNF-α)-induced cell-killing [43]; a reduction of IGF-I plasma levels has been demonstrated in CHF [44]. A significant increase of IGF-I plasma levels associated with reduced cytokine activation was observed in 25 patients after 3 months of BVP [45].

QRS duration before (wider) and during BVP (narrower) is correlated with the hemodynamic improvement with BVP [33,40,46]. However, Kass et al. [34] demonstrated in their acute study that hemodynamic improvement obtained by BVP was not correlated with the degree of QRS narrowing. Indeed one study showed that over an 8-month period of follow-up, patients not improved by BVP exhibited the same degree of QRS shortening as patients improved clinically [47]. Thus, ECG criteria do not clearly correlate with the mechanical aspect of asynchrony. In this respect, Gras et al. [48] pointed out that the QRS may be an insensitive marker for the selection of patients for BVP because a relatively short QRS may be associated with

Table 6.2 Effects of cardiac resynchronization therapy reported in controlled clinical trials.

	PATH-CHF*	MUSTIC†	MIRACLE‡
Inclusion criteria	NYHA III–IV	NYHA III	NYHA III–IV
	QRS > 120 ms	QRS > 150 ms	QRS ≥ 130 ms
	PR > 150 ms	LVEF < 35%	LVEF ≤ 35%
		LVEDD > 60 mm	LVEDD ≥ 55 mm
Follow-up (months)	12	12	6
Effects on primary endpoints			
NYHA class	+	+	+
6 min WT	+	+	+
Vo_{2max}	+	+	NS
QOL	+	+	+

PATH-CHF, pacing therapies for congestive heart failure; MUSTIC, multisite stimulation in cardiomyopathies; MIRACLE, Multicenter InSync Randomized Clinical Evaluation; PR, interval between P wave and QRS complex in ECG surface; LVEF, ejection fraction; LVEDD, left ventricle end diastolic diameter.

+, statistically significant positive change; NYHA, New York Heart Association; 6 min WT, 6-min walking test; Vo_{2max}, maximum oxygen consumption measured during exercise test; QOL, quality of life score using Minnesota Living with Heart Failure Questionnaire.

* Auricchio A, Stellbrink C, Sack S *et al.* Long-term benefit as a result of pacing resynchronization in congestive heart failure: results of the PATH-CHF trial. *Circulation* 2000; **102** (18) (Suppl. 2): 693 (A).

† Linde C, Leclercq C, Rex S *et al.* Long-term benefits of biventricular pacing in congestive heart failure: results from the Multisite Stimulation In Cardiomyopathy (MUSTIC) study. *J Am Coll Cardiol* 2002; **40**: 111–18.

‡ Abraham WT, Fisher W, Smith A *et al.* Cardiac resynchronization therapy in chronic heart failure. *N Engl J Med* 2002; **346**: 1845–53.

dyssynchrony detectable by echocardiography or other ways.

The role of echocardiography in cardiac resynchronization therapy

CRT is commonly equated only with ventricular resynchronization. However, the concept should encompass a more complex form of 'synchronism' involving important parameters such as interatrial, atrioventricular, intra-atrial, interventricular and intraventricular synchronization. The temporal sequence and reciprocal relationship of electrical and mechanical events in every cardiac cycle and in all chambers define cardiac efficiency. Cardiac pacing by acting on the timing of electrical and mechanical events can correct asynchrony and improve hemodynamics.

New roles of echocardiography are evolving in CRT:
1 evaluation of the temporal sequence of cardiac mechanical events;
2 assessment of CRT effects; and
3 identification of CRT responders.

Evaluation of the temporal sequence of cardiac mechanical events

The P wave and QRS complex are electrical phenomena with corresponding atrial and ventricular mechanical contractions. By simultaneous ECG and echocardiography recordings it is possible to measure the delay between these events, for both left and right atrium and left and right ventricle. These intervals are defined as 'electromechanical delay'. Therefore, left and right atrial electromechanical delays (L/RAED) can be measured as the interval from the onset of the P wave and the beginning of the diastolic mitral or tricuspidal A wave respectively (Figure 6.1). In the same way left and right ventricular electromechanical delays (L/RVED), can be measured as the interval between QRS onset and the beginning of aortic or pulmonary systolic flow respectively (Figure 6.2). Interatrial and interventricular delays (IAD, IVD) are expressions of interatrial and interventricular synchrony and can be measured as the difference between left and right atrial and between left and right ventricular electromechanical delays (Figures 6.1 & 6.2).

Interatrial delay (IAD) measurement

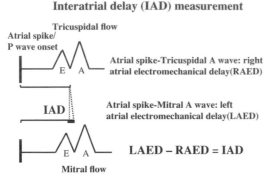

Figure 6.1 Method for the measurement of left and right atrial electromechanical delays, as the difference between atrial spike and beginning of mitral or tricuspidal A wave. Interatrial delay is obtained from the difference between left and right atrial electromechanical delays.

Interventricular delay (IVD) measurement

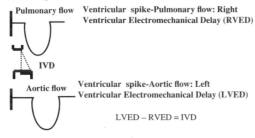

Figure 6.2 Method for the measurement of left and right ventricular electromechanical delays, as the difference between ventricular spike/QRS onset and the beginning of aortic or pulmonary systolic flows. Interventricular delay is obtained from the difference between left and right ventricular electromechanical delays.

AV synchrony is another important aspect of CRT because appropriate timing between left atrial and LV contraction, i.e. optimal AV delay, can improve CO by reducing mitral valve regurgitation and increasing mitral diastolic filling time [49]. AV delay optimization modulates the hemodynamic benefit of BVP in a way similar to traditional DDD pacing [33,34]. However, new problems with AV delay optimization have surfaced. The programmed right-sided AV delay can differ from the effective left-sided AV delay because of IAD and IVD [50], so that the left AV delay is equal to the programmed right AV delay minus IAD plus IVD [50]. Thus, the difference between left and right AV delay depends

Mechanical AV delay (MAVD) measurement

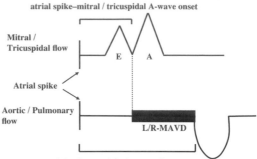

Figure 6.3 Right and left mechanical atrioventricular delay (RMAVD and LMAVD) can be calculated as the interval between the beginning of the atrial and ventricular contractions, that is, the time from mitral or tricuspid A-wave onset to aortic or pulmonary flow onset, respectively. When a partial fusion of E and A wave occurs, the beginning of A wave should be obtained by extrapolating the time of rising of A-wave velocity to the zero line. Since the mitral and aortic flows cannot be simultaneously recorded, the atrial spike should be considered as a reference point and the left and right mechanical AV delays are calculated as the difference between [atrial spike to aortic or pulmonary flow onset] interval and [atrial spike to mitral or tricuspidal A-wave onset] interval, respectively.

strictly on the balance between IAD and IVD. In dilated cardiomyopathy IVD and IAD delays frequently coexist as the same myocardial structural alterations (elongation and loss of myocytes, fibrosis and disarray of specialized and working cells) can involve both atria and ventricles [51]. BVP by reducing IVD could produce a consistent imbalance between left and right AV temporal sequences when IVD and IAD coexist.

Echo/Doppler recording of aortic/mitral and pulmonary/tricuspid flows allows measurement of the time between the beginning of the left and right atrial and ventricular contraction, i.e. left/right mechanical AV delays (L/RMAVD) (Figure 6.3).

In a previous study [52] using pulsed echo/Doppler, L/RMAVD, IAD and IVD were measured in two different combinations of atriobiventricular sequential pacing using right atrial appendage (RAA)/BVP and interatrial septum (IAS)/BVP. This was based on the hypothesis that IAS pacing, a new technique proposed to prevent atrial fibrillation by reducing IAD [53,54], could reduce the difference between left and right AV sequences. In fact, in the first combination, LMAVD was significantly shorter than the right one and IAD was simultaneously significantly longer than IVD. But when IAS pacing was combined with BVP no differences were observed between left and right AV sequences or IAD and IVD delay.

The major clinical impact of slowed interatrial conduction in BVP is a decrease in left heart AV delay and an adverse excessively short left AV interval that might impair the hemodynamic benefit of BVP. Optimal hemodynamic conditions are achieved when ventricular contraction begins after completion of the end-diastolic filling time. Atrial contraction at end-diastole allows maintenance of a low atrial pressure during early and mid-diastole while it increases preload just before ventricular contraction [55]. If the AV interval is shorter than the optimal value, there will be a relatively lower preload at the onset of ventricular contraction and stroke volume will be reduced. At very short AV intervals atrial contraction occurs against a closed mitral valve causing a further decrease in CO together with an increase in mean left atrial pressure. This effect may be even more deleterious in patients with a BVP pacemaker for severe CHF.

Chiife et al. described a case of pacemaker syndrome in a patient with BVP and a long IAD in whom lengthening of the programmed AV delay resulted in a dramatic improvement of the symptoms [56]. Because the left mechanical AV sequence might be significantly affected by IAD, all patients undergoing BVP should have a simple non-invasive evaluation of interatrial conduction time. IASP/BVP combination should be considered in order to facilitate left AV delay optimization and maximize hemodynamic benefit in patients with marked IAD.

Over the last few years tissue Doppler imaging (TDI) has been emerging as a new echocardiographic technique. It has been proven to be useful in assessing qualitatively the regional electromechanical activation pattern as well as detecting quantitatively the systolic and diastolic times and velocities within the myocardium. TDI is a variation of conventional Doppler. The velocity of moving tissue can be studied with pulsed wave tissue Doppler sampling, which displays the velocity of a selected myocardial region against time, with high temporal resolution. In addition the velocities can be calculated with time–velocity maps and displayed as color-coded velocity maps in either M-mode or two-dimensional format. Color-coded tissue Doppler resolves mean velocities with higher spatial resolution, and postprocessing analysis of digitally acquired images has been shown to be feasible and reproducible. Using surface ECG recording as a reference point, it is possible to measure the regional electromechanical delay that is the interval between QRS onset and regional systolic peak velocity. Thus, TDI allows investigation of both intraventricular and interventricular asynchrony.

Assessment of CRT hemodynamic effects

The evaluation of the hemodynamic effect of CRT involves several echo Doppler parameters:
- systolic function parameters;
- diastolic function parameters; and
- myocardial performance index.

Systolic function parameters

Systolic function parameters include:
- fractional shortening (FS);
- ejection fraction (EF);
- cardiac output (CO); and
- LV dP/dt$_{max}$ (LV dP/dt$_{max}$).

The diagnostic accuracy of EF assessment is improved by endocardial border delineation using second harmonic imaging. Kim [57] has recently proposed the use of three-dimensional echocardiography with tissue harmonic imaging for assessment of EF; the volumes evaluated by this method closely agree with those recorded by magnetic resonance imaging.

Doppler-derived CO is crucial for evaluation of the effect of CRT; this parameter is more important than EF in verifying the hemodynamic improvement in patients with dilated cardiomyopathy because CO rather than EF increases with BVP [58–60].

Breithard et al. have proposed [60] calculating CO from continuous wave (CW) Doppler imaging across the aortic valve instead of a pulsed wave (PW) sample volume in the LV outflow tract (LVOT). CO measurement by CW Doppler imaging across the aortic valve results in overestimation of true CO with less effect on relative intraindividual changes. Furthermore, the assumption that LVOT diameter remains constant during various hemodynamic states may introduce a systematic error because a rise in CO may increase aortic diameter. However, it is unlikely that the increase in maximal CO in

LV + dP/dT measurement

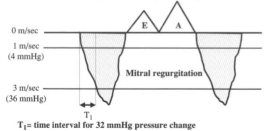

Figure 6.4 Method by which left ventricular +dP/dt can be evaluated. The time interval of the velocity increase from 1 m/s to 3 m/s is measured on continuous wave Doppler of the mitral regurgitation curve. The pressure difference of this velocity (36–4 mmHg) according to the Bernouilli equation is divided by the corresponding time interval. Care should be taken to align the imaging beam parallel to the direction of the regurgitant jet and to adjust the gain, compress, wall filter and velocity scale settings to obtain the clearest spectral Doppler trace.

such patients causes a significant change in LVOT diameter.

LV + dP/dt$_{max}$ obtained non-invasively from the CW mitral regurgitation curve with the 'rate pressure rise' method [61] (as illustrated in Figure 6.4) has been proposed by Oguz *et al.* [59] as a valid index in predicting the long-term response to BVP. The same authors showed in 16 patients that the duration of mitral regurgitation is another important parameter to identify responders to BVP. The duration of mitral regurgitation is influenced by the AV delay [27] and, particularly in the presystolic phase, by ventricular conduction disturbances [49].

Diastolic function parameters
Several aspects of diastolic function should be considered:
• left and right diastolic ventricular filling time (LVFT, RVFT) from the beginning to the end of diastolic mitral or tricuspid valvular flow respectively;
• peak flow velocity in early diastole (E peak), E wave deceleration time (DT), peak flow velocity in late diastole (A peak) and the ratio between E peak and A peak (E/A);
• isovolumetric relaxation time (IRT) which is the difference between the [QRS–onset of diastolic mitral flow] interval and the [QRS onset–end of

Left/Right IsoVolumic Relaxation Time (L/R-IRT) measurement

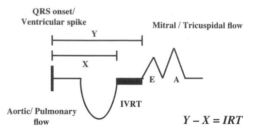

Figure 6.5 Method by which left and right isovolumetric relaxation time can be calculated. This time is the difference between the [QRS–onset of diastolic mitral/tricuspid flow] interval and the [QRS onset–end of systolic aortic/pulmonary flow] interval.

systolic aortic flow] interval. This method also allows measurement of the right IRT as the difference between [QRS onset–onset of diastolic tricuspid flow] interval and [QRS onset–end of systolic pulmonary flow] interval (Figure 6.5).

Reports of the effects of BVP on echocardiographic diastolic parameters are conflicting [35,59, 60,62]. However, the reason might be related to the coexistence of restrictive (E/A ≥ 2 or E/A 1–2 and DT ≤ 140 ms) and no restrictive (E/A ≤ 1 or E/A 1–2 and DT ≥ 140 ms) diastolic filling patterns in the same study population. In a restrictive pattern the diastolic improvement is indicated by E/A reduction and DT and IRT increase, while in the absence of a restrictive pattern the improvement is inversely indicated by E/A increase and DT and IRT reduction. The opposite variation of the diastolic parameters in the two mixed patterns could influence the validity of the results.

Myocardial performance index (MPI)
MPI is a simple Doppler-derived index [63] defined as the sum of isovolumetric contraction (ICT) and relaxation times (IRT) divided by ejection time (ET—interval from the beginning and the end of systolic aortic flow) (Figure 6.6). The index has several practical and conceptual advantages: (i) it is easily obtained from conventional Doppler recordings; (ii) it is independent of heart rate and blood pressure; and (iii) it is applicable to left and right heart function [63]. It can be conceptualized as the sum of

Left/Right MyocardialPerformance Index (L/R-MPI) measurement

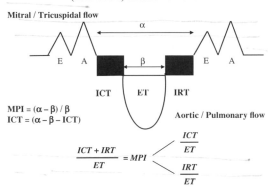

Figure 6.6 Method by which left and right myocardial performance index can be calculated by the assessment of Doppler-derived ejection time (ET), isovolumetric relaxation time (IRT) and isovolumetric contraction time (ICT) as (ICT + IRT)/ET. ET is calculated as the interval between the beginning and end of aortic/pulmonary flow. The sum of the isovolumetric contraction and relaxation times is derived from the interval from the end of mitral/tricuspid inflow to the onset of the next mitral/tricuspid inflow signal minus ET. IRT is calculated as in Figure 6.5. ICT is derived from the interval between the end of mitral/tricuspid inflow to the onset of the next mitral/tricuspid inflow minus (ET + IRT).

two ratios: ICT divided by ET (ICT/ET) and IRT divided by ET (IRT/ET) (Figure 6.5). In a study of simultaneous Doppler and high-fidelity LV pressure recordings [64], ICT/ET ratio correlated to +dP/dt obtained invasively, whereas IRT/ET ratio correlated with –dP/dt. Thus, this index reflects both systolic and diastolic function. Some studies [35,59,62] reported significant improvement of LV MPI during BVP; there is universal agreement that the reduction (i.e. improvement) involves the ICT/ET ratio with no significant difference in IRT/ET ratio, suggesting that improvement involves mainly LV systolic function. Porciani *et al.* [62] also observed reduction of the right ventricular MPI associated with no significant change in right IRT/ET. Thus BVP can also improve systolic function of the right ventricle. There is a complex ventricular interdependence by which the LV contraction contributes to RV performance [65]. The right ventricle begins and ends its ejection after that of the LV [66]. Thus, during isovolumetric contraction there is a rapid increase of LV pressure and through ventricular interdependence this increase also contributes to

a rapid increase in right ventricular pressure. Although the LV has not generated sufficient pressure to initiate its ejection it has developed sufficient pressure to help the right ventricle in starting ejection. When delayed LV contraction occurs, there is no contribution of the LV to right ventricular ejection. BVP, by anticipating LV contraction, replaces its isovolumetric contraction correspondingly with that of the right ventricle and allows the LV contribution to right ventricular performance. The effect of BVP on ventricular interdependence is another important issue of CRT that should be explored.

Identification of CRT responders

Assessment of mechanical asynchrony has been postulated as a predictor of hemodynamic improvement during BVP [37]. Tissue Doppler imaging (TDI) analysis can assess the pattern of regional electromechanical activation and detect the systolic and diastolic times and velocities within the myocardium. Thus, this technique is particularly suitable for evaluating the degree of LV asynchrony in patients with dilated cardiomyopathy before BVP, and identifying potential responders.

An increasing number of studies have reported interesting results [67–69]. Using TDI in 25 patients before BVP implantation, Yu *et al.* [67] demonstrated the presence of LV systolic dyssynchrony by the significant regional difference in time to peak myocardial sustained systolic velocity (T_s). Septal, lateral, anteroseptal, posterior, anterior and inferior LV segments were studied at both basal and mid levels. The improvement of intraventricular synchronicity after BVP was reflected by the loss of regional difference in T_s as well as by the significant reduction in T_s standard deviation. Interestingly, BVP improves LV synchronicity by homogeneously delaying those sites with early peak systolic contraction, in particular in the anteroseptal, septal, inferior and posterior segments, resulting in a later contraction of all segments with respect to QRS onset but simultaneously with respect to each other.

Ansalone *et al.* [68] studied 21 patients by standard two-dimensional echocardiography and by TDI. To assess long axis function, TDI qualitative analysis at the basal level of the interventricular septum and the inferior, posterior, lateral and anterior walls was performed in M-mode color and pulsed wave Doppler modalities before and after BVP. On the basis of evaluation of systolic and diastolic phases in the 105 basal segments studied, 4 electromechanical patterns were identified and graduated in a scale reflecting the progression from asynchronous to dyskinetic: normal (pattern I); mildly unsynchronized (pattern IIA); severely unsynchronized (pattern IIB); reversed early in systole (pattern IIIA); reversed late in systole (pattern IIIB); and reversed throughout systole (pattern IV). After CRT, 49 (46.7%) of 105 segments had unsynchronized contraction to the same degree as before, 36 (34.3%) of 105 showed unsynchronized contraction to a lesser degree and 20 (19%) showed unsynchronized contraction to a greater degree than before; a pre-excitation pattern was found in 11 (10.5%) of 105, but no segment with pattern IV was observed. According to these TDI findings, after BVP, patients were divided into group 1 (10 of 21) with less severe asynchrony than before BVP and group 2 (11 of 21) with no change or more severe LV asynchrony than before BVP. In group 1 only, the LV EF increased significantly, the NYHA class decreased and exercise tolerance increased significantly; no significant differences were found in LV EF, in NYHA class or in exercise tolerance in group 2. QRS narrowing was significant in both groups.

In a subsequent study, the same authors [69] evaluated by TDI the regional activation delay in basal segments of the LV and defined as the most delayed region that in which the time interval between the end of the A wave and the beginning of the E wave was the longest. After BVP the left pacing site was considered concordant with the most delayed site when the lead was positioned at the wall with the greatest regional delay. The patients were divided into group A (paced at the most delayed site) and group B (paced at any other site). After BVP, LV performance improved significantly in all patients; however, the greatest improvement was found in group A patients.

Previous studies had focused on IVD evaluation by traditional PW Doppler or, as more recently proposed, by TDI [70]. However, the findings of these studies [67–69] underline the importance of identification of regional LV delays by TDI. This new doppler application is a useful tool in reflecting the presence of intraventricular asynchrony that may not be detectable by surface ECG recording alone [48]. Unexpected delay in regional LV contraction evidenced by TDI analysis was recently described by Garrigue et al. [71] in patients with CHF and right bundle branch block patients who subsequently improved with BVP. Further studies need to identify intraventricular asynchrony in patients with narrow QRS who might benefit from BVP.

Conclusions

Synchrony of contraction is an important factor in cardiac performance because it results in a more effective and energetically efficient ejection.

Asynchronous contraction represents wasted work that does not contribute to ejection. CRT, by changing the timing of electrical and mechanical events to a near-normal sequence, can produce a more homogeneous regional contraction of the LV so that all regions contribute to ejection.

Thus correct timing of regional contraction rather than intrinsic muscle contraction enhancement produces systolic improvement in CRT. This may be the mechanism by which BVP results in a systolic improvement without increasing energy consumption [39].

References

1 Wiggers CJ. The muscular reactions of the mammalian ventricles to artificial surface stimuli. *Am J Physiol* 1925; **73**: 346–78.

2 Park C, Little WC, O'Rourk RA. Effect of alteration of left ventricular activation sequence on the left ventricular end-systolic pressure–volume relation in closed-chest dogs. *Circ Res* 1985; **57**: 706–17.

3 Burkhoff D, Oikawa RY, Sagawa K. Influence of pacing site on canine left ventricular contraction. *Am J Physiol* 1986; **251** (*Heart Circ Physiol* **20**): H428–H435.

4 Prinzen FR, Augustijn CH, Arts T *et al.* Redistribution of myocardial fiber strain and blood flow by asynchronous activation. *Am J Physiol* 1990; **259** (*Heart Circ Physiol* **28**): H300–H308.

5 Prinzen FW, Hunter WC, Wyman BT *et al.* Mapping of regional myocardial strain and work during ventricular pacing: experimental study using magnetic resonance tagging. *J Am Coll Cardiol* 1999; **33**: 1735–42.

6 Wyman BT, Hunter WC, Prinzen FW *et al.* Mapping propagation of mechanical activation in the paced heart with MRI tagging. *Am J Physiol* 1999; **276** (*Heart Circ Physiol* **45**): H881–H891.

7 Prinzen FW, Cheriex EC, Delhaas T *et al.* Asymmetric thickness of the left ventricular wall resulting from asynchronous electric activation: a study in dogs with ventricular pacing and in patients with left bundle branch block. *Am Heart J* 1995; **130**: 1045–53.

8 van Oosterhout MFM, Prinzen FW, Arts T *et al.* Asynchronous electrical activation induces asymmetrical hypertrophy of the left ventricular wall. *Circulation* 1998; **98**: 588–95.

9 Bourassa MG, Boiteau GM, Allenstein BJ. Hemodynamic studies during intermittent left bundle branch block. *Am J Cardiol* 1965; **10**: 792–9.

10 Takeshita A, Basta LL, Kloschos JM. Effect of intermittent left bundle branch block on left ventricular performance. *Am J Med* 1974; **56**: 251–5.

11 Wong B, Rinkenberger R, Dunn M. Effect of intermittent left bundle branch block on left ventricular performance in the normal heart. *Am J Cardiol* 1977; **39**: 459–63.

12 Grines CL, Bashore TM, Boudoulas H *et al.* Functional abnormalities in isolated left bundle branch block. The effect of interventricular asynchrony. *Circulation* 1989; **79**: 845–53.

13 Xiao HB, Brecker JD, Gibson DG. Differing effects of right ventricular pacing and left bundle branch block on left ventricular function. *Br Heart J* 1993; **69**: 166–73.

14 Tse HF, Lau CP. Long-term effect of right ventricular pacing on myocardial perfusion and function. *J Am Coll Cardiol* 1997; **29**: 744–9.

15 Murkofsky RL, Dangas G, Diamond JA *et al.* A prolonged QRS duration on surface electrocardiogram is a specific indicator of left ventricular dysfunction. *J Am Coll Cardiol* 1998; **32**: 476–82.

16 Das MK, Cheriparambil K, Bedi A. Prolonged QRS duration (QRS ≥ 170 ms) and left axis deviation in the presence of left bundle branch block: a marker of poor left ventricular systolic function? *Am Heart J* 2001; **142**: 756–9.

17 White PD. *Heart Disease*, 3rd edn. New York: The Macmillan Co., 1944.

18 Johnson RP, Messer AL, Shreenivas *et al.* Prognosis in bundle branch block. II. Factors influencing the survival period in left bundle branch block. *Am Heart J* 1951; **41**: 225.

19 Xiao HB, Roy C, Fujimoto S *et al.* Natural history of abnormal conduction and its relation to prognosis in patients with dilated cardiomyopathy. *Int J Cardiol* 1996; **53**: 163–70.

20 Venkateshawar K, Gottipaty K, Krelis P *et al.* for the VEST investigators. The resting electrocardiogram provides a sensitive and inexpensive marker of prognosis in patients with chronic congestive heart failure. *J Am Coll Cardiol* 1999; **33**: 145A.

21 Baldasseroni S, Opasich C, Gorini M *et al.* Left bundle branch block is associated with increased 1-year sudden and total mortality rate in 5517 outpatients with congestive heart failure: a report from the Italian Network on Congestive Heart Failure. *Am Heart J* 2002; **143**: 398–405.

22 Hochleitner M, Hortnagl H, Ng CK *et al.* Usefulness of physiologic dual-chamber pacing in drug-resistant idiopathic dilated cardiomyopathy. *Am J Cardiol* 1990; **66** (2): 198–202.

23 Hochleitner M, Hortnagl H, Hortnagl H *et al.* Longterm efficacy of physiologic dual-chamber pacing in the treatment of end-stage idiopathic dilated cardiomyopathy. *Am J Cardiol* 1992; **70** (15): 1320–5.

24 Brecker SJ, Xiao HB, Sparrow J *et al.* Effects of dual chamber pacing with short atrioventricular delay in dilated cardiomyopathy. *Lancet* 1992; **340**: 1308–12.

25 Linde C, Gadler F, Edner M *et al.* Results of atrioventricular synchronous pacing with optimized delay in patients with severe congestive heart failure. *Am J Cardiol* 1995; **75**: 919–23.

26 Gold MR, Feliciano Z, Gottlieb SS *et al.* Dual chamber pacing with a short atrioventricular delay in congestive heart failure: a randomized study. *J Am Coll Cardiol* 1995; **26**: 967–73.

27 Nishimura RA, Hayes DL, Holmes DR Jr *et al.* Mechanism of hemodynamic improvement by dual chamber pacing for severe left ventricular dysfunction: an acute Doppler and catheterization hemodynamic study. *J Am Coll Cardiol* 1995; **25**: 281–8.

28 Sack S, Franz R, Dagres N *et al.* Can right sided atrioventricular sequential pacing provide benefit for selected patients with severe congestive heart failure? *Am J Cardiol* 1999; **83**: 124–129D.

29 De Teresa PA, Chamoro JL. An even more physiological pacing: changing the sequence of ventricular activation. *Proceedings VIIth World Symposium of Cardiac Pacing.* Vienna, Austria: 1983, 95–100.

30 Cazeau S, Ritter P, Lazarus A *et al.* Multisite pacing for end-stage heart failure: early experience. *Pacing Clin Electrophysiol* 1996; **19**: 1748–57.

31 Blanc JJ, Etienne Y, Gilard M *et al.* Evaluation of different ventricular pacing sites in patients with severe heart failure: results of an acute hemodynamic study. *Circulation* 1997; **96**: 3273–7.

32 Leclercq C, Cazeau S, Le Breton H *et al.* Acute hemodynamic effects of biventricular DDD pacing in patients with end-stage heart failure. *J Am Coll Cardiol* 1998; **32**: 1825–31.

33 Auricchio A, Stellbrink C, Block M *et al.* Effect of pacing chamber and atrioventricular delay on acute systolic function of paced patients with congestive heart failure. The Pacing Therapies for Congestive Heart Failure Study Group. The Guidant Congestive Heart Failure Research Group. *Circulation* 1999; **99**: 2993–3001.

34 Kass DA, Chen CH, Curry C *et al.* Improved left ventricular mechanics from acute VDD pacing in patients with dilated cardiomyopathy and ventricular conduction delay. *Circulation* 1999; **99**: 1567–73.

35 Saxon LA, Kerwin WF, Cahalan MK *et al*. Acute effects of intraoperative multisite ventricular pacing on left ventricular function and activation/contraction sequence in patients with depressed ventricular function. *J Cardiovasc Electrophysiol* 1998; **9**: 13–21.

36 Kerwin WF, Botvinick EH, O'Connell JW *et al*. Ventricular contraction abnormalities in dilated cardiomyopathy: effect of biventricular pacing to correct interventricular dyssynchrony. *J Am Coll Cardiol* 2000; **35**: 1221–7.

37 Cazeau S, Leclercq C, Lavergne T *et al*. Effects of multisite biventricular pacing in patients with heart failure and intraventricular conduction delay. *N Engl J Med* 2001; **344**: 873–80.

38 Abraham WT, Fisher WG, Smith AL *et al*. Cardiac resynchronization in chronic heart failure. *N Engl J Med* 2002; **346**: 1845–53.

39 Nelson GS, Berger GD, Fetics BJ *et al*. Left ventricular or biventricular pacing improves cardiac function at diminished energy cost in patients with dilated cardiomyopathy and left bundle-branch block. *Circulation* 2000; **102**: 3053–9.

40 Hamdan MH, Zagrodzky JD, Joglar JA. Biventricular pacing decreases sympathetic activity compared with right ventricular pacing in patients with depressed ejection fraction. *Circulation* 2000; **102**: 1027–32.

41 Saxon LA, De Marco T, Chatterjee K *et al*. Chronic biventricular pacing decreases serum norepinephrine in dilated heart failure patients with the greatest sympathetic activation at baseline. *Pacing Clin Electrophysiol* 1999; **22**: 830A.

42 Sharma R, Anker SD. Immune and neurohormonal pathways in chronic heart failure. *Congest Heart Fail* 2002; **8**: 23–8.

43 Wang L, Ma W, Markovich R *et al*. Regulation of cardiomyocyte apoptotic signaling by insulin-like growth factor I. *Circ Res* 1998; **83**: 516–22.

44 Berry C, Clark AL. Catabolism in chronic heart failure. *Eur Heart J* 2000; **21**: 521–32.

45 Padeletti L, Porciani MC, Colella A *et al*. Cardiac resynchronization reverses left ventricular remodeling and reduces cytokine activation in patients with dilated cardiomyopathy and left bundle branch block. *J Am Coll Cardiol* 2002; **39**: 78A.

46 Alonso C, Leclercq C, Victor F *et al*. Electrocardiographic predictive factors of long-term clinical improvement with multisite biventricular pacing in advanced heart failure. *Am J Cardiol* 1999; **84**: 1417–21.

47 Reuter S, Garrigue S, Bordachar P. Intermediate-term results of biventricular pacing in heart failure: correlation between clinical and hemodynamic data. *Pacing Clin Electrophysiol* 2000; **23**: 1713–17.

48 Gras D, Cebron JP, Brunel P *et al*. Optimal stimulation of the LV. *J Cardiovasc Electrophysiol* 2002; **13**: S57–S62.

49 Brecker SJ, Xiao HB, Sparrow J *et al*. Effects of dual-chamber pacing with short atrioventricular delay in dilated cardiomyopathy. *Lancet* 1992; **340**: 1308–11.

50 Chirife R, Ortega DF, Salazar A. Nonphysiological left heart AV intervals as a result of DDD and AAI 'physiological' pacing. *Pacing Clin Electrophysiol* 1991; **14**: 1752–6.

51 Oakley C. Aetiology, diagnosis, investigation, and management of the cardiomyopathies. *Br Med J* 1997; **315**: 1520–4.

52 Porciani MC, Colella A, Costoli A. Left and right atrio-ventricular intervals synchronizations: a rising problem in new pacing techniques. *Pacing Clin Electrophysiol* 2000; **23**: 610A.

53 Padeletti L, Porciani MC, Michelucci A *et al*. Interatrial septum pacing: a new approach to prevent recurrent atrial fibrillation. *J Interv Card Electrophysiol* 1999; **3**: 35–43.

54 Padeletti L, Pieragnoli P, Ciapetti C *et al*. Randomized crossover comparison of right atrial appendage pacing versus interatrial septum pacing for prevention of paroxysmal atrial fibrillation in patients with sinus bradycardia. *Am Heart J* 2001; **142**: 1047–55.

55 Skinner NS, Mitchell JH, Wallace AG *et al*. Hemodynamic effects of altering the timing of atrial systole. *Am J Physiol* 1963; **205**: 499–503.

56 Chirife R, Helguera M, Elizalde G *et al*. Pacemaker syndrome during biventricular multisite DDD pacing in a patient with dilated cardiomyopathy. *Europace* 2000; **1**: D223 (Abstract.).

57 Kim WY, Søgaard P, Mortensen PT *et al*. Three dimensional echocardiography documents hemodynamic improvement by biventricular pacing in patients with severe heart failure. *Heart* 2001; **85**: 514–20.

58 Saxon LA, De Marco T, Schafer J *et al*. Effects of long-term biventricular stimulation for resynchronization on echocardiographic measures of remodeling. *Circulation* 2002; **105**: 1304–10.

59 Oguz E, Dagdeviren B, Bilsel T *et al*. Echocardiographic prediction of long-term response to biventricular pacemaker in severe heart failure. *Eur J Heart Fail* 2002; **4**: 83–90.

60 Breithard OA, Stellbrink C, Franke A. Acute effects of cardiac resynchronization therapy on left ventricular Doppler indices in patients with congestive heart failure. *Am Heart J* 2002, **143**: 34–44.

61 Bargiggia GS, Bertucci C, Recusani F *et al*. A new method for estimating left ventricular dP/dT by continuous wave Doppler echocardiography. *Circulation* 1989; **80**: 1287–92.

62 Porciani MC, Puglisi A, Colella A *et al*. Echocardiographic evaluation of the effect of biventricular pacing: the InSync Italian Registry. *Eur Heart J Suppl* 2000; **2** (Suppl J): J23–J30.

63 Tei C. New noninvasive index for combined systolic and diastolic ventricular function. *J Cardiol* 1995; **26**: 135–6.

64 Tei C, Nishimura RA, Seward JB, Tajik J. Noninvasive Doppler-derived myocardial performance index: correlation with simultaneous measurements of cardiac catheterization. *J Am Soc Echocardiogr* 1997; **10**: 169–78.

65 Hoffman D, Sisto D, Fratu RW *et al.* Left-to-right ventricular interaction with a non contracting right ventricle. *J Thorac Cardiovasc Surg* 1994; **107**: 1496–1502.

66 Wiggers CJ. *Physiology in Health and Disease.* Philadelphia: Lea and Febiger, 1954.

67 Yu CM, Chau E, Sanderson J E *et al.* Tissue doppler echocardiography evidence of reverse remodeling and improved synchronicity by simultaneously delaying regional contraction after biventricular pacing therapy in heart failure. *Circulation* 2002; **105**: 438–45.

68 Ansalone G, Giannantoni P, Ricci R *et al.* Doppler myocardial imaging in patients with heart failure receiving biventricular pacing treatment. *Am Heart J* 2001; **142**: 881–96.

69 Ansalone G, Giannantoni P, Ricci R *et al.* Doppler myocardial imaging to evaluate the effectiveness of pacing sites in patients receiving biventricular pacing. *J Am Coll Cardiol* 2002; **39**: 489–99.

70 Rouleau F, Merheb M, Geffroy S *et al.* Echocardiographic assessment of the interventricular delay of activation and correlation to the QRS width in dilated cardiomyopathy. *Pacing Clin Electrophysiol* 2001; **24**: 1500–6.

71 Garrigue S, Reuter S, Labeque JN *et al.* Usefulness of biventricular pacing in patients with congestive heart failure and right bundle branch block. *Am J Cardiol* 2001; **88**: 1436–41.

CHAPTER 7

Ventricular Resynchronization: Predicting Responders

David A. Kass

Patients with dilated cardiomyopathy and discoordinate wall motion due to intraventricular conduction delay are at an increased risk of exacerbated pump failure, arrhythmia and mortality. Both biventricular and left ventricular free-wall pacing resynchronization both acutely improve systolic ventricular function and energetic efficiency in patients with heart failure and left bundle branch-type conduction block. Chronic therapy improves heart failure symptoms and exercise capacity, and appears to inhibit and/or reverse progressive chamber remodeling. As with all therapies for heart failure, subject response can vary considerably. Given the complex invasive nature of resynchronization therapy and its medical costs, identification of candidates most likely to benefit is important. This brief review summarizes factors that have been identified to acutely predict cardiac improvement, and more chronically identify patient responders.

Introduction

Dilated cardiomyopathy (DCM) results from the consequence of abnormalities of cardiac muscle contraction coupled to pathophysiologic volume and arterial loading and potent activation of the neuroendocrine system. In addition to these changes, abnormal electrical conduction can develop that delays the timing of atrial contraction and generates discoordinate contraction of the left ventricle (LV). The latter is typically observed in individuals with a widened QRS complex and bundle branch block, which are independent risk factors for DCM mortality [1–3]. Unilateral loss of normal His–Purkinje conduction results in the separation of the heart

chamber into early and late activated regions, with the net result being a decline in systolic function and reduced energetic efficiency.

Over the past decade, various investigative groups have established that ventricular preexcitation (or pacing) of both right and left or just left ventricles—commonly referred to as resynchronization therapy—mechanically and energetically improves left ventricular function in DCM patients with discoordinate contraction [4]. Chronic studies have confirmed enhancement of clinical symptoms, increased exercise capacity, neurostimulation withdrawal, and cessation or reversal of chronic chamber remodeling [5–10]. However, as with all therapies for heart failure, individual patient response to cardiac resynchronization varies, with most series reporting about 25% nonresponder rate. Given the complexity of the instrumentation, the need for device implantation and the medical costs associated with the treatment, investigators have sought markers to best prospectively identify the patients most likely to respond. While several candidate indices to predict both acute and chronic responsiveness have been suggested, prospective proof of their predictive value remains to be obtained. In the meantime, existing data have helped identify which features are likely useful and which are not. This chapter reviews our present knowledge of this important issue.

Pathophysiology of abnormal electrical conduction

In order to understand factors associated with the clinical efficacy of cardiac resynchronization therapy (CRT), it is important to review the primary pathophysiology of altered electrical conduction. The normal cardiac conduction system modulates contraction rate, the mechanical efficacy of atrial systole and contractile coordination of ventricular chambers. Sinus node disease results in chronotropic incompetence that can prove problematic in individuals with little preload or contractile reserve. Atrioventricular (AV) nodal disease delays atrial contraction relative to onset of systole, rendering atrial systole synchronous with early passive filling and effectively removing its value as a booster pump [11,12]. Optimal atrial–ventricular delay is also important to mitral valve competence as too much delay leaves the mitral leaflets open in the midplane position as ventricular systole starts, leading to presystolic mitral regurgitation. Lastly, long AV delays shorten the diastolic filling period, limiting net filling [13].

Infranodal conduction delay—most commonly in a left bundle branch pattern—can induce discoordinate LV contraction [14,15]. As demonstrated by the tagged magnetic resonance scans in Plate 7.1a, facing p. 84 [16,17], DCM hearts with a left bundle branch block (LBBB) display early activation of the septal wall with lateral prestretch, followed by markedly delayed lateral contraction with late systolic septal stretch towards the right ventricle (RV). Cardiac discoordination induced by LBBB or by RV-ventricular pacing reduces systolic function, prolongs isovolumic relaxation [18–20], and has been coupled to widening of the QRS complex [18]. Energetic cost of contraction can increase relative to effective ejection, since the early activated myocardium largely serves to increase preload on the lateral free wall, leaving the late activated wall to contract at higher stress while wasting work by stretching the more pliable early activated territory [21–23]. Biventricular pacing or univentricular pacing of the LV lateral free wall can recoordinate contraction and is associated with systolic improvement [7,9,24–26]. Resynchronization effects are manifest abruptly (i.e. rise in dP/dt$_{max}$, arterial pressures, Plate 7.1b) occurring within one beat, and reflect increased systolic flow. Chronic non-invasive studies have reported sustained responses of similar magnitude [27]. When displayed as ventricular pressure–volume loops, the resynchronization effect can be observed as a widening of the loop (enhanced stroke volume), decline in end-systolic

wall stress (left shift of end-systolic pressure–volume point) and increased cardiac work (Plate 7.1c). Importantly, the latter is not accompanied by increases in energy consumption but, to the contrary, has been shown to be coupled with a decline in energy consumption [28].

The magnitude of systolic benefit depends in part on the AV timing delay selected [7,9]. Clearly, when atrial and ventricular activation are synchronous, there is a detrimental effect on chamber filling and increased atrial pressures. Increasing the delay time enhances atrial–ventricular mass transfer while still maintaining pre-excitation of the portion of the myocardium with delayed activation. Too long a delay reduces the efficacy of pacing as pre-excitation is lost. However, studies have found that mechanical responses are similar over a fairly broad range of AV timing intervals (typically ranging from 100 to 140 ms).

Results of recent chronic trials: what defines response?

In order to develop criteria by which to identify candidates for resynchronization, the definition of a responder vs. non-responder must be clarified. To date, several moderate-sized controlled trials have reported 6-month follow-up data in patients treated by CRT—and it is reasonable to base such a definition on these data. The first major study to be reported was the MUSTIC trial [5]. This study reported data on 48 patients with NYHA class III heart failure and a QRS duration exceeding 150 ms who were studied using a transvenous biventricular system using a single-blind, randomized, controlled crossover study. The primary clinical endpoint was the distance walked in 6 min, with secondary endpoints being quality of life as measured by questionnaire, peak oxygen consumption, hospitalizations related to heart failure, the patients' treatment preference (active vs. inactive pacing) and mortality rate. Six-minute walk distance increased by 22%, quality of life score improved by 32%, peak oxygen uptake increased by 8%, hospitalizations declined by 66%, and active pacing was preferred by 85% of the patients. All of these endpoints reached statistical significance.

While MUSTIC did not present echocardiographic remodeling data, such results were obtained by the second moderately large and placebo-controlled trial. The recently reported MIRACLE trial provided such data, extending prior observations in very important ways [6]. This was designed as a double-blind parallel treatment study of 453 patients with moderate-to-severe heart failure, and a QRS interval of 130 ms or more. Primary endpoints were NYHA class, quality of life and distance walked in 6 min. All three parameters improved significantly: e.g. 6-min walk distance (+39 vs. +10 m, $P = 0.005$), quality of life (-18.0 vs. -9.0 points, $P = 0.001$), time on the treadmill during exercise testing (+81 vs. +19 s, $P = 0.001$) and ejection fraction (+4.6% vs. -0.2%, $P < 0.001$). There was a significant decline in rehospitalization (8% vs. 15%) or need for intravenous therapy (7% vs. 15%). Chronic therapy was also associated with a decline in end-systolic and end-diastolic volumes, supporting non-controlled data indicating reverse remodeling [27] as well as single-blind crossover studies [8,10]. These data suggest another potential definition of responders—that is, objective evidence of chronic reverse remodeling.

To date, there are few published data from controlled studies beyond 6 months. One recent report of 41 patients using a single-blind crossover design has provided 1-year follow up [8]. This study (PATH-CHF I) showed similar results for both single-site LV pacing and biventricular CRT, reporting improved maximal oxygen consumption (12.5–14.3 mL/kg/min) and anerobic threshold, and 6-min walk distance 342 m at baseline to 386 m. These changes were observed during two periods where therapy was activated, but not during the 4-week intervening period where therapy had been suspended (AAI pacing). Importantly, improvements were nearly identical after the initial 3 month crossover portion of the study to those after 9 additional months of active treatment.

Together these chronic trials suggest a way to identify responders. Exercise capacity improvements based on 6-min walk distance have been used in all three studies, and average improvements have been quite similar. A patient with a response < 2 SD below the average might then be considered a non-responder. Alternatively, patients with at least a 10% reduction in cavity volume (evidence of reverse remodeling) or an improvement in peak exercise oxygen consumption might be considered responders. As new markers are defined to assess the efficacy of therapy delivery and identify responders, we will need to keep these issues in mind, and to have commonly accepted criteria by which to classify these patients.

Electrocardiographic criteria for identifying responders

The most widely used marker to identify patients with cardiac dyssynchrony has been a widened QRS complex on the surface electrocardiogram. To date, all clinical trials have entered subjects based on the presence of systolic dysfunction with dilated cardiomyopathy, and a widened QRS duration. The precise amount of widening used for entry has varied from > 120 ms to 150 ms. The notion that QRS duration could index dyssynchrony seemed logical, in that substantial LV conduction delay should result in widening, in concordance with experimental data [18]. Indeed, many studies have shown that the wider the basal QRS duration, the greater the systolic improvement from biventricular (BiV) or LV pacing. Figure 7.1(a) shows such data from two populations [9,26]. A threshold of a QRS > 150 ms has been consistently found to better discriminate between a majority of responders vs. non-responders (Figure 7.1b). However, the relationship to QRS duration to even this acute mechanical response displays considerable scatter, so that both responsive patients with narrow complexes and less responsive ones with wide ones exist. Figure 7.1(c) provides further evidence for this correlative and indirect nature of basal QRS width vs. response to resynchronization. Despite substantial systolic improvement with LV or BiV pacing, QRS duration does not consistently narrow, with many subjects displaying no change or even widening of the duration [26]. This may reflect the fact that one is still relying on intramyocardial conduction, and abnormal wall geometry (dilatation) as well as gap junction and ion channel abnormalities can slow this process further. These data highlight the notion that QRS duration is at best an indirect correlate but not a direct reflection of mechanical synchrony—which is the real substrate that causes a decline chamber function.

Some improvement in predicting acute response has been achieved by combining QRS width with data regarding basal mechanical function (Figure 7.1d). Patients with cardiac failure have reduced dP/dt_{max} and published values show remarkable concordance (near 1000 mmHg/s. vs. 1500–2000

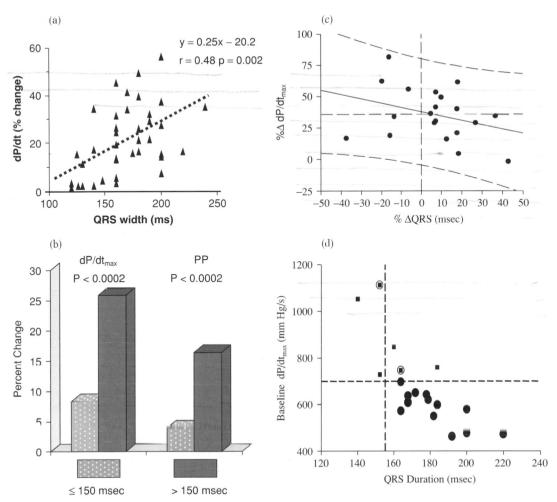

Figure 7.1 Electrocardiographic correlates of mechanical response to biventricular (or left ventricular-only) pacing. (a) QRS duration correlates with the acute mechanical response, although there is considerable scatter in these data, raising questions as to their predictive value. (b) Threshold of QRS duration > 150 ms identifies a majority of responders, but there are still individuals with shorter or longer durations who do not respond. (c) Correlation between QRS duration change from biventricular or left ventricular-only pacing and mechanical response. While mechanical changes are substantial, there is no correlation between them and QRS duration change. (d) Combined analysis of resting dP/dt_{max} and QRS duration to better identify acute responders. This bidiscriminate analysis provides better specificity and sensitivity. Patients with both a rise in pulse pressure > 10% and dP/dt_{max} of > 25% are displayed by open square surrounded by solid circle symbols. These individuals all have resting dP/dt_{max} < 750 mmHg/s, and QRS duration > 150 ms.

in controls). Individuals with dyssynchrony typically display significantly lower values of resting dP/dt_{max} (averaging 600–700 mmHg/s). Nelson *et al.* [26] first reported that bidiscriminate analysis, combining a QRS duration ≥ 150 ms with a basal dP/dt_{max} of < 750 mmHg/s, identified essentially all responders with no false positives, and few false negatives. This approach can be used non-invasively in many patients (e.g. Yu *et al.* [27]) due to the presence of mitral regurgitation which enables estimation of dP/dt_{max}.

Recent studies have begun to examine the utility of QRS duration in predicting the chronic response to CRT. These data have generally confirmed acute results—showing a general correlation between basal QRS duration with efficacy [29], but the discriminative value for identifying responders from non-responders appears to be poor. For example, baseline NYHA function class, age, sex, QRS duration and ejection fraction (EF) were no different between responsive and non-responsive subjects in a recent study of 45 subjects [30]. In a larger cohort of 102 consecutive patients, both responders and non-responders had similar basal QRS duration, and both displayed near-identical shortening of complex duration [31], a finding mirrored by other recent reports [32]. Patients with reduced dP/dt_{max} that display > 22% acute improvement have been reported to be consistent responders (with very few false negatives) [29], concordant with the acute observations of Nelson *et al.* [26].

Mechanical dyssynchrony as a predictor

The use of QRS duration has been generally recognized as a surrogate for mechanical discoordination, its value residing in its clinical simplicity. However, as electrical markers have been proving disappointing, recent studies have begun to quantify mechanical dyssynchrony directly, and test this as a prognostic index. Dyssynchrony was first comprehensively examined by means of tagged magnetic resonance imaging (MRI) (Figure 7.2a) [26]. This approach provided full three-dimensional strain measurements throughout the left ventricle, and allowed calculation of a variety of synchrony indexes from these maps. As shown in the figure, normal hearts contract with nearly all parts of the wall being synchronous, whereas in a DCM heart with LBBB, there is marked regional discordance of contraction times, with delayed lateral shortening. Importantly, dyssynchrony correlated with acute mechanical response (Figure 7.2b) to biventricular and LV-only pacing better than electrical parameters.

This type of complex analysis has limited clinical use, and simpler echo-based methods have been

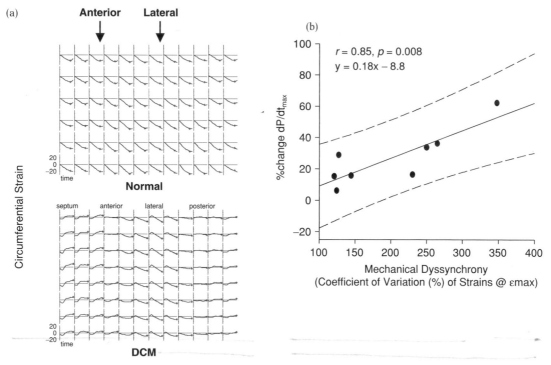

Figure 7.2 Assessment of mechanical dyssynchrony derived from tagged MRI imaging in humans. Maps of circumferential strain are displayed, with the anterior–lateral wall (left to right) and base–apex (top to bottom) regions shown. In a normal contracting ventricle (a—top), all of the regions develop similar levels of circumferential strain at approximately the same time. In contrast, the dilated cardiomyopathy patient with left bundle branch block delay shows marked dyssynchrony (a—bottom), with early septal shortening and late stretch, and the opposite pattern in the lateral wall. Analysis of the overall variance of strain at the time of maximal shortening yields a dyssynchrony index, which is more strongly correlated with systolic improvement generated by resynchronization pacing (b).

developed. The most widely applied to date is Doppler tissue velocity imaging to determine longitudinal wall velocity. This measure is applied to the septum vs. lateral wall, and the time of maximal velocity can be measured at multiple sites and then plotted. An example of this analysis is shown in Plate 7.2(a) (facing p.84) from Yu *et al.* [27]. The color-coded image shows regions of the left ventricle at a given time point, demonstrating disparate velocities in septal and lateral walls during systole. The lower panel shows the same heart after initiation of biventricular pacing, demonstrating greater concordance of velocity magnitude (and direction) accompanying synchronization. The lower panel displays the time of peak velocity at various regions around the ventricle in both the discoordinate and CRT-treated ventricle. There is considerable variability in times in the native condition, and this curve flattens with greater consistency of timing with the implementation of therapy.

Dysynchrony assessed by tissue Doppler has been reported to predict acute hemodynamic improvement from biventricular pacing—reflected by enhanced EF and reduced cardiac volumes [33]. More importantly, several groups have reported preliminary evidence that clinical outcome (i.e. responders) is also best predicted by baseline tissue Doppler dyssynchrony analysis. If true, then this relatively simple approach may be combined with electrocardiographic screening to better target responders.

Tissue Doppler generally examines longitudinal wall velocity which, while correlated to shortening, is not necessarily the most direct motion relevant to chamber ejection. Radial shortening has been studied using a novel echo-contrast enhancement method [34]. As shown in Plate 7.2b, this approach yields two-dimensional echo images with blood-pool contrast much like that of a radioventriculogram or MRI cine-scan. Improved delineation of the wall facilitates quantitative analysis of radial displacements, yielding strain patterns that are similar to those based on tagged MRI. From such analyses, Kawaguchi *et al.* [34] developed dyssynchrony indexes analogous to those obtained by tissue Doppler, and demonstrated their utility for predicting acute hemodynamic response. The value of this method for predicting chronic responders awaits larger-scale studies.

Lastly, very simple measures have also been proposed that determine *inter-* rather than *intraventric*-ular discoordination. The time from the peak of the QRS to the onset of pulmonary vs. aortic flow can be used to assess delay between contraction of the RV and LV. A delay of greater than 40 ms is considered compatible with significant dyssynchrony. This was first examined by high-fidelity pressure measurements in each ventricle (Plate 7.2c), where a loop containing positive area indicated a phase delay between the pressures. Quantitation of this area directly correlated with the delay, and could be used to predict acute responders. An analogous measure that can be derived noninvasively is the time delay between the onset of aortic versus pulmonary outflow, and is currently an entry criterion for a large multicenter trial ongoing in Europe (CARE-HF).

Summary

Biventricular and left ventricular pre-excitation to resynchronize a discoordinate heart have been established as a novel method to enhance systolic function in a subset of patients with dilated cardiomyopathy. Optimal identification of candidates remains a high priority. While initially focusing on electrical markers, recent data have highlighted the value of more direct assessment of mechanical discoordination by means of tissue Doppler, echo Doppler or MRI. Ongoing efforts to prospectively test the utility of these measures to predict responders will likely provide a major advance in targeting this therapy to those most likely to benefit.

References

1 Xiao HB, Roy C, Fujimoto S, Gibson DG. Natural history of abnormal conduction and its relation to prognosis in patients with dilated cardiomyopathy. *Int J Cardiol* 1996; **53**: 163–70.

2 Murkofsky RL, Dangas G, Diamond JA, Mehta D, Schaffer A, Ambrose JA. A prolonged QRS duration on surface electrocardiogram is a specific indicator of left ventricular dysfunction [see comment]. *J Am Coll Cardiol* 1998; **32**: 476–82.

3 Hamby RI, Weissman RH, Prakash MN, Hoffman I. Left bundle branch block: a predictor of poor left ventricular function in coronary artery disease. *Am Heart J* 1983; **106**: 471–7.

4 Leclercq C, Kass DA. Retiming the failing heart: principles and current clinical status of cardiac resynchronization. *J Am Coll Cardiol* 2002; **39**: 194–201.

5 Cazeau S, Leclercq C, Lavergne T *et al.* Effects of multisite biventricular pacing in patients with heart failure

and intraventricular conduction delay. *N Engl J Med* 2001; **344**: 873–80.

6 Abraham WT, Fisher WG, Smith AL *et al.* Cardiac resynchronization in chronic heart failure. *N Engl J Med* 2002; **346**: 1845–53.

7 Kass DA, Chen CH, Curry C *et al.* Improved left ventricular mechanics from acute VDD pacing in patients with dilated cardiomyopathy and ventricular conduction delay. *Circulation* 1999; **99**: 1567–73.

8 Auricchio A, Stellbrink C, Sack S *et al.* Long-term clinical effect of hemodynamically optimized cardiac resynchronization therapy in patients with heart failure and ventricular conduction delay. *J Am Coll Cardiol* 2002; **39**: 2026–33.

9 Auricchio A, Stellbrink C, Block M *et al.* Effect of pacing chamber and atrioventricular delay on acute systolic function of paced patients with congestive heart failure. The Pacing Therapies for Congestive Heart Failure Study Group. The Guidant Congestive Heart Failure Research Group. *Circulation* 1999; **99**: 2993–3001.

10 Stellbrink C, Breithardt OA, Franke A *et al.* Impact of cardiac resynchronization therapy using hemodynamically optimized pacing on left ventricular remodeling in patients with congestive heart failure and ventricular conduction disturbances. *J Am Coll Cardiol* 2001; **38**: 1957–65.

11 Meisner JS, McQueen DM, Ishida Y *et al.* Effects of timing of atrial systole on LV filling and mitral valve closure: computer and dog studies. *Am J Physiol* 1985; **249**: H604–H619.

12 Yellin EL, Nikolic S, Frater RWM. Left ventricular filling dynamics and diastolic function. *Prog Cardiovasc Dis* 1990; **32**: 247–71.

13 Brecker SJ, Xiao HB, Sparrow J, Gibson DG. Effects of dual-chamber pacing with short atrioventricular delay in dilated cardiomyopathy. *Lancet* 1992; **340**: 1308–12.

14 Prinzen FW, Hunter WC, Wyman BT, McVeigh ER. Mapping of regional myocardial strain and work during ventricular pacing: experimental study using magnetic resonance imaging tagging. *J Am Coll Cardiol* 1999; **33**: 1735–42.

15 Wyman BT, Hunter WC, Prinzen FW, McVeigh ER. Mapping propagation of mechanical activation in the paced heart with MRI tagging. *Am J Physiol* 1999; **276**: H881–H891.

16 Curry CC, Nelson GS, Wyman BT *et al.* Mechanical dyssynchrony in dilated cardiomyopathy with intraventricular conduction delay as depicted by 3-D tagged magnetic resonance imaging. *Circulation* 2000; **101**: E2.

17 McVeigh ER, Prinzen FW, Wyman BT, Tsitlik JE, Halperin HR, Hunter WC. Imaging asynchronous mechanical activation of the paced heart with tagged MRI. *Magn Reson Med* 1998; **39**: 507–13.

18 Burkhoff D, Oikawa RY, Sagawa K. Influence of pacing site on canine left ventricular contraction. *Am J Physiol* 1986; **251**: H428–H435.

19 Park RC, Little WC, O'Rourke RA. Effect of alteration of the left ventricular activation sequence on the left ventricular end-systolic pressure–volume relation in closed-chest dogs. *Circ Res* 1985; **57**: 706–17.

20 Liu L, Tockman B, Girouard S *et al.* Left ventricular resynchronization therapy in a canine model of left bundle branch block. *Am J Physiol Heart Circ Physiol* 2002; **282**: H2238–H2244.

21 Baller D, Wolpers HG, Zipfel J, Bretschneider HJ, Hellige G. Comparison of the effects of right atrial, right ventricular apex and atrioventricular sequential pacing on myocardial oxygen consumption and cardiac efficiency: a laboratory investigation. *Pacing Clin Electrophysiol* 1988; **11**: 394–403.

22 Owen CH, Esposito DJ, Davis JW, Glower DD. The effects of ventricular pacing on left ventricular geometry, function, myocardial oxygen consumption, and efficiency of contraction in conscious dogs. *Pacing Clin Electrophysiol* 1998; **21**: 1417–29.

23 Prinzen FW, Augustijn CH, Arts T, Allessie MA, Reneman RS. Redistribution of myocardial fiber strain and blood flow by asynchronous activation. *Am J Physiol* 1990; **259**: H300–H308.

24 Blanc JJ, Etienne Y, Gilard M *et al.* Evaluation of different ventricular pacing sites in patients with severe heart failure: results of an acute hemodynamic study. *Circulation* 1997; **96**: 3273–7.

25 Leclercq C, Cazeau S, Le Breton H *et al.* Acute hemodynamic effects of biventricular DDD pacing in patients with end-stage heart failure. *J Am Coll Cardiol* 1998; **32**: 1825–31.

26 Nelson GS, Curry CW, Wyman BT *et al.* Predictors of systolic augmentation from left ventricular preexcitation in patients with dilated cardiomyopathy and intraventricular conduction delay. *Circulation* 2000; **101**: 2703–9.

27 Yu CM, Chau E, Sanderson JE *et al.* Tissue Doppler echocardiographic evidence of reverse remodeling and improved synchronicity by simultaneously delaying regional contraction after biventricular pacing therapy in heart failure. *Circulation* 2002; **105**: 438–45.

28 Nelson GS, Berger RD, Fetics BJ, Talbot M, Hare JM, Spinelli JCKDA. Left ventricular or biventricular pacing improves cardiac function at diminished energy cost in patients with dilated cardiomyopathy and left bundle-branch block. *Circulation* 2000; **102**: 3053–9.

29 Oguz E, Dagdeviren B, Bilsel T *et al.* Echocardiographic prediction of long-term response to biventricular pacemaker in severe heart failure. *Eur J Heart Fail* 2002; **4**: 83–90.

30 Krahn AD, Snell L, Yee R, Finan J, Skanes AC, Klein GJ. Biventricular pacing improves quality of life and exercise tolerance in patients with heart failure and intraventricular conduction delay. *Can J Cardiol* 2002; **18**: 380–7.

31 Reuter S, Garrigue S, Barold SS *et al.* Comparison of characteristics in responders versus non-responders with biventricular pacing for drug-resistant congestive heart failure. *Am J Cardiol* 2002; **89**: 346–50.

32 Lunati M, Paolucci M, Oliva F *et al.* Patient selection for biventricular pacing. *J Cardiovasc Electrophysiol* 2002; **13**: S63–S67.

33 Sogaard P, Kim WY, Jensen HK *et al.* Impact of acute biventricular pacing on left ventricular performance and volumes in patients with severe heart failure. A tissue Doppler and three-dimensional echocardiographic study. *Cardiology* 2001; **95**: 173–82.

34 Kawaguchi M, Murabayashi T, Fetics BJ *et al.* Quantitation of basal dyssynchrony and acute resynchronization from left or biventricular pacing by novel echo-contrast variability imaging. *J Am Coll Cardiol* 2002; **39**: 2052–8.

CHAPTER 8

Electrocardiography of Multisite Ventricular Pacing

Stéphane Garrigue, S. Serge Barold and Jacques Clémenty

Introduction

Multisite ventricular pacing refers to stimulation techniques that change the degree of ventricular electromechanical asynchrony in patients with major intra- or interventricular conduction disorders [1–9]. The latter includes the inter- and intraventricular conduction delay induced by conventional right ventricular pacing as well as patients with congestive heart failure (CHF), dilated cardiomyopathy and complete left bundle branch block. The change in electrical activation produced by multisite ventricular pacing which has no positive inotropic effect as such, is translated into mechanical improvement from a more coordinated ventricular contraction [10–18]. In other words, stimulation can affect only electrical conduction which, in turn, leads to the desired hemodynamic [10,11] and/or antiarrhythmic effect [12–16]. It is therefore conceivable that the surface electrocardiogram (ECG) during biventricular pacing (BVP) or left ventricular pacing (LVP) could be useful to identify criteria predictive of clinical improvement.

Multisite ventricular pacing can be accomplished from one or more pacing sites in the ventricular myocardium considered as a single electrical chamber. Observations that single-site LVP may be hemodynamically equivalent or even superior to BVP in selected patients with CHF raise crucial issues about basic electrophysiology [10,17].

Effect of left ventricular and biventricular pacing on the surface ECG

It has been thought that the wider the QRS complex,

the longer the conduction delay in a particular electrical chamber [19,20]. Indeed, Figure 8.1(a) identifies the terminal part of the QRS as originating from the LV but in Figure 8.1(b), apical right

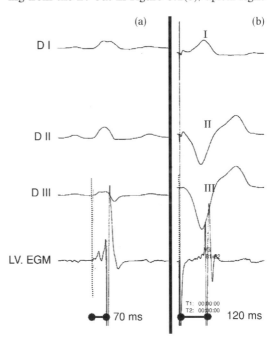

Figure 8.1 Recordings from a patient who presented with a complete left bundle branch block and a left ventricular (LV) ejection fraction of 28% (idiopathic cardiomyopathy). (a) ECG recorded simultaneously with the bipolar electrogram (EGM) from the proximal part of the LV free wall. The bipolar electrogram shows LV activation at the end of the surface QRS complex. The delay from the onset of the QRS to the bipolar signal reaches 70 ms. (b) During right ventricular apical pacing, the delay from the onset of the QRS complex to the bipolar signal at the same site as in (a) jumps to 120 ms.

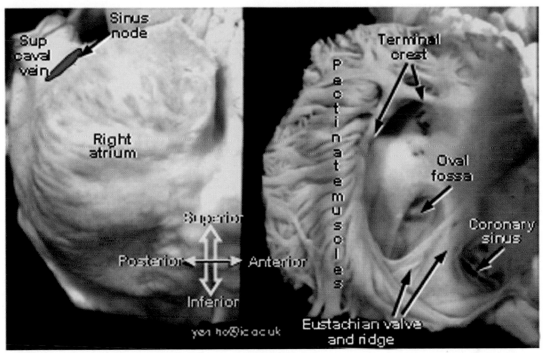

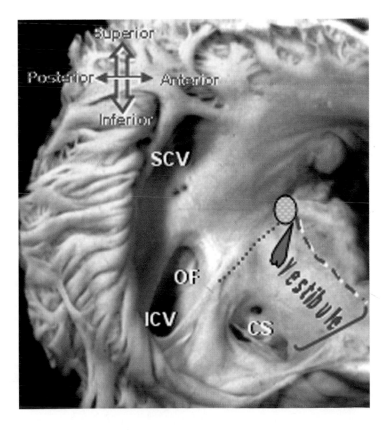

Plate 1.1 (a) Right anterior view of the right atrium from outside showing the relationship of the superior vena cava and atrial appendage. The right atrium (RA) is thin-walled with a rough texture. The sinus node is shown. (b) Interior of the right atrium as seen from the right anterior oblique view. The RA free wall is retracted posteriorly. The septal aspect and venous components are visible. The pectinate muscles arise from the terminal arch of the crista terminalis. The Eustachian ridge and valve, and a fenestrated thesbesian valve are seen. (Reproduced with permission from [20], with permission from Greycoat Publishing.)

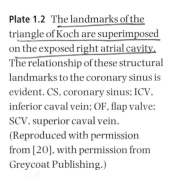

Plate 1.2 The landmarks of the triangle of Koch are superimposed on the exposed right atrial cavity. The relationship of these structural landmarks to the coronary sinus is evident. CS, coronary sinus; ICV, inferior caval vein; OF, flap valve; SCV, superior caval vein. (Reproduced with permission from [20], with permission from Greycoat Publishing.)

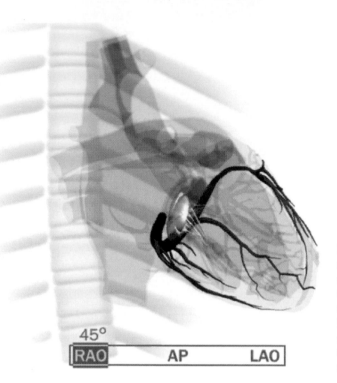

45°

RAO   AP   LAO

Plate 1.3 Coronary sinus (CS)
seen in the right anterior oblique
projection. The plane of the CS is
vertical with the branch tributaries
at a right angle. In this view all the
branches come of the CS at nearly a
right angle and are directed slightly
inferiorly and to the left. Courtesy of
Guidant Corporation.

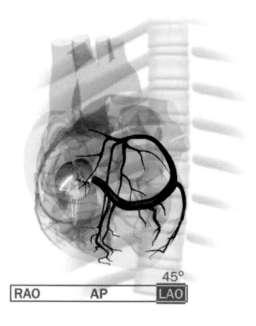

45°

RAO   AP   LAO

Plate 1.4 Coronary sinus (CS) in the left anterior oblique
projection. The plane of the CS is more horizontal and
posterior. The posterior and lateral branches are directed
inferiorly and to the left while the anterior branches are
directed superiorly and to the right. Courtesy of Guidant
Corporation.

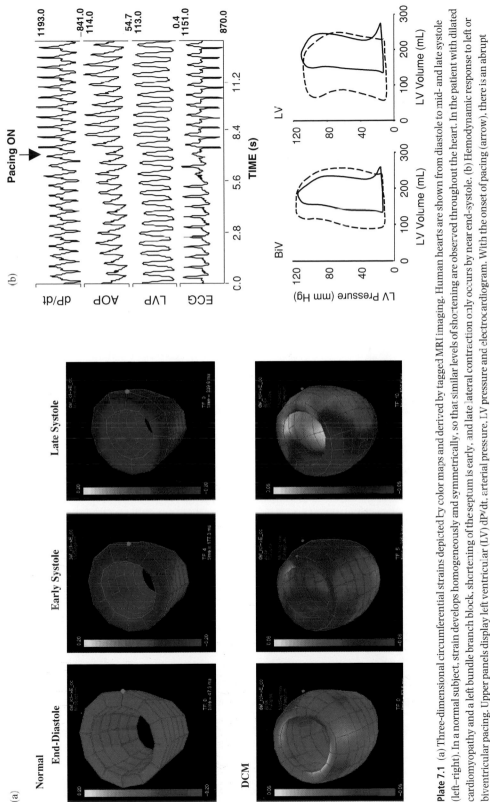

Plate 7.1 (a) Three-dimensional circumferential strains depicted by color maps and derived by tagged MRI imaging. Human hearts are shown from diastole to mid- and late systole (left–right). In a normal subject, strain develops homogeneously and symmetrically, so that similar levels of shortening are observed throughout the heart. In the patient with dilated cardiomyopathy and a left bundle branch block, shortening of the septum is early, and late lateral contraction only occurs by near end-systole. (b) Hemodynamic response to left or biventricular pacing. Upper panels display left ventricular (LV) dP/dt, arterial pressure, LV pressure, and electrocardiogram. With the onset of pacing (arrow), there is an abrupt increase in systolic function indexed by the rise in dP/dt$_{max}$, aortic pulse pressure and LV pressure. Bottom panels display data as pressure–volume loops showing increased stroke volume (loop width), stroke work (loop area), and decline in end-systolic pressure–volume point.

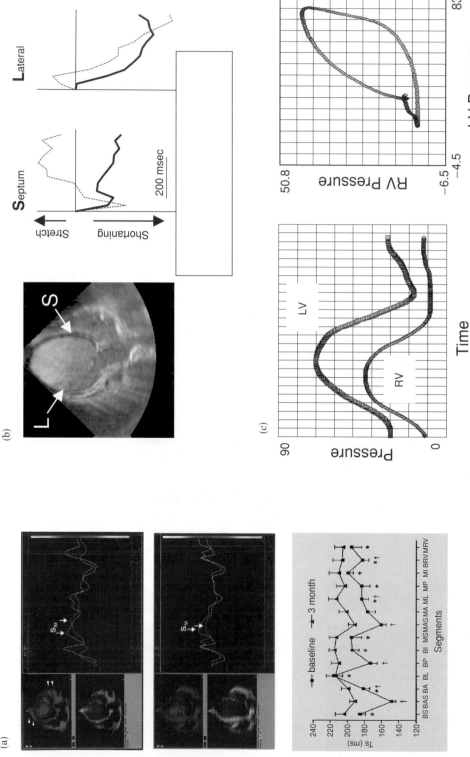

Plate 7.2 Assessment of mechanical dyssynchrony derived by non-invasive Doppler/echo analysis. (a) Example figures of tissue velocity Doppler and timing analysis showing heterogeneous contraction timing in dyssynchronous heart that is improved with biventricular pacing. (From Yu *et al.* [27], with permission.) (b) Examples of contrast variability echo-contrast wall motion analysis which provides quantitative measures of radial shortening times and dyssynchrony. The strain plots from septal (midpanel) and lateral (right panel) walls are shown with pacing off (dashed) and on (solid). Patterns from this analysis are similar to those obtained by MRI [25]. (c) Analysis of intraventricular synchrony by RV pressure–LV pressure plots. Phase delay appears as an open loop of a P–P plot, whereas synchronous contraction produces a near-straight line.

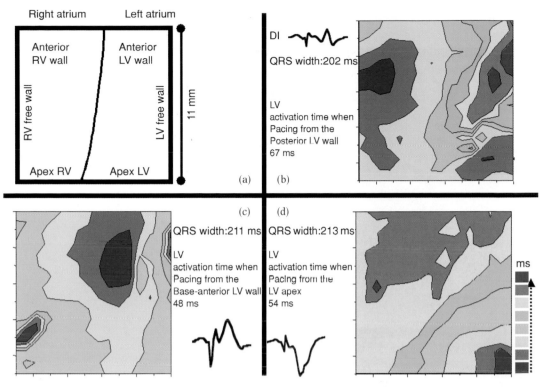

Plate 8.1 (a) Representation of the squared window used for optical mapping in guinea-pig heart preparations during ischemia (see text for details). (b–d) Isochronal maps and left ventricular (LV) activation times during LV pacing from three different sites. Output propagation is depicted inside the window. An inset shows the corresponding QRS complex. The earliest depolarized window area is shown in purple and the latest one in red. Notice that the longest QRS duration (d) does not correspond to the longest LV activation time (b).

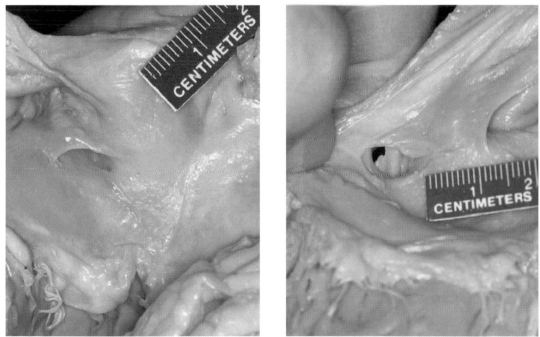

Plate 10.1 (a–f) Human heart specimens demonstrating variation in coronary sinus size and variant anatomic structures that are potentially obstructing at or near the level of the coronary sinus ostium. The arrows indicate areas or structures of interest around the coronary sinus os. TV identifies level of the tricuspid valve, oriented toward the bottom of all figures. This specimen shows a superior flap valve. (b) Internal flap valve.

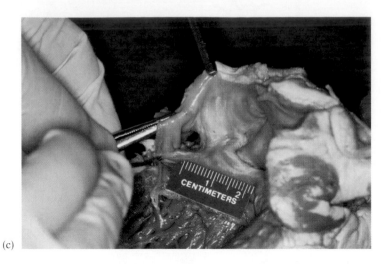

(c)

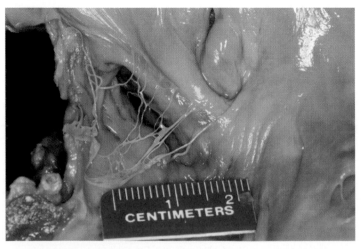

(d)

(e)

Plate 10.1 (*cont'd*) (c) Internal coronary sinus os structures. (d) Dilated right atrium and large unobstructed coronary sinus os. (e) Dilated right atrium with Chiari's network at coronary sinus os.

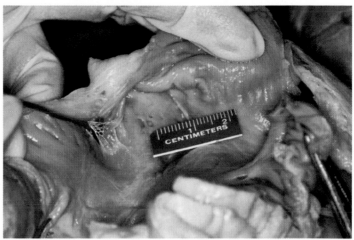

Plate 10.1 (*cont'd*) (f) Membranous Chiari's network with fenestrations.

(f)

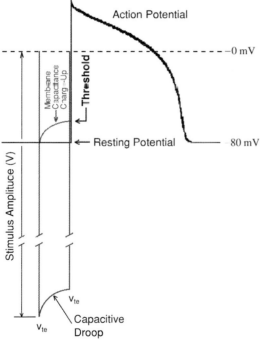

Plate 10.2 (Not to scale) Plates 10.2–10.4 show a proposed theory on the effect of impedance from the combined electrode surface areas on the trailing edge pulse amplitude and the resultant observed 'threshold' increase when larger surface area electrodes are combined. A pacing pulse (blue) begins charge-up of the membrane's equivalent capacitor (red) at the leading edge and completes it at the trailing edge to reach threshold, resulting in an action potential (black).

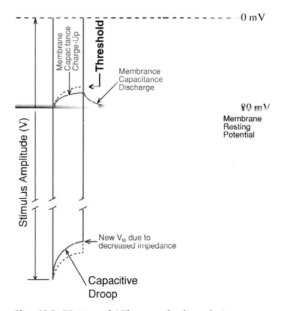

Plate 10.3 (Not to scale) The same (leading edge) amplitude pacing pulse as in Plate 10.2 (blue) now has a decreased trailing edge due to impedance decrease. The membrane's equivalent capacitor (red) cannot complete charge-up to threshold so no action potential results.

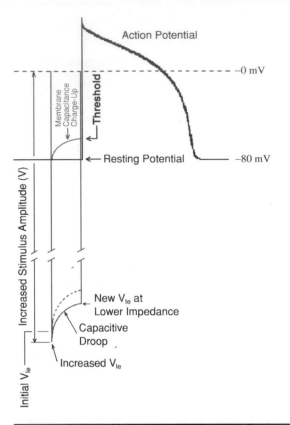

Plate 10.4 (Not to scale) The amplitude of the lower impedance pacing pulse in Plate 10.3 must be increased to increase the trailing edge so the membrane's equivalent capacitor can fully charge to threshold, resulting in an action potential.

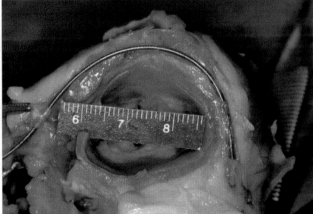

Plate 10.5 Superior aspect of the mitral valve with roof of coronary sinus removed. This demonstrates typical canine encapsulation of cardiac vein lead at 12 weeks.

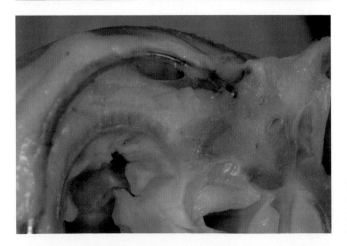

Plate 10.6 Example of typical encapsulation after 2 years of implantation, demonstrating progressive encapsulation in the canine heart.

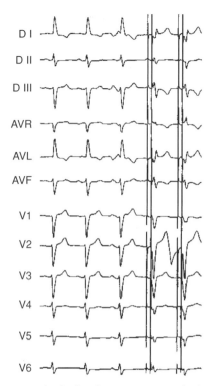

D I

D II

D III

AVR

AVL

AVF

V1

V2

V3

V4

V5

V6

Figure 8.2 Twelve-lead surface ECG in a sinus rhythm patient with severe congestive heart failure (LV ejection fraction 24%) showing QRS shortening with biventricular pacing (118 ms) compared with a duration of 145 ms during spontaneous rhythm.

ventricular pacing (RVP) substantially prolongs the interval between the onset of RVP (stimulation spike) and LV depolarization (from 70 to 120 ms). Accordingly, it might be suggested that RVP should be hemodynamically and electrophysiologically detrimental to CHF patients without a long PR interval. The mortality rate appears proportional to the QRS duration in CHF patients, especially in the setting of left bundle branch block [21]. This observation underscores the close relationship between hemodynamics and electrophysiology, and highlights the importance of conduction block in the clinical evaluation of patients with heart failure. In this context, the question arises as to what is the significance of QRS shortening during BVP. Figure 8.2 shows the 12-lead ECG of a patient (LV ejection fraction 24%) with complete left bundle branch block (QRS = 145 ms). In this patient, BVP resulted in major shortening of the QRS to 118 ms. The mean frontal plane QRS axis shifted from left to right, suggesting that most ventricular activation

was produced by the LV lead. The patient had sustained clinical improvement, suggesting a potential relationship between clinical status and QRS shortening [22]. In this respect, Alonso *et al.* [22] reported in a population of 26 patients that QRS shortening during BVP was closely related to clinical improvement at 1 year after pacemaker implantation, particularly because 7 patients with a prolonged QRS duration during BVP were not clinically improved. However, the sample size of the study was too small to make meaningful conclusions. In addition, LVP alone was not assessed in the patients that improved with BVP. It is possible that LVP alone could have been beneficial despite generating a wider QRS complex than BVP. Indeed, there are other studies suggesting that the concept proposed by Alonso *et al.* [22] is not applicable from patient to patient (Table 8.1). Two randomized controlled studies showed the absence of close relationship (i.e. patient to patient) between the paced QRS duration and the degree of clinical and/or hemodynamic improvement. These observations indicate that some patients improve with BVP without systematic QRS narrowing [7,27].

Left ventricular pacing

Blanc *et al.* [17] first suggested the benefit of isolated or monochamber LV pacing in CHF by showing significant acute hemodynamic improvement with a single LV lead. Several other acute experiments and two midterm studies have supported the concept of monochamber LV pacing for the treatment of severe CHF [10,28–30]. Not surprisingly, LVP is characterized on the surface ECG by an obvious increase in QRS duration with right axis deviation. In Figure 8.3 (taken from a patient who had undergone AV junctional ablation for chronic atrial fibrillation with rapid ventricular response), the QRS duration with spontaneous rhythm (i.e. before ablation) is 165 ms compared with 240 ms with LVP (after ablation). Yet, the patient exhibited significant clinical improvement. Although increased QRS duration is often considered to reflect the presence of ventricular areas with slow conduction resulting in more heterogeneous myocardial activation, with LVP, there is an obvious discrepancy between QRS duration (compared with baseline) and hemodynamic and clinical improvement [10,17,28–30]. Thus in CHF patients the paced QRS duration cannot be assumed to reflect a more

Table 8.1 Studies with left ventricular and/or biventricular pacing in patients with intraventricular delay.

Studies	Study date/no. patients	Mean follow-up	Mean QRS width change with biventricular pacing	Mean QRS axis change	Clinical and hemodynamic improvement	Relationship between the QRS shortening and clinical improvement from patient to patient
Gras et al. [23]	1998/68	3 months	−16%	–	Yes	No
Alonso et al. [22]	1999/26	12 months	−14%	+33°	Yes	Yes
Leclercq et al. [24]	2000/50	15 months	−18%	+36°	Yes	Yes
Cazeau et al. [7]	2001/67	6 months	−10%	–	Yes	No
Reuter et al. [9]	2002/102	12 months	−9%	+19°	Yes	No
Ansalone et al. [25]	2002/31	1 month	−24%	–	Yes	No
Yu et al. [26]	2002/25	1 month	−12%	–	Yes	–
Abraham et al. [27]	2002/228	6 months	−12%	–	Yes	No
			With left ventricular pacing			
Kass et al. [10]	1999/18	Acute study	+12%	–	Yes	No
Touiza et al. [28]	2001/18	6 months	+2%	–	Yes	No
Garrigue et al. [29]	2002/13	2 months	−2%	+42°	Yes	No

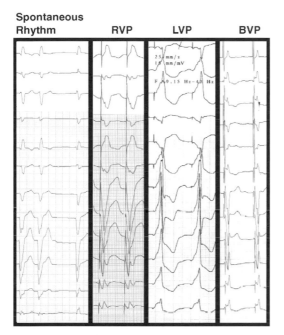

Figure 8.3 Twelve-lead surface ECG showing QRS morphology and duration with spontaneous rhythm (SR), right (RVP), left (LVP) and biventricular pacing (BVP) in a patient with severe congestive heart failure, chronic atrial fibrillation and complete left bundle branch block. The QRS width measures 165 ms, 220 ms, 240 ms and 120 ms respectively (see text for details).

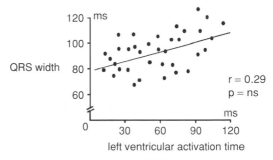

Figure 8.4 Correlation between QRS duration and ventricular activation time by using the optical mapping system. This correlation is not significant so that the QRS duration from the surface ECG does not reflect the true left ventricular activation time.

heterogeneous propagation pattern of activation [31–34]. This concept was verified experimentally in guinea-pig heart preparations during ischemia using optical mapping with the *in vitro* application of voltage-sensitive dye to compare the temporal sequence of ventricular activation by pacing at different LV sites [31]. Plate 8.1, facing p. 84, panel A shows a square in which the apex, and the anterior and free walls of the RV and LV are represented [31]. Panel B illustrates the propagation of activation when pacing is applied at the posterior LV wall. LV activation time is 67 ms with a QRS duration in lead I reaching 202 ms. Panel C depicts the same ventricular isochronal map with pacing at the base–anterior LV wall; LV activation time is 48 ms with a QRS duration in lead I reaching 211 ms, whereas in panel D, it was 54 ms with a QRS of 223 ms during apical LVP. Not only is the QRS duration different from site to site but so is the QRS morphology (Plate 8.1). Note that the shortest QRS duration (202 ms) was not associated with the shortest LV ventricular activation time (48 ms) but the longest

one (67 ms) (Plate 8.1). This indicates that LV activation time is substantially different from and much shorter than the total duration of the QRS complex. Consequently, despite a longer QRS duration, LVP may electrically resynchronize the LV with the same hemodynamic effect as BVP. The lack of correlation between the LV activation time (recorded by optical mapping) and the QRS duration on the surface ECG ($r = 0.29$; $P = NS$) in our guinea-pig experiments is likely to be similar in patients (Figure 8.4) [31]. Prinzen *et al.* [32] also showed that the sequence of LV electrical activation rather than QRS shortening determines whether or not BVP results in improved LV wall mechanical synchronization. This was confirmed by further studies showing that the ultimate benefit of BVP is mechanical (or electromechanical), an effect that does not necessarily correlate with alterations in ventricular activation [33,34].

Figure 8.5 shows the QRS morphology and duration when two LV pacing sites were assessed in a patient with severe CHF. Compared to baseline (a), pacing from the LV free wall resulted in an increased QRS duration (from 175 ms to 242 ms) and a rightward shift of the QRS axis (b). Pacing at the base–anterior LV wall (c) yielded a lesser increase in QRS duration (from 175 ms to 231 ms) and a right shift of the QRS axis with a much less fragmented QRS component. This observation illustrates that there is no reliable electrocardiographic criterion to determine the optimal LV pacing site. In this respect several recent studies found no ECG criteria (the QRS axis, duration and morphology) predictive of clinical improvement with BVP [9,25,27,28]. Such observations raise questions about the reliability of the surface ECG in the assessment of pacing-induced

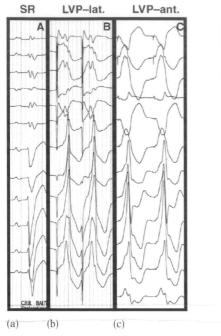

SR   LVP–lat.   LVP–ant.

(a)   (b)   (c)

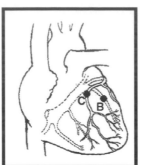

(d)

Figure 8.5 Different patterns of depolarization according to left ventricle (LV) stimulation site. (a) Twelve-lead surface ECG during spontaneous rhythm (SR) showing a non-specific bundle branch block in a patient with severe congestive heart failure. (b) Surface ECG during LV pacing (LVP) from the lateral (lat) wall. (c) Surface ECG during LV pacing from the anterior (ant) wall. (d) Shows LV pacing lead locations for (b) and (c) in the coronary venous system.

ventricular activation times. However, the predictive role of the surface ECG in identifying optimal pacing sites, perhaps in combination with vectorcardiography, requires more extensive investigation.

Frontal plane axis

Besides QRS duration, the change in the frontal plane QRS axis may provide useful data because it depends upon which pacing lead depolarizes the majority of the ventricular mass (i.e. the right or left pacing lead). Accordingly, the QRS axis moves from left to right if the ventricular mass is predominantly depolarized by the LV pacing lead. Conversely, an LV pacing lead depolarizing only a small ventricular mass will induce a slight shift in the QRS axis, compared with spontaneous rhythm in the case of left bundle branch block. It might be useful to determine whether the degree of axis change is predictive of clinical improvement. Ricci et al. [35] recently showed that, more than the QRS width, multisite ventricular pacing axis variability over time may play a determinant role if correlated with an electrical remodeling of the ventricles.

Q or q wave in lead I

Georger et al. [36] observed a q wave in lead I in 17 of 18 patients during biventricular pacing. A q wave in lead I during uncomplicated RV pacing is rare

and these workers observed it in only 1 patient. Loss of the q wave in lead I was 100% predictive of loss of LV capture [36]. It therefore appears that analysis of the q wave in lead I may be a reliable way to assess LV capture (Figure 8.6).

Associated interatrial conduction delay

In rare cases, the benefit of ventricular resynchronization is limited in the presence of associated interatrial conduction block (Figure 8.7a). Even though BVP-induced ventricular ejection phase is more homogeneous, excessively late left atrial activation alters LV filling. Consequently this problem can be addressed with biatrial pacing by implantation of a second atrial lead into the proximal coronary sinus, an arrangement that enhances the effect of BVP (Figure 8.7b). In a four-chamber device, a pacemaker with specific software can sense spontaneous right atrial depolarization and from this event, can trigger left atrial stimulation: on the surface ECG, a pacemaker stimulus becomes visible in the middle of the P wave in association with substantial shortening of the atrial depolarization, followed by a BVP-induced QRS shortening (Figure 8.7b).

Permanent atrial fibrillation

Patients with atrial fibrillation (i.e. irregular and relatively fast ventricular rate) who are candidates for

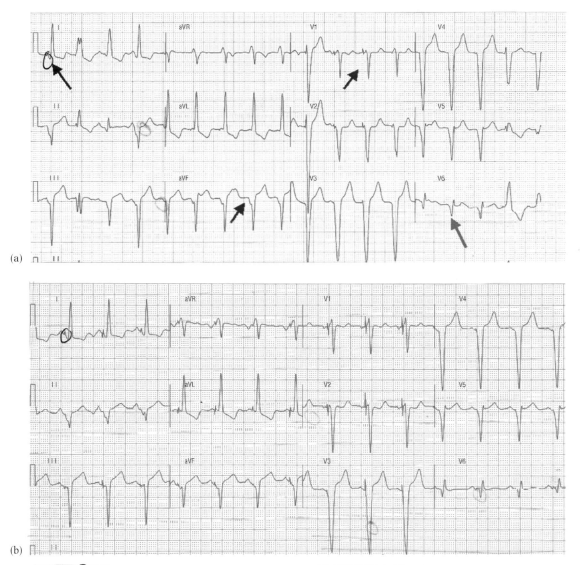

Figure 8.6 (a) Biventricular pacing in the VOO mode. The arrows point to QRS complexes without a preceding P wave. These complexes therefore do not represent ventricular fusion. Note the typical q wave in lead I during pure biventricular pacing. (b) Biventricular DDD pacing in the same patient as in (a). The configuration of the paced QRS complexes is identical to that in (a) with appropriate programming of the atrioventricular delay.

BVP should undergo a His bundle ablation to permit continuous BVP [7,24,29,30]. Because the atria need not be stimulated, implanting a dual-chamber device allows several pacing configurations that can be assessed on the surface ECG. Indeed, in the case of a conventional dual-chamber pacemaker, connecting the LV pacing lead to the atrial port and the RV pacing lead to the ventricular port offers three types of ventricular stimulation: RVP, LVP

and BVP with the shortest 'atrioventricular' delay possible (i.e. between 10 and 30 ms). The surface ECG will provide the QRS pattern of each pacing configuration (Figure 8.3). With BVP mode, two spikes are visible, the first one originating from LV stimulation and the second one from RV stimulation. In Figure 8.3, the QRS axis changed from an obvious left axis during spontaneous ventricular activation to normalization with BVP (here, 58°).

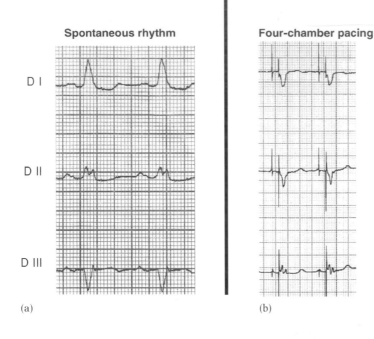

Spontaneous rhythm

D I

D II

D III

(a)

Four-chamber pacing

(b)

Figure 8.7 (a) Surface ECG showing interatrial conduction block (wide P wave) with left bundle branch block in a congestive heart failure patient (left ventricular ejection fraction 18%). (b) Surface ECG after the patient received a four-chamber pacing device. The pacemaker is equipped with software that allows sensing of right atrial depolarization which triggers left atrial stimulation. Accordingly, an atrial spike is visible in the middle of the P wave followed by a BVP-induced QRS shortening.

Ventricular fusion beats

In patients with sinus rhythm and a relatively short PR interval, a ventricular fusion phenomenon may lead to misinterpretation of the ECG. Figure 8.8(a) shows a surface ECG in a patient with dilated idiopathic cardiomyopathy and a spontaneous QRS duration of 125 ms. After implantation of a BVP device, the QRS was considered shortened to 115 ms (Figure 8.8b). However, the QRS morphology was similar to that of the spontaneous ventricular rhythm except for lead III. Figure 8.8(c) illustrates a BVP tracing with complete ventricular capture, indicating that (b) represents ventricular fusion. Consequently, the true QRS duration during BVP is 130 ms and longer than that during spontaneous rhythm. This example illustrates a frequent pitfall of apparent QRS shortening with BVP when the possibility of a ventricular fusion beat is not considered in the presence of a relatively short PR interval. Despite prolongation of the QRS duration with BVP compared to the QRS during fusion, the patient was clinically improved on a long-term basis.

Figure 8.9 illustrates the same phenomenon during LVP. The QRS duration with spontaneous rhythm (Figure 8.9a) is 130 ms with a PR interval of 140 ms. In Figure 8.9(b), the atrioventricular delay was programmed to 100 ms with LVP. The QRS axis changed from −6° towards +92° with a

QRS duration reaching 160 ms. When the atrioventricular delay was further shortened down to 70 ms (Figure 8.9c), the QRS axis became similar to that obtained with a 100-ms atrioventricular delay, but the QRS duration was substantially increased to 200 ms. In the latter case, the QRS duration was similar to that generated with LV pacing in the VVI mode (not shown in the figure), confirming complete ventricular capture. Consequently, complete LV pacing must be carefully verified (if the device allows) before assessing hemodynamics. It is likely that a fusion QRS pattern between spontaneous ventricular activation and LVP results in a particular type of BVP; comparison of these two types of BVP might be interesting in some patients to determine whether a certain degree of fusion enhances the hemodynamic benefit of the pacemaker.

Electrocardiographic follow-up of multisite ventricular pacing

A baseline 12-lead ECG should be recorded at the time of implantation during assessment of the independent capture thresholds of the RV and LV to identify the specific morphology of the paced QRS complexes in a multiplicity of leads. This requires having the patient connected to a multichannel 12-lead ECG during the implantation procedure.

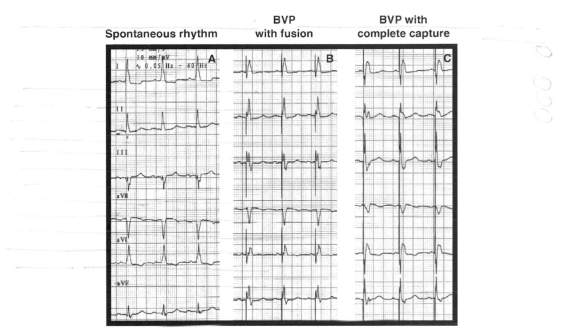

Spontaneous rhythm   **BVP with fusion**   **BVP with complete capture**

Figure 8.8 Ventricular fusion during biventricular pacing (BVP). (A) Spontaneous ventricular depolarization. Surface ECG from a patient with severe congestive heart failure showing sinus rhythm, complete left bundle branch block and QRS duration of 125 ms. (B) Ventricular fusion. ECG from the same patient after receiving a BVP device. The atrioventricular (AV) delay was fixed at 120 ms and the paced QRS shortened to 115 ms. The slight change in QRS morphology strongly suggests a fusion phenomenon with spontaneous ventricular depolarization. (C) Pure biventricular depolarization. The AV delay was programmed to 80 ms, resulting in a longer QRS duration of 130 ms. The QRS morphology is quite different from that in (B) and similar to that obtained with biventricular VVI pacing, confirming complete biventricular capture. The shorter AV delay therefore eliminated ventricular fusion with spontaneous ventricular depolarization.

Spontaneous rhythm   **LVP with fusion**   **LVP with complete capture**

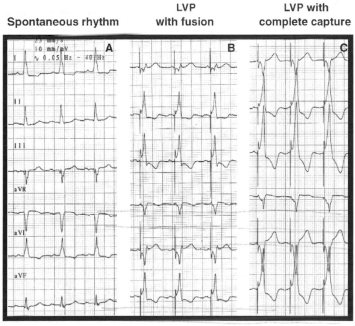

Figure 8.9 Ventricular fusion during left ventricular pacing (LVP). (A) Surface ECG of a congestive heart failure patient during spontaneous rhythm: prolonged QRS complex duration and PR interval of 140 ms. (B) LVP with fusion between the spontaneous QRS complex and LVP by programming a relatively long atrioventricular (AV) delay (100 ms). (C) Complete capture with LVP (AV delay programmed to 70 ms) (see text for details).

A total of four 12-lead ECGs are required as shown in Figure 8.3:

① intrinsic rhythm and QRS complex prior to any pacing;
② paced QRS associated with RV pacing;
③ paced QRS associated with LV pacing; and
④ paced QRS associated with biventricular pacing.

The four tracings should be examined to identify the lead configuration that best demonstrates a discernible and obvious difference between the four pacing states (inhibited, RV only, LV only and biventricular). This ECG lead should then be used as the surface monitoring lead for subsequent evaluations. Loss of capture in one ventricle will cause a change in the morphology of ventricular paced beats in the 12-lead ECG to that of either single-chamber RVP or single-chamber LVP. A shift in the frontal plane axis may be useful to corroborate the loss of capture. If both the native QRS and the biventricular paced complex are relatively narrow, then a widening of the paced QRS complex will identify loss of capture in one chamber with effective capture in the other. In questionable cases, loss of capture requires monitoring the ECG with telemetered markers and the intracardiac electrogram (Figure 8.10). When there is intact capture in both the RV and LV, the evoked response on the ventricular electrogram will show a monophasic complex in contrast to two distinct depolarizations during spontaneous conduction if the native QRS is wide (left intraventricular conduction delay). With loss of capture in one of the ventricles, the ventricular lead which is still effective will cause a depolarization of that ventricle. The impulse will then have to be conducted via the native pathways to the other ventricle in an manner identical to single ventricular systems with standard pacing. If there is a significant left intraventricular conduction delay, the ventricular electrogram will change from a monophasic complex to two discrete complexes similar but not identical to that registered by the spontaneous conducted QRS complex (Figure 8.10).

Many studies have shown that QRS duration does not vary over time as long as the LV pacing lead does not move from its initial site [9,22–24,37]. Yet surface ECGs should be performed periodically because the LV lead may become displaced in a collateral branch of the coronary sinus as active fixation leads are not used. Dislodgement of the LV lead may result in loss of LV capture; in this case, the ECG will reveal an RV pacing QRS pattern with an increased QRS duration and a left axis deviation.

Far-field atrial oversensing

A slight dislodgement of the LV lead may cause sensing of left atrial activity [38–41]. In dual cathodal systems, with simultaneous sensing from both ventricular leads, this phenomenon can deactivate BVP as the LV lead senses P waves as a far-field signal. This form of oversensing counteracts the effect of BVP and may precipitate recurrent congestive heart failure (Figure 8.11). Far-field atrial oversensing is more devastating in patients with atrial fibrillation following atrioventricular (AV) junctional ablation. Figure 8.12 illustrates an example of P-wave sensing by the ventricular channel. The patient complained of repeated syncope. The marker annotations clearly show that the P wave was initially sensed by the atrial channel and 80 ms later by the ventricular channel. The P wave was not followed by a spontaneous ventricular depolarization because of complete AV block from AV ablation performed for drug-resistant paroxysmal atrial fibrillation. The chest X-ray showed only slight dislodgement of the LV lead; the P-wave amplitude was 3 mV in the ventricular channel whereas premature ventricular beats generated a ventricular electrogram of 11 mV. The ventricular sensitivity was decreased to 6 mV (initially programmed to 2.5 mV) with apparent correction of oversensing. One month later, the patient was rehospitalized again for repeated syncope. The ECG now revealed the presence of atrial pacing not followed by ventricular stimulation (Figure 8.13a). Figure 8.13(b) shows the corresponding marker annotations confirming that, despite a correct postatrial ventricular blanking period, the paced atrial event was sensed by the ventricular channel and, most importantly, beyond the ventricular safety pacing window. Consequently ventricular safety pacing was not activated. A repeat chest X-ray revealed further displacement of the LVP lead toward the great cardiac vein. The lead was therefore repositioned to its initial location (proximal part of a lateral branch) with resolution of the disturbance.

Atrial undersensing

Loss of P-wave sensing by the atrial channel can also cause progressive clinical deterioration. This phenomenon can precipitate heart failure symp-

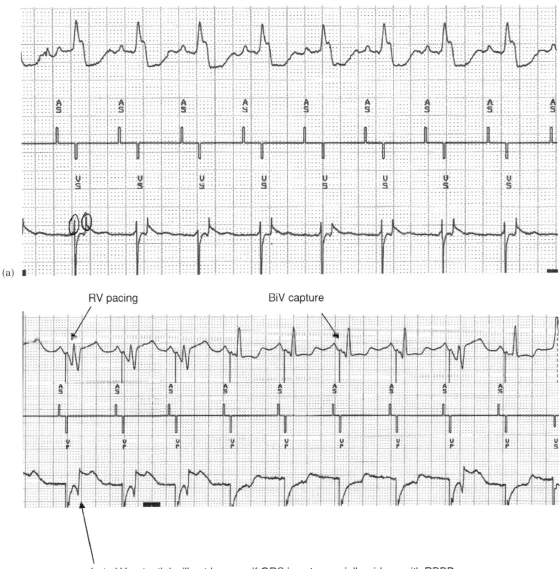

(a)

(b)

Figure 8.10 (a) Simultaneous recording of the ECG and telemetered ventricular electrogram during spontaneous rhythm in a patient with left bundle branch block and a biventricular pacemaker. The ventricular electrogram shows two components corresponding to right ventricular and delayed left ventricular (LV) activation. (b) Simultaneous recording of the ECG and telemetered ventricular electrogram in a patient with left bundle branch block and a biventricular pacemaker. The ventricular electrogram displays a monophasic pattern during biventricular capture. With loss of LV pacing, the ventricular electrogram shows a late deflection which represents delayed LV activation through ordinary myocardium.

toms as the patient no longer derives benefit from BVP. From these observations, we recommend periodic analysis of the ECG to avoid sensing problems. Furthermore, heart failure decompensation in a patient with a BVP device requires meticulous investigation to determine whether pacemaker malfunction or suboptimal operation is responsible for clinical deterioration.

Anodal stimulation

Although anodal capture may occur with high output traditional RV pacing, this phenomenon is

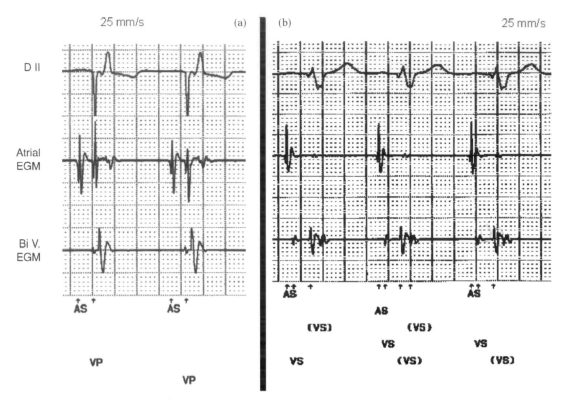

Figure 8.11 Sensing of left atrial activity by the left ventricular (LV) pacing lead in a patient with sinus rhythm and complete left bundle branch block. (a) The spontaneous P wave is sensed by the right atrial lead (AS symbol in the atrial channel) and after a programmed atrioventricular (AV) delay of 140 ms, the ventricle is paced (VP symbol in the ventricular channel—dual cathodal biventricular pacing mode). (b) Same patient as in (a). The first and third group of deflections show the following: 40 ms after the right atrial lead senses the spontaneous P wave (AS symbol: first potential), the ventricular channel senses the P wave (VS symbol in the ventricular channel: second potential) interpreted as spontaneous ventricular activation following the P wave. The ventricular channel then senses the third potential originating from true right ventricular (RV) activation (VS in parentheses in the ventricular channel; sensed in the ventricular refractory period beyond the blanking period). Note that the interval between VS and (VS) exceeds the ventricular blanking period of the device. LV activation is not recorded and presumably falls in the ventricular blanking period initiated by sensing RV activity. The second group of deflections shows sensing of LV activity (VS) in the ventricular refractory period beyond the ventricular blanking period generated by RV sensing. This generates three sequential ventricular sensed events.

almost always not discernible electrocardiographically. Biventricular pacing systems generally utilize a unipolar lead for LV pacing via a coronary vein. The tip electrode of the LV lead is the cathode and the proximal electrode of the bipolar RV lead often provides the anode for LV pacing. This arrangement creates a common anode for RV and LV pacing. A high current density (from two sources) at the common anode during biventricular pacing may cause anodal capture manifested as a paced QRS complex with a different configuration from that of pure biventricular pacing [42, 43] (Figure 8.14). Anodal

capture disappears by reducing the output of the pacemaker or when the device (even at high output) is programmed to a true unipolar system with the common anode on the pacemaker can. Anodal capture was recognized in first generation transvenous biventricular pacemakers (without separately programmable RV and LV outputs) when 3 distinct pacing morphologies were observed exclusive of fusion with the spontaneous QRS complex: biventricular with anodal capture (at a high output), biventricular (at a lower output), and RV (with loss of LV capture). Anodal capture involving the ring

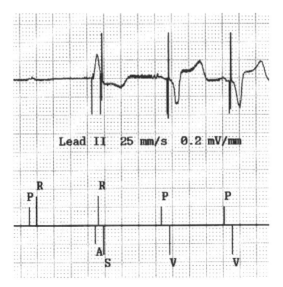

Figure 8.12 Far-field atrial oversensing during biventricular pacing. Recording of the ECG and markers during biventricular pacing in a pacemaker-dependent patient. The first P wave is not followed by ventricular stimulation. The markers indicate that 70 ms after the atrial channel senses the P wave (P symbol), the ventricular channel identifies the P wave as a ventricular event (R symbol). This phenomenon is intermittent, suggesting that the left ventricular pacing lead is unstable in a position close to the left atrium. The first spontaneous QRS complex induces ventricular safety pacing (S symbol). The following ventricular events are paced (V symbol) with atrial sensing and AV synchronization (P symbol).

electrode of the bipolar RV lead can also occur during monochamber LV pacing at a relatively high output when the QRS complex may be identical to that obtained with biventricular pacing. Anodal stimulation should not be misinterpreted as pacemaker malfunction.

Right bundle branch block and multisite ventricular pacing

Recently, complete right bundle branch block was suggested as an independent predictor of mortality in patients with congestive heart failure with the same weight as left bundle branch block [44]. In patients with severe congestive heart failure and complete right bundle branch block, it is likely that a concomitant left-sided intraventricular conduction disorder is concealed from the surface ECG. This

should perhaps be suspected when the ECG exhibits an atypical right bundle branch block frequently encountered with a left axis deviation of the QRS in ischemic disease (Figure 8.15a) [45]. Patients with common and even rare types of right bundle branch block in severe heart failure might also be improved with BVP [45] since it causes a rightward shift of the axis and shortening of the QRS complex in such patients (Figure 8.15b,c).

A pilot study involving heart failure patients (*n* = 12) with complete right bundle branch block followed their progress for over 1 year after ventricular resynchronization [46]. Figure 8.16 illustrates how right, left and biventricular pacing can modify the surface ECG in this situation. Although all patients presented with major interventricular delay, only nine (75%) who demonstrated important intra-LV electromechanical disorders characterized by Doppler tissue imaging improved with biventricular pacing by reduction of the degree of intra-LV delay. Three patients who had no left intraventricular delay during spontaneous rhythm did not benefit from BVP. No surface ECG criteria could characterize this category of patients with complete right bundle branch block and no intra-LV delay. Here, sophisticated techniques of echocardiography (such as Doppler tissue imaging for evaluation of electromechanical delays) rather than a simple surface ECG should be performed to identify potential responders. These observations are consistent with data suggesting that patients with advanced heart failure and major left intraventricular conduction delay (with or without interventricular delay) might be the optimal candidates for biventricular pacing regardless of the presence of right or left bundle branch block [10,46–48]. However, this concept remains to be verified in a larger population.

Conclusion

The surface ECG appears helpful in the follow-up of patients with multisite ventricular pacing, particularly in terms of QRS duration and frontal axis shifts. It permits the diagnosis of dislodgement of the LV pacing lead with or without loss of LV stimulation. However, the QRS morphology and duration do not accurately correlate with clinical and hemodynamic improvement so that the QRS width is not a predictive factor of efficient biventricular pacing in heart failure patients.

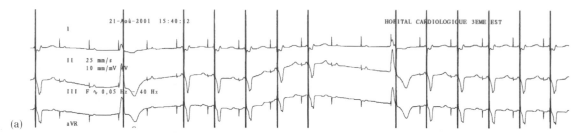

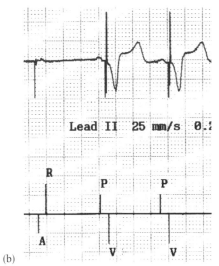

(a)

(b)

Figure 8.13 Far-field atrial oversensing during biventricular pacing. Same patient as Figure 8.12. (a) The ECG shows prolonged ventricular inhibition induced by atrial stimulation. The postatrial ventricular blanking period was fixed at 36 ms. Note that ventricular inhibition occurs in conjunction with successful atrial capture. Reprogramming the pacemaker to DDD mode with pacing only the right ventricle eliminated the abnormality. (b) The annotation channel confirms ventricular detection of atrial activity during atrial stimulation. The atrial stimulus is accompanied by an 'A' symbol. It is then followed by an 'R' symbol indicating that atrial activity is sensed by the ventricular channel (in biventricular mode) beyond the blanking period and the ventricular safety window.

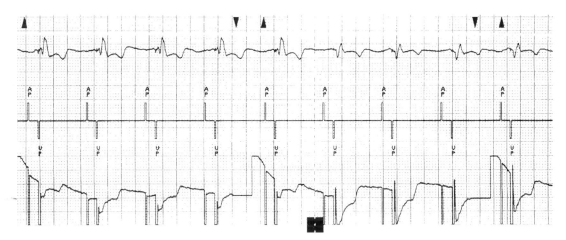

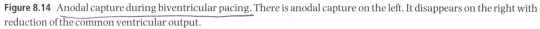

Figure 8.14 Anodal capture during biventricular pacing. There is anodal capture on the left. It disappears on the right with reduction of the common ventricular output.

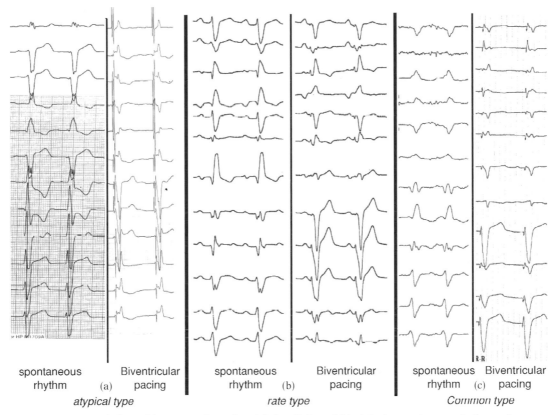

Figure 8.15 QRS morphology of three types of complete right bundle branch block during spontaneous rhythm and biventricular pacing (see text for details).

References

1 Cazeau S, Ritter P, Bakdach S *et al.* Four chamber pacing in dilated cardiomyopathy. *Pacing Clin Electrophysiol* 1994; **17**: 1974–9.

2 Barold SS, Cazeau S, Mugica J *et al.* Permanent multisite cardiac pacing. *Pacing Clin Electrophysiol* 1997; **20**: 2725–9.

3 Linde C. Biventricular pacing in patients with severe heart failure: has the time come? *Heart* 2000; **84**: 123–4.

4 Kay GN, Bourge RC. Biventricular pacing for congestive heart failure: questions of who, what, where, why, how, and how much. *Am Heart J* 2000; **140**: 821–3.

5 Barold SS. Biventricular cardiac pacing: promising new therapy for congestive heart failure. *Chest* 2000; **118**: 1819–21.

6 Leclercq C, Kass DA. Retiming the failing heart: principles and current clinical status of cardiac resynchronization. *J Am Coll Cardiol* 2002; **39**: 194–201.

7 Cazeau S, Leclercq C, Lavergne T *et al.* Effects of multisite biventricular pacing in patients with heart failure and intraventricular conduction delay. *N Engl J Med* 2001; **344**: 873–80.

8 Daubert JC, Leclercq C, Alonso C, Cazeau S. Long-term experience with biventricular pacing in refractory heart failure. In: Ovsyshcher IE, ed. *Cardiac Arrhythmias and Device Therapy: Results and Perspectives for the New Century.* Armonk NY: Futura, 2000: 385–92.

9 Reuter S, Garrigue S, Barold SS *et al.* Comparison of characteristics in responders versus nonresponders with biventricular pacing for drug resistant congestive heart failure. *Am J Cardiol* 2002; **89**: 346–50.

10 Kass DA, Chen HC, Curry C *et al.* Improved left ventricular mechanics from acute VDD pacing in patients with dilated cardiomyopathy and ventricular conduction delay. *Circulation* 1999; **99**: 1567–73.

11 Nelson GS, Berger RD, Fetics BJ *et al.* Left ventricular or biventricular pacing improves cardiac function at diminished energy cost in patients with dilated cardiomyopathy and left bundle branch block. *Circulation* 2000; **102**: 3053–9.

12 Daubert JC, Revault d'Allonnes G, Pavin D, Mabo P. Prevention of atrial fibrillation by pacing. In:

Spontaneous rhythm	RV pacing	LV pacing	BV pacing
QRS width: 165 ms	155 ms	180 ms	126 ms

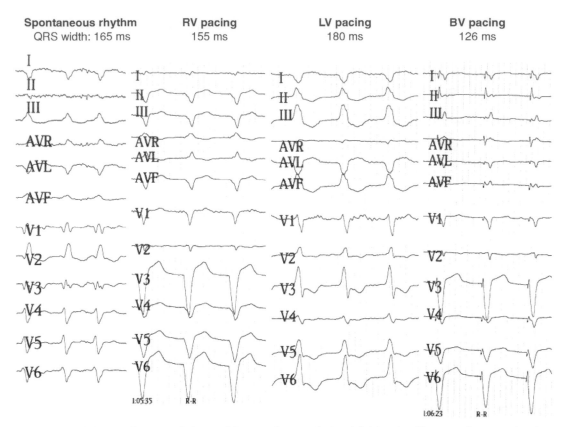

Figure 8.16 Modification of QRS morphology and duration during right (RVP), left (LVP) and biventricular pacing (BVP) in a congestive heart failure patient (LV ejection fraction 21%) with complete right bundle branch block and chronic atrial fibrillation. With spontaneous rhythm, the QRS morphology in V1 shows a common type of right bundle branch block. LVP results in right axis shift with a QS pattern in leads I and aVL, and increased QRS duration. BVP provides a substantial narrowing of the QRS complex along with a smaller amplitude and a right axis shift (compared with spontaneous rhythm and RVP). This suggests that the LV pacing lead might depolarize most of the LV (QS aspect of the QRS complex in leads 1 and aVL).

Ovsyshcher IE, ed. *Cardiac Arrhythmias and Device Therapy: Results and Perspectives for the New Century.* Armonk, NY: Futura, 2000: 155–66.

13 Daubert JC, Mabo P. Atrial pacing for the prevention of postoperative atrial fibrillation: how and when to pace. *J Am Coll Cardiol* 2000; **35**: 147.

14 Ramaswamy K, Zagrodsky JD, Page RL *et al.* Biventricular pacing decreases the inducibility of sustained monomorphic ventricular tachycardia [abstract]. *Pacing Clin Electrophysiol* 2000; **23**: 748.

15 Garrigue S, Barold SS, Hocini M *et al.* Treatment of drug-refractory ventricular tachycardia by biventricular pacing. *Pacing Clin Electrophysiol* 2000; **23**: 1700–2.

16 Higgins SL, Yong P, Sheck D *et al.* Biventricular pacing diminishes the need for implantable cardioverter defibrillator therapy. Ventak CHF Investigators. *J Am Coll Cardiol* 2000; **36**: 824–7.

17 Blanc JJ, Etienne Y, Gilard M *et al.* Evaluation of different ventricular pacing sites in patients with severe heart failure. Results of an acute hemodynamic study. *Circulation* 1997; **96**: 3273–7.

18 Auricchio A, Stellbrink C, Block M *et al.* Effect of pacing chamber and atrioventricular delay on acute systolic function of paced patients with congestive heart failure. The Pacing Therapies for Congestive Heart Failure Study Group. The Guidant Congestive Heart Failure Research Group. *Circulation* 1999; **99**: 2993–3001.

19 Leclercq C, Cazeau S, Le Breton H *et al.* Acute hemodynamic effects of biventricular DDD pacing in patients with end-stage heart failure. *J Am Coll Cardiol* 1998; **32**: 1825–31.

20 Xiao HB, Roy C, Gibson DG. Nature of ventricular activation in patients with dilated cardiomyopathy: evidence for bilateral bundle branch block. *Br Heart J* 1994; **72**: 167–74.

21 Gottipaty VK, Krelis SP, Lu F *et al.* The resting electrocardiogram provides a sensitive and inexpensive marker of prognosis in patients with chronic congestive heart failure [abstract]. *J Am Coll Cardiol* 1999; **33**: 145A.

22 Alonso C, Leclercq C, Victor F *et al.* Electrocardiographic predictive factors of long-term clinical improvement with multisite biventricular pacing in advanced heart failure. *Am J Cardiol* 1999; **84**: 1417–21.

23 Gras D, Mabo P, Tang T *et al.* Multisite pacing as a supplemental treatment of congestive heart failure: preliminary results of the Medtronic, Inc. Insync study. *Pacing Clin Electrophysiol* 1998; **21**: 2249–55.

24 Leclercq C, Victor F, Alonso C *et al.* Comparative effects of permanent biventricular pacing for refractory heart failure in patients with stable sinus rhythm or chronic atrial fibrillation. *Am J Cardiol* 2000; **85**: 1154–6.

25 Ansalone G, Giannantoni P, Ricci R *et al.* Doppler myocardial imaging to evaluate the effectiveness of pacing sites in patients receiving biventricular pacing. *J Am Coll Cardiol* 2002; **39**: 489–99.

26 Yu C M, Chau E, Sanderson JE *et al.* Tissue Doppler echocardiographic evidence of reverse remodeling and improved synchronicity by simultaneously delaying regional contraction after biventricular pacing therapy in heart failure. *Circulation* 2002; **105**: 438–45.

27 Abraham WT, Fisher WG, Smith AL *et al.* Cardiac resynchronization in chronic heart failure. The MIRACLE prospective study. *N Engl J Med* 2002; **346**: 1845–53.

28 Touiza A, Etienne Y, Gilard M *et al.* Long-term left ventricular pacing: assessment and comparison with biventricular pacing in patients with severe congestive heart failure. *J Am Coll Cardiol* 2001; **38**: 1966–70.

29 Garrigue S, Bordachar P, Reuter S *et al.* Comparison of permanent left ventricular and biventricular pacing in patients with heart failure and chronic atrial fibrillation: prospective hemodynamic study. *Heart* 2002; **87**: 529–34.

30 Etienne Y, Mansourati J, Gilard M *et al.* Evaluation of left ventricular based pacing in patients with congestive heart failure and atrial fibrillation. *Am J Cardiol* 1999; **83**: 1138–40.

31 Garrigue S, Efimov IR, Jaïs P, Haïssaguerre M, Clémenty J. Voltage-sensitive dye mapping technique applied to biventricular pacing during ischemia: role of the voltage output, the interventricular delay, pacing sites on ventricular arrhythmias occurrence [abstract]. *Pacing Clin Electrophysiol* 2001; **24**: 539.

32 Prinzen FW, Van Oosterhout MF, Vanagt WY, Storm C, Reneman RS. Optimization of ventricular function by improving the activation sequence during ventricular pacing. *Pacing Clin Electrophysiol* 1998; **21**: 2256–60.

33 Wyman BT, Hunter WC, Prinzen FW, McVeigh EA. Mapping propagation of mechanical activation in the paced heart with MRI tagging. *Am J Physiol* 1999; **276**: H881–H891.

34 Prinzen FW, Hunter WC, Wyman BT, Mc Veigh ER. Mapping of regional myocardial strain and work during ventricular pacing: experimental study using magnetic resonance imaging tagging. *J Am Coll Cardiol* 1999; **33**: 1735–42.

35 Ricci R, Pignalberi C, Ansalone G *et al.* Early and late QRS morphology and width in biventricular pacing: relationship to lead site and electrical remodeling. *J Interv Card Electrophysiol* 2002; **6**: 279–85.

36 Georger F, Scavee C, Collet B *et al.* Specific electrocardiographic patterns may assess left ventricular capture during biventricular pacing [abstract]. *Pacing Clin Electrophysiol* 2002; **25**: 561.

37 Linde C, Leclercq C, Rex S *et al.* Long-term benefits of biventricular pacing in congestive heart failure: results from the Multisite Stimulation in Cardiomyopathy (MUSTIC) study. *J Am Coll Cardiol* 2002; **40**: 111–18.

38 De Cock CC, Van Campen CMC, Vos DHS, Visser CA. Left atrial- and left ventricular-based single lead DDD pacing. *Pacing Clin Electrophysiol* 2001; **24**: 486–8.

39 Ricci R, Ansalone G, Toscano S *et al.* Cardiac resynchronization: materials, technique and results. The InSync Italian Registry. *Eur Heart J* 2000; **2**: J6–J15.

40 Lipchenca I, Garrigue S, Glikson M, Barold SS, Clémenty J. Inhibition of biventricular pacemakers by oversensing of farfield atrial depolarization. *Pacing Clin Electrophysiol* 2002; **25**: 365–7.

41 Taieb J, Benchaa T, Foltzer E *et al.* Atrioventricular cross talk in biventricular pacing: a potential cause of ventricular standstill. *Pacing Clin Electrophysiol* 2002; **25**: 929–35.

42 Steinhaus D, Suleman A, Vlach K, Germanson N, Hebert K, McVenes R. Right ventricular anodal capture in biventricular stimulation for heart failure: a look at multiple lead models. (Abstract.) *J Am Coll Cardiol* 2002; **39**: Supplement A.

43 Van Gelder BM, Bracke FA, Pilmeyer A, Meijer A. Triple-site ventricular pacing in a biventricular pacing system. *Pacing Clin Electrophysiol* 2001; **24**: 1165–67.

44 Hesse B, Diaz LA, Snader CE, Blackstone EH, Lauer MS. Complete bundle branch block as an independent predictor of all-cause mortality: report of 7073 patients referred for nuclear exercise testing. *Am J Med* 2001; **110**: 318–9.

45 Richman JL, Wolff L. Left bundle branch block masquerading as right bundle branch block. *Am Heart J* 1954; **47**: 383–92.

46 Garrigue S, Reuter S, Labeque JN *et al.* Usefulness of biventricular pacing in patients with congestive heart failure and right bundle branch block. *Am J Cardiol* 2001; **88**: 1436–41.

47 Garrigue S, Lafitte S, Hocini M, Jaïs P, Haïssaguerre M, Clémenty J. Mechanisms of left ventricular walls resynchronization during multisite ventricular pacing: direct effects on the variations of the regional electromechanical delays and wall motion velocities [abstract]. *Eur Heart J* 2000; **21**: 119.

48 Kerwin WF, Botvinick EH, O'Connell JW *et al.* Ventricular contraction abnormalities in dilated cardiomyopathy: effect of biventricular pacing to correct interventricular dyssynchrony. *J Am Coll Cardiol* 2000; **35**: 1221–7.

CHAPTER 9

Arrhythmias of Biventricular Pacemakers and Implantable Cardioverter Defibrillators

S. Serge Barold, Stéphane Garrigue, Carsten W. Israel, Ignacio Gallardo and Jacques Clémenty

Dual-site or multisite ventricular pacing (resynchronization) with or without a combined implantable cardioverter-defibrillator (ICD) has emerged as promising therapy for patients with dilated cardiomyopathy and congestive heart failure (CHF) associated with major left intra- and interventricular conduction disorders. Cardiac resynchronization is an important new therapy but not without technical issues related to pacemaker timing that have created new problems in the interpretation of pacemaker function and arrhythmias [1]. Implanted systems can be effective with proper programming of pacemaker timing to avoid some of the pitfalls described in this chapter.

Wenckebach upper rate response

In a traditional Wenckebach upper rate response, a dual-chamber pacemaker (where upper rate interval > total atrial refractory period) delivers its ventricular stimulus only at the completion of the (atrial-driven) upper rate interval. The atrioventricular (AV) delay initiated by a sensed P wave increases progressively because the ventricular channel waits to deliver its output at the end of the upper rate interval. Eventually a P wave falls in the postventricular atrial refractory period, a pause occurs and the ventricular *paced* sequence repeats itself (Figure 9.1). In patients with pacemakers implanted for CHF, the Wenckebach upper rate response (or more precisely the manifestation of upper rate > total atrial refractory period) assumes

a form that is not immediately recognizable because no paced beats are evident [2–4].

In patients with normal or near-normal sinus node function and AV conduction, a pacemaker Wenckebach upper rate response takes the form of a repetitive pre-empted process which consists of an attempted Wenckebach upper rate response with each cycle, associated with continual *partial* or *incomplete* extension of the programmed AV interval (Figure 9.1). The conducted spontaneous QRS complex continually occurs before completion of the upper rate interval. It is therefore sensed by the pacemaker, and ventricular pacing is pre-empted. In other words, the pacemaker cannot complete the upper rate interval and thus cannot emit a ventricular stimulus at its completion. This form of upper rate response tends to occur in patients with relatively normal AV conduction, a short programmed AV delay, a relatively slow programmed (atrial-driven) upper rate, and a sinus rate faster than the programmed (atrial-driven) upper rate. It is therefore more likely to emerge on exercise or during times of distress when adrenergic tone is high. Consequently the pre-empted Wenckebach upper rate response has become important recently because pacemakers are now implanted in patients with CHF (or hypertrophic cardiomyopathy) where there is usually relatively normal sinus node function and AV conduction. The occurrence of a pre-empted Wenckebach response in such patients defeats the very purpose of this type of cardiac stimulation. Hence, in patients with CHF susceptible to

Normal upper rate response of the Wenckebach type

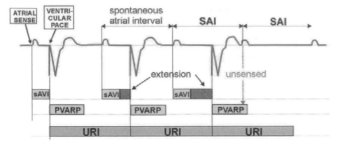

The pre-empted Wenckebach behavior with short sAVI

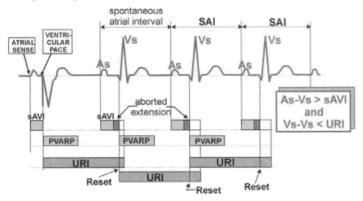

Figure 9.1 (Top) Normal pacemaker Wenckebach upper rate response. (Bottom) Repetitive pre-empted Wenckebach upper rate response (courtesy of A. Sinnaeve and R Stroobrandt). See text for details. As, atrial sense; Vs, ventricular sense; sAVI, AV delay after sensing; PVARP, postventricular atrial refractory period; URI, upper rate interval; SAI, spontaneous atrial interval.

sinus tachycardia (despite beta-blocker therapy and especially during decompensation), it is important to program a relatively fast upper rate during biventricular pacing to avoid a pre-empted Wenckebach upper rate response with resultant loss of cardiac resynchronization manifested by the emergence of the patient's own QRS in the electrocardiogram (ECG) (Tables 9.1 & 9.2).

In summary, a pre-empted Wenckebach upper rate response has *no paced events* and is characterized by three features [2–4] (Figure 9.1):

1 Vs–Vs interval < atrial-driven upper rate interval (Vs, ventricular sensed event).

2 PR interval (As–Vs) > programmed As–Vp. The spontaneous PR interval remains relatively constant (Vp, ventricular paced event; As, atrial sensed event).

3 There are no unsensed (or refractory sensed) P waves as in a typical Wenckebach upper rate response in the presence of AV block.

P-wave tracking will not be restored until the atrial cycle length exceeds the duration of the intrinsic total atrial refractory period (intrinsic PR + postventricular atrial refractory period, PVARP).

Double counting of the ventricular electrogram

In first generation biventricular pacemakers with parallel dual cathodal biventricular systems, the pacemaker paces and senses from the two ventricles simultaneously. Double counting of the ventricular complex may involve the spontaneous conducted QRS complex (as most patients do not have AV block) or may occur when there is loss of left ventricular (LV) capture with preservation of right ventricular (RV) pacing [5–12]. Both situations produce temporal separation of RV and LV electrograms. The degree of separation depends on the severity of the interventricular conduction delay and the location of the electrodes. The LV electrogram may therefore be sensed some time after detection of the RV electrogram if the LV signal extends beyond the relatively short ventricular blanking period initiated by RV sensing. With ventricular rhythms, the LV electrogram may precede that from the RV. The circumstances leading to the emergence of the spontaneous QRS complex and the perpetuation of double QRS counting must be understood because

Table 9.1 Recommended parameters for the Medtronic InSync biventricular DDDR pacemaker.

Parameter	InSync recommended settings
Mode	DDDR or as indicated
Mode switch	OFF (optionally ON for AF patients)
Lower rate	< Intrinsic rate unless otherwise indicated
Upper tracking rate	140 b.p.m.
SAV	As optimized
Rate-adaptive AV	ON
Start rate	100 b.p.m.
Stop rate	140 b.p.m.
Minimum SAV	30 ms
PVARP	250 ms
Ventricular refractory period	> Intraventricular conduction delay
ELT intervention	ON
PVC response	OFF
Ventricular sensitivity	> P wave amplitude
Atrial polarity	Bipolar
Ventricular polarity	Bipolar (if at least one V lead is bipolar)
Diagnostics	Rate histogram for first month, then high rate episode monitor

AF, atrial fibrillation; SAV, sensed atrioventricular delay; PVARP, postventricular atrial refractory period; ELT, endless loop tachycardia; PVC, premature ventricular complex; V, ventricular.

Table 9.2 Optimal programming of biventricular pacemakers with biventricular or common sensing.

Parameter	Management
AV delay	Shortening of the sensed AV delay alone does not prevent DC. A long AV delay should not be used in ventricular resynchronization. Use the optimized sensed AV delay and avoid fusion with spontaneous activation.
Atrial sensing and PVARP	1 Shorter PVARP can prevent DC (250 ms). 2 Program off the post-VPC PVARP extension. 3 Automatic mode switching off in devices with a relatively long PVARP mandated by the mode-switching algorithm.
Upper rate	DC can often be prevented by programming a relatively fast upper rate (140 p.p.m.) so the patient does not have 'breakthrough' ventricular sensing within their exercise zone.
AV conduction	Use drugs that impair AV conduction. In refractory cases, slow VT, SVT: 1 consider ablation of the AV junction with the production of AV block; 2 replace the device with one that senses only from the RV.
Ventricular sensitivity	1 Reduction may mitigate DC. 2 Ventricular sensitivity < P-wave amplitude.
Sensed ventricular blanking period.	1 Pacemaker: not presently programmable. Will be programmable to a longer duration in future pacemakers. 2 ICD: not generally programmable by design.
LV lead position	Repositioning the LV lead at a site with less RV–LV conduction delay may eliminate DC.

AV, atrioventricular; DC, double counting; ICD, implantable cardioverter defibrillator; LV, left ventricle; PVARP, postventricular atrial refractory period; RV, right ventricle; SVT, supraventricular tachycardia; VPC, ventricular premature complex; VT, ventricular tachycardia.

the problem can often be corrected by appropriate programming of the pacemaker. Future devices will allow programming of the sensing function of the ventricular channels individually to prevent double counting (RV and LV electrograms) or triple counting (far-field P wave, RV and LV electrograms). Theoretically (but unlikely), lack of LV sensing could result in competitive pacing and arrhythmia induction. This might occur if a premature ventricular complex originates near the LV sensing site and at a specific time before the P wave. If ventricular activation initiated by the ventricular premature complex (VPC) conducts to the RV sensing site with a marked delay, it will be unable to inhibit the scheduled ventricular pacing pulse (triggered by the P wave) and the stimulus may fall beyond the absolute myocardial refractory period.

Isolated loss of LV pacing

The pacemaker interprets delayed LV activation (initiated by RV pacing) as a VPC beyond the ventricular blanking period but still in the pacemaker refractory period. In other words, the pacemaker interprets LV activation as a ventricular refractory

sensed event (VR). This signal reinitiates a PVARP with automatic extension (if this function is programmed). The subsequent sinus P wave can then easily fall within this reinitiated and extended PVARP related to VR. An unsensed sinus P wave within the PVARP then generates a conducted QRS complex with two distinct RV and LV electrographic components. The process becomes self-perpetuating and inhibits cardiac resynchronization pacing [12]. The pacemaker continually defines the LV electrogram as a VPC and continually induces automatic PVARP extension (according to design) that prevents sensing of the P waves, giving rise to the conducted spontaneous QRS complexes.

Activation of the automatic PVARP extension by a pacemaker-defined ventricular extrasystole

Double sensing of the QRS may occur by the same mechanism as above when a pacemaker-defined VPC (sensed once) activates automatic extension of the PVARP, an algorithm designed to prevent endless loop tachycardia (Figure 9.2a). The PVARP extension algorithm should therefore be turned off during biventricular pacing in parallel dual

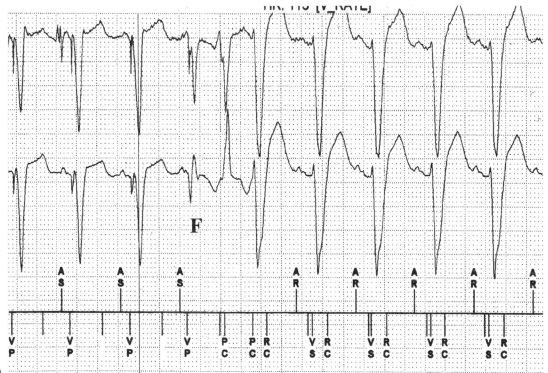

(a)

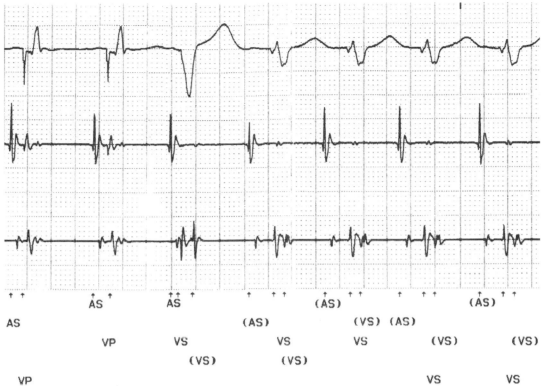

AS   AS   (AS)   (VS) (AS)   (AS)

AS   (AS)   (VS) (AS)

VP   VS   VS   VS   (VS)   (VS)

(VS)   (VS)

(b)   VP   VS   VS

Figure 9.2 (a) (Opposite) Biventricular pacing (Medtronic) showing loss of resynchronization after a sensed ventricular premature complex (VPC). Basic postventricular atrial refractory period (PVARP) = 300 ms. There are two consecutive VPCs. The first causes ventricular fusion (F). The second VPC correctly identified by the pacemaker (PC) exhibits double counting of its ventricular electrogram with the second component falling in the pacemaker ventricular refractory period. The device also identifies the second component as a VPC (RC). The device activates PVARP extension to 400 ms after a sensed ventricular event (even in the ventricular refractory period) defined as a VPC. The second component (RC) therefore initiates a 400-ms PVARP. The succeeding sinus P wave falls in the postventricular atrial blanking period and is unsensed and no marker is emitted. This promotes AV conduction with a left bundle branch block (LBBB) pattern. The LBBB-conducted beats also induce double counting with only the second component interpreted as a VPC by the pacemaker which again extends its PVARP so that the next sinus P wave (AR) falls in the PVARP and cannot initiate an AV delay. The conducted LBBB beat is again doubly sensed and with PVARP extension (initiated by the second component), the process perpetuates itself with loss of atrial sensing and resynchronization. The tracing illustrates the importance of avoiding the PVARP extension algorithm during resynchronization with this pacemaker as recommended by the manufacturer. In Guidant devices PVARP extension occurs only with alternate beats whenever the pacemaker continually senses VPC-defined events without other intervening ventricular events so that the type of locking shown in this tracing is minimized. AS, atrial sensed event; AR, atrial sensed event in the refractory period; VP, ventricular paced event; VS, ventricular sensed event; PC, VPC; RC, VPC sensed in the ventricular refractory period. The vertical bars without annotations represent the termination of the PVARP and clearly show how the sinus P waves (AR) fall in the extended PVARP (courtesy of Medtronic, Inc.). (b) Biventricular pacing (Guidant) in the DDDR mode showing loss of resynchronization after a sensed ventricular premature complex (VPC) in the setting of a long PVARP used to limit the upper rate because of cardiac ischemia (25 mm/s). The device senses a VPC but it does not interpret it as a pacemaker-defined VPC because it is preceded by an atrial sensed event (AS). The VPC exhibits double sensing with the second component falling in the ventricular refractory period. The next sinus P wave falls in the long programmed PVARP and cannot initiate the programmed AV delay. The ventricular channel double counts the conducted QRS complex (left bundle branch block) first from the right ventricle as VS and then from the left ventricle as (VS) in the ventricular refractory period. The second component reinitiates the PVARP and the process perpetuates itself. AS, atrial sensed event; (AS), atrial event sensed in the atrial refractory period; VP, ventricular paced event. Note the absence of VPC markers used by this device upon sensing a pacemaker-defined VPC.

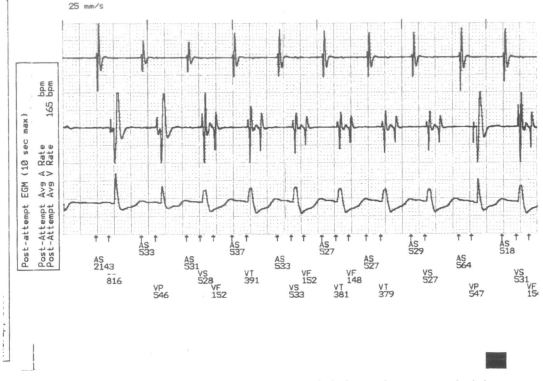

Figure 9.3 Double counting of the ventricular electrogram of a patient who had received inappropriate shocks by an implanted Guidant Contak CD biventricular implantable cardioverter defibrillator that senses from both ventricles simultaneously. The atrial and ventricular electrograms are on top. The first two ventricular complexes are paced. The atrial rate then exceeds the programmed upper rate and a repetitive pre-empted Wenckebach sequence starts. The device then senses the conducted QRS twice (ventricular electrogram in the middle recording). The second last cycle terminates with a paced ventricular beat because of slight sinus slowing. AS, atrial sensed event; VP, ventricular paced event; VS, ventricular sensed event; VT, ventricular tachycardia; VF, ventricular fibrillation.

cathodal systems (Tables 9.1 & 9.2). Figure 9.2(b) shows the importance of programming a relatively short basic PVARP. The same mechanism as in Figure 9.2(a) can also occur, with double sensing of a VPC when the LV and RV components of the electrogram are sufficiently separated. T-wave oversensing by an implantable cardioverter defibrillator (ICD) may also cause double counting, because it creates timing cycles similar to those induced by a VPC and pushes the succeeding P wave into the PVARP initiated by the T-wave signal.

Atrial premature beats may also promote spontaneous AV conduction and, in turn, double counting and inappropriate ICD firing.

Upper rate response and sinus tachycardia

In devices that sense from the RV and LV simultaneously, double counting of the spontaneous QRS complex may occur during a pre-empted Wenckebach sequence (as well as during supraventricular tachycardia (SVT) or ventricular tachycardia (VT) faster than the programmed upper rate) if the interval between the RV and LV electrograms exceeds the duration of the ventricular blanking period [5–9] (Figures 9.3 & 9.4). This phenomenon is particularly important in patients with biventricular ICDs that sense from both ventricles simultaneously (either by design or through the use of a Y-adapter with a conventional device) as discussed below.

Double counting by biventricular ICDs

The consequences of double sensing in biventricular ICDs may be serious and include ventricular inhibition (with denial of beneficial resynchronization) and inappropriate shocks (excluding double counting resulting from lack of LV capture). The Guidant Contak CD system is a biventricular dual cathodal

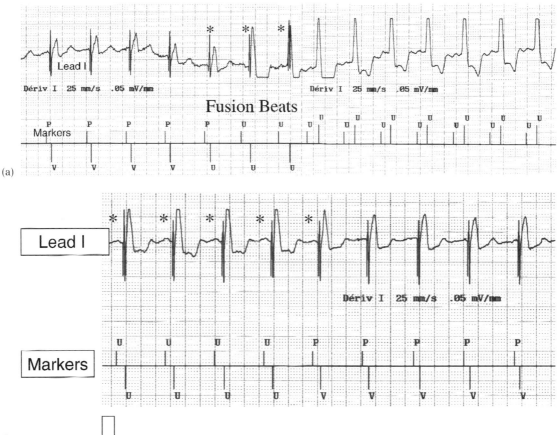

Figure 9.4 (a) Biventricular pacing (Sorin) with an excessively low programmed upper rate in a 54-year-old patient with ischemic cardiomyopathy (left ventricular ejection fraction 28%). The upper rate was programmed to 90 p.p.m. because the patient presented with chest pain at a sinus rate of 100 b.p.m. The spontaneous QRS duration measures 145 ms. This tracing was obtained during a rapid walking test with biventricular pacing. Despite beta-blockers (small doses due to the low blood pressure), the sinus rate increases progressively beyond 90 b.p.m. ('U' as upper rate was reached), biventricular pacing gives way to fusion beats (asterisks), and a conducted wide QRS emerges because the spontaneous sinus rate exceeds the programmed upper rate of 90 b.p.m. The patient consequently no longer benefited from biventricular pacing on exercise and developed dyspnea. The markers indicating sensing point upwards with different heights for atrial and ventricular events. V, ventricular pacing. (b) Same patient as in (a). As soon as the spontaneous sinus rate falls to 90 b.p.m. and lower, the patient benefits from biventricular pacing. As the beta-blockers could not be increased, the upper rate was programmed to 110 p.p.m., and the patient was clinically improved on exercise without chest pain suggesting that pacing reduced the MV_{O_2} (asterisks depict fusion beats).

ICD that senses from both ventricles simultaneously so that double counting of ventricular depolarizations may occur. This was observed in about 7% of patients during the Contak CD clinical trial in the US [13] (Figure 9.3). Its successor the Renewal Contak CD permits selective sensing from the RV to prevent double counting.

Standard dual-chamber ICDs modified with a Y connector have also been used in an 'off-label' fashion for biventricular pacing. In such an unmatched ICD/pacer system, double counting and

inappropriate firing of the ICD may occur during sinus tachycardia, and supraventricular and ventricular tachycardia at rates below the cut-off point (Figures 9.5 and 9.6). Prolongation of the ventricular blanking period is generally not an option in an ICD because the timing cycles are designed to optimize sensing of ventricular tachycardia and fibrillation and such devices incorporate a non-programmable ventricular blanking period after sensing. St. Jude DDDR devices allow programming of the postsense ventricular blanking up to

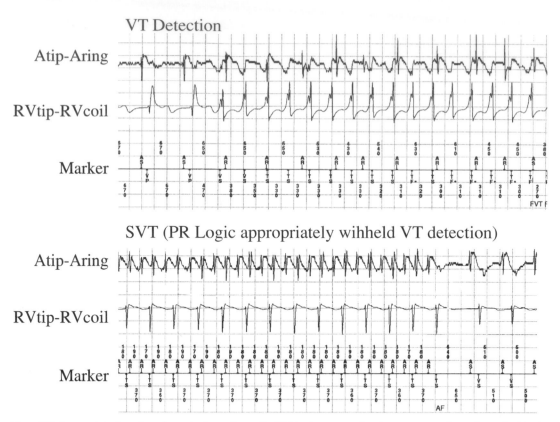

Figure 9.5 Appropriate detection of ventricular tachycardia (VT) in the top panel and supraventricular tachycardia (SVT) in the bottom panel by a Medtronic InSync biventricular implantable cardioverter defibrillator that senses ventricular activity only from the right ventricle. The atrial and ventricular electrograms are on top and the annotated markers at the bottom of each panel (courtesy of Medtronic, Inc.).

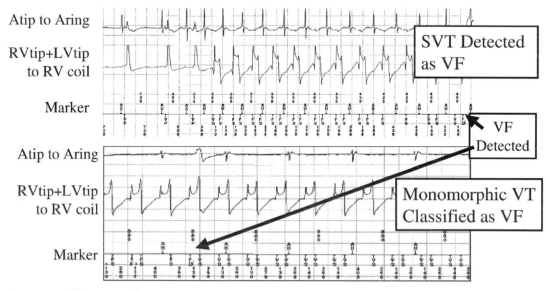

Figure 9.6 Double counting of supraventricular tachycardia (SVT) by an 'off-label' biventricular implantable cardioverter defibrillator (ICD) system using a conventional ICD and a Y-adapter to produce a dual cathodal system. The atrial and ventricular electrograms are on top and the annotated markers at the bottom. (Top panel) The device interprets the SVT as ventricular fibrillation (VF). (Bottom panel) The device interprets slow VT as ventricular fibrillation (courtesy of Medtronic, Inc.).

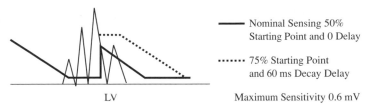

——— Nominal Sensing 50%
Starting Point and 0 Delay

······· 75% Starting Point
and 60 ms Decay Delay

LV   Maximum Sensitivity 0.6 mV

Figure 9.7 Prevention of double counting in an off-label label biventricular implantable cardioverter defibrillator (ICD) consisting of a St. Jude ICD and a Y-adapter. The QRS signal would be doubly counted at the nominal sensing parameters (50% Starting Point and 0 ms Decay Delay). The Postsense Starting Point and Decay Delay are changed to 75% and 60 ms respectively (broken line). This alteration to the sensing algorithm still allows the device to reach the programmed maximum sensitivity of 0.6 (mV). The combination of these modifications can eliminate double counting if the LV component is smaller than the RV contribution.

157 ms. The longer blanking decreases the chance of double counting and makes the device more attractive when a standard dual-chamber ICD with a Y-adapter is used. On the other hand, the short (120-ms) postventricular sense blanking in Medtronic devices makes them more prone to double counting when used with a Y-adapter. In the Photon family of ICDs (St. Jude) used with a Y-adapter, the sensing algorithm can be modified to prevent double counting sensing, provided the second component of the ventricular electrogram is smaller than the first one. The system allows changes in the postsensed decay delay and postsensed threshold starting point, features specifically designed to prevent T-wave sensing (Figure 9.7). There are several options in difficult cases of double counting with ICDs: (i) ablation of the AV junction [9] (discussed later); (ii) replacement of the device with one that functions with univentricular (RV) sensing; or (iii) repositioning of the LV at a site where less RV–LV conduction delay might eliminate double counting at least during supraventricular rhythms. Biventricular pacemakers without an ICD function should all have the capability of univentricular sensing and a programmable blanking period after ventricular sensing.

Device design to prevent double counting

The Medtronic biventricular InSync ICD, InSync III ICD Marquis (under clinical investigation in the US), and the recently released InSync III biventricular pacemaker (without defibrillation capability) permit sensing only from the RV (i.e. univentricular sensing), to avoid double ventricular sensing [14–16] (Figure 9.5). The InSync III pacemaker is designed with two new functions to enhance ventricular resynchronization.

1 Ventricular Sense Response: This feature is intended to provide cardiac resynchronization in the presence of ventricular sensing by allowing a ventricular *sensed* event to trigger a biventricular *paced* event under certain circumstances during biventricular pacing. When this feature is enabled, the detected signal will trigger an immediate output delivered to both ventricles (Figure 9.8). The triggered output will be ineffective in the chamber where sensing was initiated, as the myocardium will be physiologically refractory. The triggered mode will result in an output pulse being delivered to the other ventricle thereby synchronizing activation in the setting of intraventricular conduction delay as long as the maximum rate response value is not exceeded. This function which effectively prevents double counting has also been incorporated in the InSync III ICD Marquis.

2 Interventricular Refractory Period: This prevents restarting the ventricular refractory period, postventricular atrial blanking and refractory periods, and upper rate timers when a second sensed depolarization is seen following a sensed or paced event (Figure 9.9). When the second sensed depolarization occurs within the interventricular refractory period, the refractory periods and timing intervals are not reset, thus preventing the second sensed depolarization from initiating periods of functional atrial undersensing periods (i.e. AR-VS) and loss of cardiac resynchronization in patients with a long PR interval (Figure 9.9). This function is not required during monochamber sensing but may be useful with programmed biventricular sensing which is an option in the InSync III pacemaker. Consequently the InSync III ICD Marquis that must sense only from the RV does not require this function.

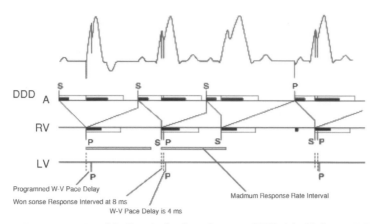

Figure 9.8 Diagrammatic representation of the Ventricular Sense Response (VSR) in the Medtronic InSync III pacemaker. This function is intended to provide cardiac resynchronization in the presence of ventricular sensing. A ventricular sensed event during the AV delay (initiated by a paced atrial event) triggers immediate biventricular pacing with a V-V delay of 4 ms between the ventricular stimuli. A ventricular sensed event preceded by a non-refractory atrial sensed event will also trigger immediate biventricular pacing pulses provided the stimuli do not violate the programmed upper rate interval. In the VSR function, the triggered pulse is delivered according to the programmed ventricular setting, one option being biventricular pacing. A = atrium, RV = right ventricle, LV = left ventricle, P = paced event, S = non-refractory sensed event. Note the short P-P intervals representing the V-V delay or the timing difference between LV and RV stimulation. (Courtesy of Medtronic).

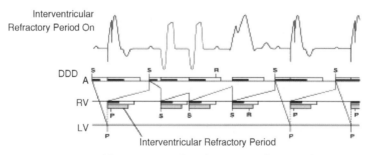

Figure 9.9 Diagrammatic representation of the interventricular refractory period (IRP) in the Medtronic InSync III pacemaker. The IRP prevents sensing of a second ventricular depolarization when the right and left ventricles do not depolarize simultaneously. Thus, a sensed event in the IRP (either following a ventricular paced event or a non-refractory sensed event) does not initiate new timing cycles. A = atrium, RV = right ventricle, LV = left ventricle, S = non-refractory sensed event, P = paced event, R = refractory sensed event. Note the short P-P intervals representing the V-V delay or the timing difference between LV and RV stimulation. (Courtesy of Medtronic).

Prevention of pre-empted Wenckebach upper rate response with resultant loss of resynchronization [3]

1 *Upper rate.* The upper rate should be programmed to a value so that the patient does not have 'break-through' ventricular sensing within their exercise zone or at a rate potentially possible during decompensation in CHF patients (Tables 9.1 & 9.2).

2 *Shortening of the pacemaker AV delay.* 'Forced ventricular pacing' will not prevent a pre-empted

Wenckebach upper rate response and may actually be hemodynamically detrimental if it critically shortens ventricular filling. In this respect, a recent report of double QRS counting by a biventricular ICD in the setting of a pre-empted Wenckebach upper rate response suggested that abbreviation of the AV delay (if tolerated hemodynamically) could prevent double QRS counting without changing the upper rate [7]. This concept applied to upper rate limitation is incorrect because a pre-empted Wenckebach sequence cannot be prevented by this maneuver and the shorter programmed AV delay will simply generate the same maximal duration of the (extended) AV delay during upper rate limitation (Table 9.2).

3 *Drug therapy.* Beta-blockers may prevent the sinus rate from attaining a relatively fast programmed upper rate, but are not always effective or tolerated.

4 *Depression of AV conduction.* Prevention of a pre-empted Wenckebach response can be achieved through appropriate drug therapy or ablation of the AV junction but there is an important trade-off that consists of a traditional Wenckebach upper rate response with its attendant hemodynamic disadvantage whenever the AV delay prolongs unphysiologically [9]. However, this approach may be useful in patients with a biventricular ICD to eliminate double counting of the QRS complex.

When using drugs to delay AV conduction for the prevention of a pre-empted Wenckebach response, it is important to ensure the absence of ventricular fusion of the conducted QRS complex with the right ventricular or biventricular paced beat during a traditional Wenckebach sequence. Fusion of the spontaneous QRS complex and right or biventricular pacing (sometimes inapparent on the surface ECG) compounds the hemodynamic disadvantage of suboptimal AV synchrony during the Wenckebach ventricular paced upper rate response. Lowering the upper rate in this situation would only aggravate the problem of unphysiological AV delays that would occur at lesser levels of activity. On the other hand, increasing the upper rate to prevent a traditional Wenckebach response carries the risk of rapid ventricular pacing with sensing of atrial tachyarrhythmias.

Far-field sensing of atrial depolarization in biventricular pacemakers with simultaneous sensing from both ventricles

An LV lead located in one of the coronary veins may sense the far-field P wave because of electrode proximity to the left atrium, especially if anatomic constraints prevent placement of the lead in a desirable distal site away from the AV groove [5,6 17–20]. Moreover, the higher dislocation rates of LV leads towards the AV groove increase the likelihood of sensing relatively large atrial signals from the cor-

onary sinus (Figure 9.10). Far-field atrial sensing by the ventricular channel can inhibit biventricular pacing and withhold therapy for CHF. Far-field P-wave sensing by a displaced lead in the coronary sinus can be devastating in pacemaker-dependent patients who have undergone ablation of the AV junction for atrial fibrillation (Figure 9.11).

Indicators for far-field P-wave sensing

1 Recurrence or development of symptoms of CHF.

2 Inappropriately short As–Vp delay on surface ECG.

3 Unexpected inhibition of ventricular output (DDD mode) with a PR (As–Vs) interval > programmed As–Vp delay (at rates *below* the maximum tracking rate).

4 Event markers recorded with simultaneously telemetered ventricular electrogram and surface ECG.

Management of atrial far-field oversensing in biventricular pacemakers with simultaneous sensing from both ventricles

1 Prophylaxis. Some cases of far-field P sensing may be prevented by repositioning the LV lead at the time of implantation if the LV or biventricular electrogram registers a large atrial deflection.

2 Reduce ventricular sensitivity while monitoring the rhythm using the programmer and marker channel.

3 Use the DOO mode in selected cases.

4 Obtain 24-h Holter monitoring looking for undersensing of ventricular premature beats and competition to determine whether the reduced sensitivity should be maintained.

5 If far-field sensing of the P wave cannot be eliminated by programming or reducing the sensitivity, the LV needs to be repositioned or a new generation pacemaker with univentricular sensing from the RV can be implanted without lead manipulation.

Far-field atrial sensing in biventricular ICDs with simultaneous sensing from both ventricles

Far-field atrial sensing can cause inappropriate discharge of a biventricular ICD with simultaneous sensing from both ventricles in one of three ways: (i) double counting of a far-field atrial and near-field ventricular signal; (ii) triple counting of a far-field

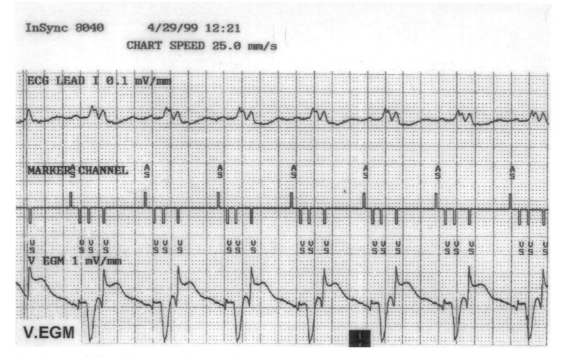

Figure 9.10 Far-field atrial sensing resulting in triple counting. Simultaneous recordings (from top to bottom) of the ECG, a marker channel and telemetered ventricular electrogram of a (dual cathodal) Medtronic InSync DDDR biventricular pacemaker programmed to the ODO mode (25 mm/s). There is sinus rhythm with 1 : 1 atrioventricular conduction with ventricular inhibition. The LV lead detects the late portion of the P wave because of its proximity to the coronary sinus and left atrium (VS follows each AS closely), resulting in complete inhibition of ventricular pacing. Every P wave is conducted and produces a wide QRS sequentially sensed by the RV lead, then by the LV lead, as a function of the distance between the leads and the long interventricular conduction time. Therefore, there are three ventricular sensed markers associated with each QRS complex: the first VS is the far-field atrial signal; the second VS and third VS are the two near-field components of the ventricular electrograms originating from the RV and LV leads, respectively. In the DDDR mode, the two signals generated by ventricular depolarization were recorded as VR events (refractory sensed) by the marker channel. VS, ventricular sensed event; AS, atrial sensed event. (Reproduced from [17] with permission.)

atrial signal together with double counting of the QRS complex; and (iii) repeated counting of far-field atrial fibrillation (in patients who generally undergo AV nodal ablation to permit resynchronization) causing ventricular asystole because of inhibition of the ventricular stimulus by oversensing a situation compounded by the delivery of an inappropriate shock [21]. With an ICD repositioning the LV lead is preferable to decreasing ventricular sensitivity which may compromise the detection of ventricular fibrillation. In special circumstances in the presence of an acceptable LV pacing threshold, replacement of the ICD with a device that ignores LV activity might even be considered without repositioning a slightly displaced LV lead in the coronary venous system.

Sensing of ventricular repolarization: cross-ventricular endless loop tachycardia

A variant of endless loop tachycardia (ELT) can occur with a standard DDDR pacemaker functioning in the biventricular pacing VVIR mode [22, 23]. This 'cross-ventricular' ELT is sustained by ventricular pacing and ventricular sensing of the T wave (with a probable contribution from the afterpotential) without atrial participation (Figure 9.12). A 'cross-ventricular' ELT can be prevented by appropriate programming of the pacemaker (as discussed later). The mechanism and electrocardiographic appearance of this ELT is similar to the tachycardia induced by single-channel VVT pacing associated with T-wave sensing. In the latter, ventricular

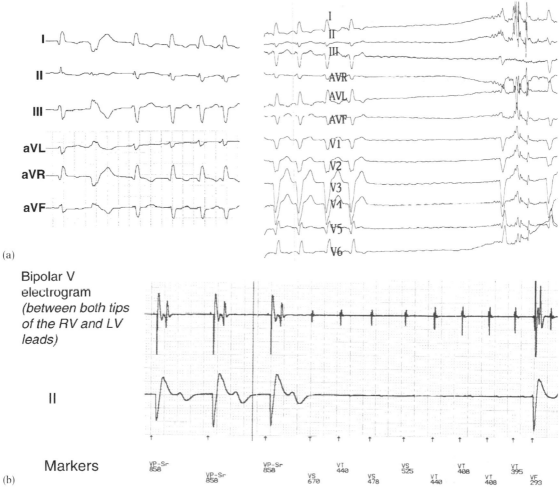

Figure 9.11 Far-field atrial sensing. (a) Inhibition of a biventricular implantable cardioverter defibrillator (ICD) from far-field atrial sensing in a patient who had undergone atrioventricular junctional ablation for drug-refractory paroxysmal atrial fibrillation. A single-chamber ICD with a Y-adapter in a split bipolar arrangement was implanted for syncopal ventricular tachycardia. (b) Same patient as in (a). Far-field atrial sensing of irregular atrial tachycardia by Guidant ICD shown in a simultaneous recording of the ventricular electrogram, surface ECG and annotated markers. The left ventricular lead was slightly displaced from its original position.

pacing is triggered without delay at the time of T-wave sensing.

Biventricular pacing with conventional pacemakers

With presently available technology several pacing systems may be used for biventricular pacing in patients with permanent atrial fibrillation where an atrial channel is unnecessary. Single-chamber devices include: (i) dedicated first and second genera-tion biventricular DDD(R) pacemaker with capping of the atrial port; (ii) a conventional VVIR pace-maker with an external Y-adapter because there are presently no dedicated VVIR devices for cardiac resynchronization approved by the Food and Drug Administration; and (iii) a conventional DDDR pacemaker suitably connected for biventricular pacing (Table 9.1). Dual-chamber sequential bivent-ricular devices capable of altering the timing of RV and LV stimulation (with so-called V–V timing) are now available in the US [14–16].

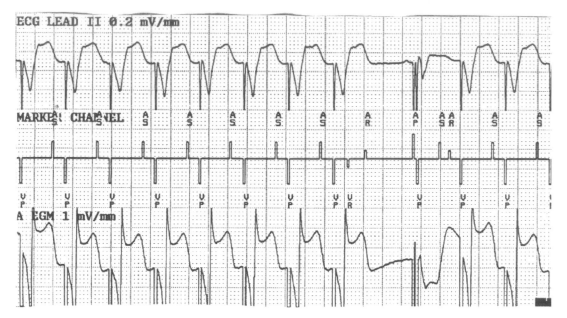

Figure 9.12 Cross-ventricular endless loop tachycardia at the programmed upper rate of 130 p.p.m. during biventricular pacing with a conventional DDDR pacemaker. The tracing shows the ECG, marker channel and LV electrogram (labeled A) at 1 mV/mm (25 mm/s). The 'atrial' channel senses the T wave which triggers a ventricular stimulus after a delay that coincides with the termination of the upper rate interval. The tachycardia terminates when the QRS complex of a paced beat (VR) is sensed in the ventricular refractory period beyond the ventricular blanking period. The succeeding T wave falls in the 'postventricular atrial refractory period' initiated by VR and the tachycardia terminates. The tachycardia is followed by biventricular pacing associated with double sensing of the T wave. The first T-wave signal (AS) restarts the tachycardia. The second T-wave signal falls in the unblanked portion of the 'AV delay' initiated by AS. (Reproduced from [22] with permission.)

Although conventional dual-chamber pacemakers are not designed for biventricular pacing and generally do not allow programming of an AV delay of zero or near zero, they are being increasingly used with their shortest 'AV delay' (0–30 ms) for ventricular resynchronization in patients with permanent atrial fibrillation [24]. Their advantages include programming flexibility, avoidance of a cumbersome Y-adapter (required for conventional VVIR devices), protection against far-field sensing of atrial activity (an inherent risk of dual cathodal devices with simultaneous sensing from both ventricles) and cost considerations (Table 9.3).

When a conventional dual-chamber pacemaker is used for biventricular pacing, the 'atrial' channel is generally connected to the LV and the 'ventricular' channel to the RV. This arrangement provides: (i) LV stimulation before RV activation (LV pre-excitation); and (ii) protection against ventricular asystole related to oversensing far-field atrial activity by dual cathodal devices in case of displacement of the LV lead towards the AV groove. With this system in the 'DDD' or 'DDDR' mode, a signal first sensed by the RV lead will inhibit the output of the ventricular channel. In contrast, a signal sensed first by the LV channel will induce a triggered output from the RV channel after a very short delay (shortest possible programmable 'AV delay') provided the programmed upper rate interval is relatively brief and RV sensing does not occur within the short 'AV delay'. This response provides ventricular resynchronization almost immediately upon sensing. However, such immediate ventricular resynchronization upon sensing cannot be achieved in the 'DDD' or 'DDDR' mode if the programmed upper rate interval is relatively long. This constraint is related to the Wenckebach upper rate response that mandates extension of the 'AV delay' (corresponding to the interval from LV sensing to triggered RV stimulation) to conform to upper rate limitation.

Table 9.4 outlines the response of conventional dual-chamber pacemakers used for biventricular pacing under a variety of circumstances when programmed to the DDDR, DDIR and DVIR modes. The

Table 9.3 Response of the various modes of conventional dual-chamber pacemakers used for biventricular pacing in patients with permanent atrial fibrillation.

Circumstance	DDD	DDI	DVI
RV sensing before LV. The LV signal falls in the 'PVARP' and is unsensed	Inhibits RV and LV channels Initiates normal AEI	Inhibits RV and LV channels Initiates normal AEI	Inhibits RV and LV channels Initiates normal AEI
LV sensing followed by RV sensing within the short 'AV delay'	As above	As above	As above Note that LV sensing cannot occur
LV sensing followed by RV sensing beyond the 'AV delay'	Triggers RV channel Initiates normal AEI	Inhibits RV and LV channels Initiates normal AEI	Inhibits RV and LV channels Initiates normal AEI
LV sensing but not RV	Triggers RV channel Initiates normal AEI	Inhibits 'atrial' or LV channel but not RV channel (see below)	LV sensing cannot occur
Apparent AEI shortening following a QRS complex	No	Interval from QRS sensed exclusively by LV channel to succeeding single RV ventricular stimulus < AEI Ensuing RV stimulus may fall on the T wave of LV sensed QRS complex	No
Potential of far-field sensing of atrial activity	Yes	Yes	Nil
Response to far-field atrial sensing by LV channel	Triggering: Pacing rate may be fast with pacing solely by LV output	LV stimulus inhibited RV stimulus delivered at completion of AEI	Sensing cannot occur
Number of stimuli. (The 2 stimuli will be fused on the ECG if the 'AV delay' is very short)	1 or 2 according to circumstance	1 or 2 according to circumstance	Always 2

The atrial channel of a conventional dual-chamber pacemaker is connected to the LV and the ventricular channel to the RV. RV, right ventricle; LV, left ventricle; AEI, atrial escape interval. The AEI can only be initiated by RV sensing or pacing with this arrangement. (Reproduced from [24] with permission.)

DDDR and DDIR modes provide no real advantages over the DVIR mode and may create difficulty in the electrocardiographic interpretation of pacemaker function with the presence according to the pacing mode of one or two closely coupled stimuli in the same strip, single stimuli within the QRS complex (with triggering), apparent shortening of the atrial escape interval and potential interference from far-field atrial sensing (Table 9.2). In contrast, the DVIR mode behaves like the VVIR mode except that there are always two closely coupled stimuli (or electrocardiographically fused stimuli if the 'AV delay' is very short) thereby facilitating evaluation of pacemaker function. Furthermore the DVIR mode pro-

vides absolute protection against far-field sensing of atrial activity in the case of LV lead displacement and other forms of oversensing related to biventricular stimulation such as cross-ventricular ELT.

The short delay between LV and RV stimulation imposed by the shortest 'AV delay' may not be a significant limitation in many patients because it is LV pacing that generally provides the salutary effect of biventricular pacing [25]. In this respect, a conventional dual-chamber pacemaker may permit a trial of unichamber LV pacing in selected patients to determine whether this modality might be hemodynamically superior to biventricular pacing. At this juncture, manufacturers should be encouraged to

Table 9.4 Characteristics of pacemakers used for biventricular stimulation in patients with permanent atrial fibrillation.

Function	Conventional single-chamber pulse generator converted to a dual cathodal system* External Y-adapter	Dual chamber with dual cathodal ventricular output* and capped atrial port No external Y-adapter	Conventional dual-chamber pulse generator No external Y-adapter
Delay between RV and LV stimulation	0	0	Duration of shortest 'AV delay' 0–30 ms
Individual programmability of output	No	No	Yes
Capability of increasing device longevity by individual programming of output	No	No	Yes
Individual telemetry of RV and LV lead impedance	No	No	Yes
Programmability of isolated LV pacing for troubleshooting	No	No	Yes
Committed simultaneous sensing from RV and LV	Yes	Yes	No. See below
Capability of sensing only from RV	No	No	Yes, when the device is programmed to the 'DVI' mode
Response to sensing far-field atrial activity	Inhibition and risk of asystole from loss of pacing	Inhibition and risk of asystole from loss of pacing	No loss of pacing (see Table 9.1)
Cost	+	+++	++

* Divided pacemaker output with the leads connected in parallel. This uses a Y-connector (which is incorporated into the pacemaker header in the case of dedicated dual-chamber devices) to produce a unipolar–unipolar or bipolar–bipolar system so that there is a connection between the two cathodes. (Reproduced from [24] with permission.)

refine conventional dual-chamber pacemakers with AV delays programmable by very small increments including zero and even negative values for sequential biventricular stimulation in patients with permanent atrial fibrillation. Such devices could even become standard cost-effective therapy for cardiac resynchronization in the 'DVI' mode for patients with permanent atrial fibrillation without the need for costly further developments in technology. Indeed, such devices would function as biventricular units with two independent ports and V–V timing. When programmed to the 'DVI' mode they would serve the growing population of patients with permanent atrial fibrillation and CHF, including those with permanent RV pacemakers that require upgrading.

References

1 Wang P, Kramer A, Estes NA III *et al*. Timing cycles for biventricular pacing. *Pacing Clin Electrophysiol* 2002; **25**: 62–75.
2 Barold SS. Wenckebach upper rate response in dual chamber pacemakers: a reappraisal and proposed new terminology. *Pacing Clin Electrophysiol* 1995; **18**: 244–52.
3 Barold SS, Sayad D, Gallardo I. Upper rate response of pacemakers implanted for nontraditional indications: the other side of the coin. *Pacing Clin Electrophysiol* 2002; **25**: 1283–4.
4 Leung SK, Lau CP, Leung WH *et al*. Apparent extension of the atrioventricular interval due to sensor-based algorithm against supraventricular tachyarrhythmias. *Pacing Clin Electrophysiol* 1994; **17**: 321–30.

5 Betts TR, Allen S, Roberts PR, Morgan JM. Inappropriate shock therapy in a heart failure defibrillator. *Pacing Clin Electrophysiol* 2001; **24**: 238–40.

6 Ricci R, Ansalone G, Toscano S *et al.* Cardiac resynchronization: materials, technique and results. The InSync Italian Registry. *Eur Heart J* 2000; **2** (Suppl J): J6–J15.

7 Garcia-Moran E, Mont L, Brugada J. Inappropriate tachycardia detection by a biventricular implantable cardioverter defibrillator. *Pacing Clin Electrophysiol* 2002; **25**: 123–4.

8 Schreieck J, Zrenner B, Kolb C *et al.* Inappropriate shock delivery due to ventricular double detection with a biventricular pacing implantable cardioverter defibrillator. *Pacing Clin Electrophysiol* 2001; **24**: 1154–7.

9 Kanagaratnam L, Pavia S, Schweikert R *et al.* Matching approved 'nondedicated' hardware to obtain biventricular pacing and defibrillation: feasibility and troubleshooting. *Pacing Clin Electrophysiol* 2002; **25**: 1066–71.

10 Liu BC, Villareal RP, Hariharan R, Rasekh A, Massumi A. Inappropriate shock delivery and biventricular pacing cardiac defibrillators. *Tex Heart Inst J* 2003; **30**: 45–49.

11 Srivathsan K, Bazzell JL, Lee RW. Biventricular implantable cardioverter defibrillator and inappropriate shocks. *J Cardiovasc Electrophysiol* 2003; **14**: 88–89.

12 Akiyama M, Kaneko Y, Taniguchi Y, Kurabayashi M. Pacemaker syndrome associated with a biventricular pacing system. *J Cardiovasc Electrophysiol.* 2002; **13**: 1061–62.

13 Sanders R. Guidant, St Paul. Personal communication 1992.

14 Leon AR, Brozena S, Liang CS, Roach A, Abraham W. Effect of resynchronization therapy with sequential biventricular pacing on Doppler-derived left ventricular stroke volume. Functional status and exercise capacity in patients with left ventricular dysfunction and conduction delay. The US InSync III Trial [abstract]. *Pacing Clin Electrophysiol* 2002; **25**: 558.

15 Sogaard P, Egeblad H, Pedersen AK *et al.* Sequential versus simultaneous biventricular resynchronization for severe heart failure: evaluation by tissue Doppler imaging. *Circulation* 2002; **106**: 2078–84.

16 Technical manual, InSync III Device. Model 8042. Medtronic Inc., Minneaplis MN 2003.

17 Lipchenka I, Garrigue S, Glikson M *et al.* Inhibition of biventricular pacemakers by oversensing of farfield atrial depolarization. *Pacing Clin Electrophysiol* 2002; **25**: 365–7.

18 Taieb J, Benchaa T, Foltzer E *et al.* Atrioventricular cross-talk in biventricular pacing: a potential cause of ventricular standstill. *Pacing Clin Electrophysiol* 2002; **25**: 929–35.

19 Oguz E, Akyol A, Okmen E. Inhibition of biventricular pacing by far-field left atrial sensing: Case report. *Pacing Clin Electrophysiol* 2002; **25**: 1517–19.

20 Vollman D, Luthje L, Gortler G *et al.* Inhibition of bradycardia pacing and detection of ventricular fibrillation due to far-field atrial sensing in a triple chamber implantable cardioverter defibrillator. *Pacing Clin Electrophysiol* 2002; **25**: 1513–16.

21 Garrigue S, Barold SS, Clémenty J. Double jeopardy in a patient with a biventricular ICD. *J Cardiovasc Electrophysiol* 2003; **14**: 784.

22 Barold SS, Byrd CL. Cross-ventricular endless loop tachycardia during biventricular pacing. *Pacing Clin Electrophysiol* 2002; **24**: 1821–3.

23 Van Gelder BM, Bracke FA, Meijer A. Pacemaker-mediated tachycardia in a biventricular pacing system. *Pacing Clin Electrophysiol* 2002; **25**: 1819–20.

24 Barold SS, Sayad D, Gallardo I. The DVI mode of cardiac pacing: a second coming. *Am J Cardiol* 2002; **90**: 521–3.

25 Touiza A, Etienne Y, Gilard M, Fatemi M, Mansourati J, Blanc JJ. Long-term left ventricular pacing in patients with severe congestive heart failure. *J Am Coll Cardiol* 2001; **38**: 1966–70.

PART III
Advances in Technology

CHAPTER 10

Left Ventricular Stimulation: Epicardial, Transvenous or Endocardial?

Rick McVenes

Introduction

Cardiac pacing started with the implantation of rudimentary temporary epicardial leads, generally on the left ventricle (LV). These early systems were adapted for permanent epicardial pacing, requiring up to 4 h of surgery [1,2]. The renewed interest in pacing for ventricular resynchronization via biventricular, multisite or single-chamber stimulation in patients with severe LV dysfunction was inspired by small initial studies. These studies suggested improved functional capacity in patients with left-sided intraventricular delay coupled with mechanical dyssynchrony [3,4]. The early results have now been validated in large clinical trials [5–7]. The challenges and surgical complications of multisite ventricular implantation resemble those experienced at the inception of permanent cardiac pacing over 40 years ago. At the present stage of development, no single surgical approach or lead design for LV stimulation has yet achieved the same degree of success as transvenous right ventricular (RV) pacing. Thus, we are faced with the crucial question as to what the optimal implantation approach is for LV stimulation in patients with heart disease of various etiologies. Is it epicardial (standard or modified), transvenous or endocardial?

Epicardial stimulation of the left ventricle

The first successful long-term epicardial lead (Hunter–Roth, Figure 10.1) was initially implanted on the RV. The site was changed to the LV because of laceration of the thin-walled RV [1,2]. The LV remains the chamber of choice for better electro-

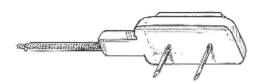

Figure 10.1 Hunter–Roth bipolar epicardial lead.

physiologic performance in terms of stimulation thresholds and electrogram amplitudes, provided the LV apex is avoided where the wall may be as thin as 2 mm [8–16]. Other LV sites to avoid include vascularized or infarcted areas, fat or locations that would result in postsurgical rubbing of the electrode head on the sternum, ribs, diaphragm or pericardium [10,16–20]. Early epicardial leads required substantial surgical exposure to accommodate suturing the leads directly to the epicardium (Figure 10.2a–d). Eventually, 'sutureless' designs were introduced, requiring much smaller surgical exposure (Figure 10.3) [8,21]. This was followed by further improvement with the addition of an application tool that allowed insertion of the lead with one hand, without other instruments [22]. A temporary mapping tool was also used to determine acceptability of implantation sites prior to final deployment of the lead [17].

Early epicardial LV implants had long-term survival of about 90% at 2 years in an analysis from seven centers performed by Lawrie in 1979 (range 70–88%) [23]. This competed favorably with transvenous RV lead technology of the same era with an average survival of 80% at 2 years. Lack of dislodgement contributed to the early success of epicardial leads compared to transvenous RV leads, prior to improvements we now take for granted.

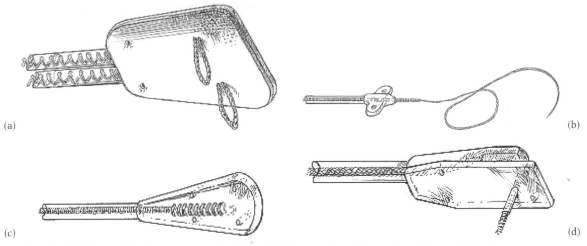

(a)

(b)

(c)

(d)

Figure 10.2 (a) General Electric suture-on epicardial lead. (b) Telectronics stitch-on epicardial lead. (c) Cordis nine-turn suture-on epicardial lead. (d) Medtronic Model 5815 stab-in suture-on epicardial lead.

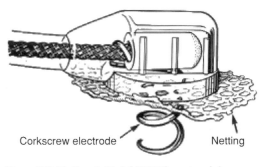

Corkscrew electrode   Netting

Figure 10.3 Medtronic Model 6917 three-turn left ventricular sutureless screw-in epicardial lead.

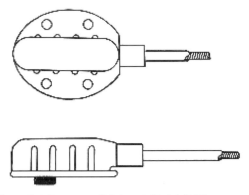

Figure 10.4 Prototype of Medtronic Model 4965 suture-on steroid-eluting epicardial lead.

Eventually, transvenous RV lead designs were improved with the addition of tines and screws in combination with better conductor coils and insulation materials so that the transvenous RV approach supplanted epicardial LV pacing. The nearly universal migration to transvenous RV implantation put the engineering development of epicardial leads low on the priority list for manufacturers and implanters. Eventually, a steroid-eluting epicardial lead, requiring suture fixation, was produced around 1990 (Figure 10.4). Steroid elution has decreased the major complication of epicardial LV and RV leads by reducing the previously high incidence of elevated pacing thresholds. Despite improved long-term electrical results, stimulation sites on the posterior and posterolateral aspects of the LV are presently not easily accessed by conventional surgical procedures, nor by the minimally invasive techniques under development.

The future of epicardial leads

Manufacturers have had little incentive to develop better epicardial leads because the majority of implants are transvenous. Early experience with epicardial leads in biventricular systems demonstrated shortcomings with available devices [24]. Investigations currently in progress using epicardial mapping for hemodynamic improvement at the time of implantation are showing much promise. Thus, improvements in epicardial leads and implantation tools are likely to take on renewed importance. Improvements in surgical positioning tools are under development as a near-term solution. For example, an implantation tool for currently available sutureless epicardial leads has been developed to improve access to the posterior and posterolateral

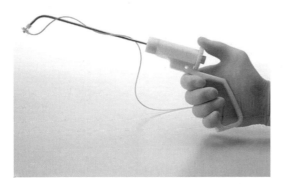

Figure 10.5 Malleable implantation tool for sutureless epicardial lead, Medtronic Model 10626.

aspect of the LV through conventional thoracotomy approaches (Figure 10.5). Many less invasive procedures today use thoracoscopes, laparoscopes, etc. Tools can be inserted through these instruments to provide many functions, such as clear visualization and identification of blood vessels, and confirmation that all bleeding from surgical manipulation and electrode implantation is controlled prior to closure. Combining these technologies should theoretically produce an implantation system that would require only a small puncture. A subxiphoid puncture could avoid the need for endotracheal intubation during surgery. With visualization and sensing capabilities incorporated in the delivery system, one could design epicardial leads and implantation tools actually within the delivery system itself to locate appropriate tissues and insert sutureless electrodes safely anywhere on the heart. With the appropriate designs, the insertion of epi- or myocardial leads could become as easy and atraumatic as transvenous implantation, and possibly more versatile.

Transvenous stimulation of the left ventricle

LV stimulation via the coronary sinus and veins

Transvenous implantation on the LV requires cannulation of the coronary sinus (CS) and passage of a lead into a peripheral cardiac vein (CV). Prior to the mid-1990s, most reported cases of long-term LV stimulation from the cardiac venous system consisted of unrecognized malpositioned leads intended for RV stimulation [25–32]. Deliberate LV stimulation from the coronary venous system was performed only in unusual situations such as the presence of a prosthetic tricuspid valve or when

placement of epicardial leads was contraindicated [33,34].

Transvenous LV stimulation has evolved rapidly since the emergence of biventricular pacing for the treatment of congestive heart failure. The hardware requirements have been established as follows [35,36]:

1 successful CS cannulation;
2 ability to select the best stimulation site in the cardiac veins;
3 acute and chronic electrode fixation;
4 acceptable stimulation thresholds and sensing function; and
5 ability to manage complications, including extraction of chronic leads.

Cannulation of the coronary sinus

While the CS is routinely cannulated during standard electrophysiologic studies, accessing it from a superior approach in patients with LV and/or right atrial enlargement can be challenging. The CS exhibits marked anatomic variability. Recent investigations have identified a significant change in CS location and angulation secondary to severe LV enlargement. In this respect, Potkin *et al.* described an approximate doubling of CS size in both ischemic and idiopathic cardiomyopathy hearts [37]. Desai *et al.* demonstrated a trend of increased angulation of the proximal CS from the horizontal plane with an increase in LV end-diastolic diameter [38]. Additionally, a variety of well-known anatomic structures in humans can impede the engagement of a lead or delivery sheath in the CS os (Plate 10.1, facing p. 84).

Two approaches to promote CS cannulation have been intensely investigated.

1 *Lead design.* A continuous curve in the distal lead was incorporated in the Medtronic Model 2187 to facilitate CS engagement with adjustment of the central stylet (Figure 10.6). A subanalysis of the early experience demonstrated a decreased implantation time with a specifically designed CS lead, compared with a standard RV lead (Table 10.1) [39].
2 *Delivery system design.* The first development to engage the CS involved multiple fixed-shape catheters (Figure 10.7) to accommodate the wide variety of CS anatomic variations. This also facilitated the superior approach to accommodate pectoral implantation of the pulse generator. More recently, a delivery catheter was developed with the

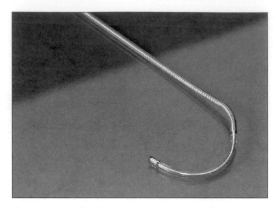

Figure 10.6 Lead with continuous curve to aid introduction into coronary sinus os. Medtronic Model 2187.

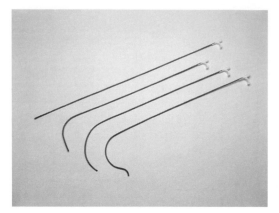

Figure 10.7 Straight and fixed-shape catheters: straight, MB2; multipurpose, Amplatz.

capability of altering its shape while in place. This decreased the need to completely withdraw the catheter from the venous system and replace it with another fixed-shape catheter to achieve the necessary angulation for CS cannulation (Figure 10.8).

Selection of site for LV stimulation

In some anatomic studies, about 10% of the population presented no suitable vein for LV pacing via the CS [40]. Tortuosity or acute angulation of a tributary from the coronary sinus or cardiac vein, or valves at the tributary os can prevent access to a posterior or lateral branch [41,42]. This technical challenge has fostered advances in the design of both lead and delivery systems. Reducing the length of the rigid distal electrode assembly of standard lead designs was established as a requirement for leads intended for the coronary venous system. The steroid elution mechanisms of conventional leads required a finite volume to hold the steroid reservoir, which contributed to the overall length of the

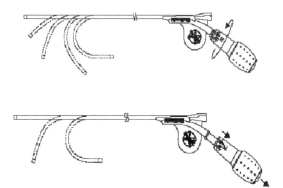

Figure 10.8 Steerable/deflectable catheter, Medtronic Model 10600.

electrode assembly. Elimination of the steroid reservoir offered a lead design with the most flexible tip assembly possible for better performance during implantation (Table 10.1). Some lead designs incorporated shaping the distal end of the lead to facilitate introduction into CV tributaries (Figure 10.9). The

Table 10.1 First-generation left ventricular (LV) lead decreases implant time (min).

	Total procedure time	LV lead placement time	Total fluoroscopy time
Standard right ventricular leads implanted in cardiac veins ($n = 30$)	157 ± 55	72 ± 54	44 ± 27
Model 2187 ($n = 64$)	124 ± 44 $P < 0.01$	45 ± 38 $P < 0.015$	26 ± 19 $P < 0.002$
Percentage reduction in implant time	21%	38%	41%

Analysis of early experience cardiac vein implantation times (c. 1999) of standard right ventricular leads implanted in cardiac veins vs. the Medtronic Model 2187 lead designed for cardiac vein implantation.

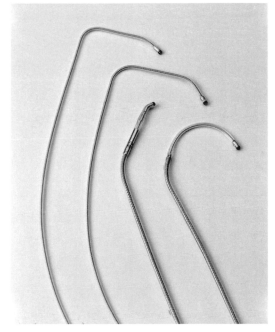

Figure 10.9 A 'tool box' approach to transvenous left ventricular lead implantation. Examples of shaped leads offered by a single manufacturer, left to right: Medtronic Models 4189, 4193, 2188 and 2187.

addition of guidewire, or combined guidewire and stylet delivery, was also investigated to improve implantation success (Figures 10.10 & 10.11). Availability of more than one type of lead has enhanced the ability to achieve the posterolateral and lateral positions commonly associated with optimal effectiveness of biventricular stimulation (Table 10.2) [43].

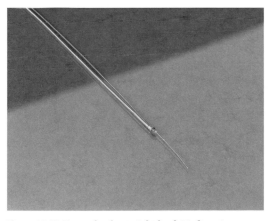

Figure 10.10 Example of a straight lead, Medtronic Model 4191.

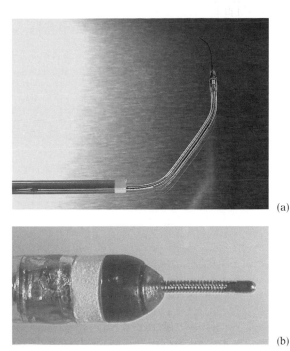

(a)

(b)

Figure 10.11 (a) Over-the-wire closed-lumen lead design with dual bend distal end for site selection and fixation. (b) Lead tip with guidewire protruding from the tip seal, black electrode area, and white steroid elution ring designed to provide the shortest distal rigid section for implantability and site selection, while providing steroid elution and preventing gross blood leakage into the central stylet/guidewire lumen. Medtronic Model 4193.

Table 10.2 Improvements in preferred site selection success using Medtronic Models 4191, 2187 and 2188.

Final position	n	%
Posterior lateral CV	47	40.5
Lateral or marginal CV	48	41.4
Posterior CV	7	6.0
Great (anterior) CV	8	6.9
Middle CV	2	1.7
Other	4	3.5

CV, cardiac vein.
With three lead models available in this human clinical study; the posterior and lateral implantation sites were achieved in approximately 90% of all implants. Medtronic Model 4191 Clinical Report, $n = 116$.

The design of delivery systems has also improved. The balloon catheter for CS venography has enhanced the identification of potential implantation sites. More distal advancement of the delivery

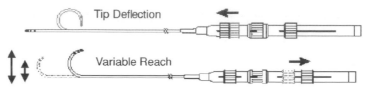

Figure 10.12 The functionality of an electrophysiologic catheter when used in a soft-tipped sheath provides both access versatility for the coronary sinus and the ability to subselect a coronary vein through advancement of the soft-tipped catheter to the level of the desired venous tributary with decreased risk of dissection.

sheath into the CS and proximal venous system facilitates passage of the guidewire or lead tip to the level of the target cardiac venous tributary. One approach involves the addition of a soft distal section to the delivery sheath to allow advancement deeper into the CS or proximal cardiac veins while reducing the potential for CS dissection and perforation (see Figure 1.6a in Chapter 1). This sheath, when combined with the functionality of a steerable electrophysiologic catheter, should provide both tip deflection and reach for engagement within a cardiac vein tributary (Figure 10.12). Such improvements of delivery systems may produce a very versatile tool to access the desired implantation site, safely and quickly.

Improvements in CS cannulation and CV site selection will most probably not be achieved by any one lead design or delivery system. Rather, combinations of technical advancements in both areas will be required. Both lead design and implant delivery system accessories contribute to increased success rates and decreased procedure time. Gurley *et al.* compared the procedure time and success rate of 571 implants in the MIRACLE trial to 264 in the InSync III clinical trial [44]. The MIRACLE trial utilized two fixed-shape catheters and two lead designs. The InSync III clinical trial utilized three lead designs and the soft-tip sheath with an optional, steerable catheter added to the delivery system options. They concluded that the availability of multiple LV lead designs and delivery systems was associated with a trend toward a higher success rate and significantly reduced median implantation times.

Stable acute and chronic fixation

CV leads for LV stimulation require low chronic dislodgement rates, and the ability to be acutely repositionable. To date, the most widely used leads for cardiac vein implantation fall into two categories: curved or shaped leads, and straight leads

Table 10.3 Variation in vein diameter at implantation site.

Vein diameter at final distal electrode implantation position	n	%
≤ 4 French	24	21.4
5 French	40	35.7
6 French	23	20.5
7 French	14	12.5
8 French	5	4.5
9 French	4	3.6
≥ 10 French	2	1.8

A poststudy analysis using width of the venography fluoroscopy images, converted to diameter in French size, demonstrates widely varying diameters of veins at the final implantation sites. Thus, the leads designed for left ventricular stimulation in the cardiac veins must accommodate stable fixation of many venous diameters and angulations. Model 4191 Clinical Report, $n = 112$; three lead models available.

with protruding profiles such as tines, eccentric tips or helical channels (Figs 10.10 & 10.11). Continued reduction in dislodgement rates has occurred with each clinical trial of evolving lead types. However, a decrease in the chronic dislodgement rate close to that of RV leads has not yet been demonstrated. The optimal lead design will need to accommodate the marked variations in vein size and anatomic orientations at the implantation site to achieve successful long-term stability (Table 10.3) [43,45]. It will also require improvements in the design of lead fixation. In addition, several techniques may also contribute to improvement in the overall dislodgment rate. These include techniques that minimize the postimplantation interaction of multiple lead bodies, and surgical tiedown techniques to secure three lead bodies at the venous insertion site.

Acceptable stimulation and sensing performance

Acceptable performance of a biventricular system in terms of stimulation thresholds and sensing is somewhat different from that of leads for traditional antibradycardia therapy. Greater priority has been given to LV lead design for successful implantation rather than pulse generator longevity, because many early investigators considered that a 2–3-year pulse generator is of less consequence to this patient population, given their poor survival rate.

The early systems for cardiac resynchronization employed Y-adapters for biventricular stimulation. The first Y-adapters made one ventricular lead the cathode and the other the anode in a 'split bipole' configuration. Failure to maintain capture at both sites occurred commonly, primarily on the lead connected to the anodal terminal. Reoperation to change or adjust the adaptors was often required [46]. Subsequent Y-adapters and first-generation pulse generator connectors shorted the two leads together to yield a 'dual cathode' configuration. In these systems, individual pacing thresholds can not be measured independently or directly. This arrangement has been used with acceptable results. Our canine experience has evaluated the perform-

ance of dual cathodal systems compared to split bipoles [47]. Our 12-week canine data from early prototype LV leads used in various configurations for biventricular stimulation help to demonstrate threshold relationships and establish guidelines for programming pulse generator safety factors. This canine study implies that adequate 2 : 1 chronic safety margins can be achieved for > 98% of the population with dual cathodal systems programmed at or below the maximum output of commercially available cardiac resynchronization pulse generators. It is important to recognize that Y-adapters used in configurations creating anodal stimulation from the left ventricular cardiac vein (LVCV) electrode will likely have high thresholds, and patients implanted with adapters that create the split bipole configuration should be managed carefully to assure dual site capture is achieved and maintained. The various published human reports are consistent with this animal experience. However, there is no published human experience that compares these various configurations, or establishes safety factor considerations (Figure 10.13).

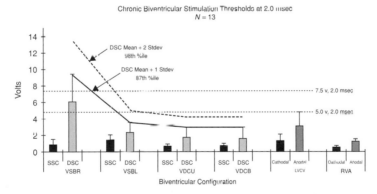

Figure 10.13 Comparison of split bipole (SB) and dual cathodal (DC) biventricular pacing thresholds to illustrate the implications for determining a safety margin. The data come from 13 canines at week 12 after receiving early prototype left ventricular cardiac vein (LVCV) leads used in various configurations for biventricular stimulation. The four pairs of bar graphs on the left show the relationship of dual site capture (DSC) for the mean and standard deviation X_1 and standard deviation X_2 to outline where the 98th percentile of the population will be served by a 5 V and 7.5 V, 2.0 ms pacing output. This canine study implies that adequate 2 : 1 chronic safety margins (in volts) can be achieved for ≥ 98% of the population with dual cathodal systems programmed at or below the maximum output of commercially available cardiac resynchronization pulse generators. The two pairs of bar graphs on the right demonstrate the relationship of cathodal and anodal thresholds from the tip electrode of the RV and the tip of the LV lead. Configurations creating anodal stimulation from the left cardiac vein (LVCV) electrode will commonly register high thresholds. Stdev, standard deviation; DSC, dual site capture (gray); SSC, single site capture (black). *Ventricular split bipole (VSB):* **VSBR**, right ventricular cathode, left ventricular anode; **VSBL**, left ventricular cathode, right ventricular anode. *Ventricular Dual Cathodal (VDC):* **VDCU**, both right and left ventricular electrodes are cathodes, with an extracardiac indifferent electrode as the anode; **VDCB**, both right and left ventricular electrodes are cathodes with an intracardiac electrode as the anode, by convention bipolar, i.e. all electrodes are intracardiac. On the right, cathodal (black) and anodal (diagonal) threshold relationship of the tip electrode of left ventricular cardiac vein (LVCV) and right ventricular apical (RVA) leads.

We also found that the sensing function of dual cathodal systems has performed satisfactorily in canines. The intrinsic electrogram of the dual cathodal system is uniformly longer in duration and lower in amplitude and slew rate than that from either single LV site or spilt bipole configuration. However this has not been demonstrated in human experience to date. In the absence of large population data on sensing performance, the first Medtronic biventricular implantable cardioverter defibrillator (ICD) involved sensing only from an independent RV channel, thus maintaining the known ICD performance for arrhythmia detection from the RV chamber. This decreases the probability of double counting the wide dual cathodal electrogram.

The impedance of individual leads used in dual cathodal systems has raised interesting questions. Reports by Puglisi *et al.* suggested that high-impedance RV leads contributed to lower biventricular pacing thresholds [48]. In a dual cathodal system, the voltage on both electrodes should be the same, thus this effect seemed to contradict theory. Upon further analysis we determined that the effect was related to increased total combined electrode impedance and improvement in maintaining the trailing edge of the stimulus pulse in a capacitively coupled output device. While threshold amplitude is usually *estimated* in terms of leading edge peak values, the actual threshold of the tissue is the total voltage (area under the waveform, sometimes approximated by a 'midpoint' value). Increased impedance causes the trailing edge of the waveform to increase. Thus, higher impedance causes the mean (area under the waveform) voltage to increase with no change in the leading edge value. The result is that more voltage is applied with no change in the measured (leading edge) voltage, which is interpreted as 'lower threshold' (Plates 10.2–10.4, facing p. 84).

Because LV thresholds cannot be obtained in a dual cathodal system, the performance of LV leads has not been well characterized. More recent systems that provide independent channels for both ventricular outputs have yielded preliminary experience with various leads used in clinical trials. The Medtronic Model 4193 (Figure 10.11) was studied in the clinical trial of a pulse generator with independent RV and LV output channels. Stable mean voltage thresholds at 0.5 ms were 1.3 ± 1.2 V at prehospital discharge, 1.4 ± 1.1 V at 1 and

3 months postimplantation and 1.6 ± 1.4 V after 6 months ($n = 220$ patients). The median implantation time was < 10 min with a range of < 1–270 min. The total dislodgement rate was 3% [49]. Comprehensive comparative studies of multiple leads used in clinical practice on these newer pulse generators have not yet been reported. Experience to date suggests that RV electrode technology adapted for LV use has higher threshold variations when used in cardiac venous sites. This difference may be due to several factors. The epicardial tissue of the LV with advanced cardiomyopathy may have intrinsically higher thresholds. The cardiac vein electrode is separated from stimulable tissue by the non-stimulable vein wall and epicardium, overlying myocardial cells. In comparison, the transvenous electrode is separated from the subendocardium (Purkinje fibers) by a single non-stimulable endocardial membrane. Thus, different tissues may also produce intrinsically higher thresholds. Orientation of the electrodes in the cardiac veins is parallel with the epicardial surface, resulting in an orientation different from that seen in endocardial systems. This may result in a less optimum alignment of the stimulating electric field relative to myocardial fiber orientation [50]. Some areas surrounding the cardiac veins are suffused with non-stimulable fat. Sustained local movement of the electrodes in cardiac veins may impede the maturation process at the electrode site, and even override the beneficial effects of steroid elution.

Successful clinical management of complications, including chronic removal of CV leads

Historically, the few reported complications related to thrombosis or perforation from devices or procedures involving cannulation of the CS and CV came from acute and temporary procedures. These were typically related to the use of relatively stiff catheters or accessories [27]. Only one case involving a chronic device, a cerebral shunt for hydrocephalus requiring five reoperative manipulations over 5 years, demonstrated CS thrombosis [51]. More recently, the clinical trials of cardiac resynchronization therapy (CRT) demonstrated a low level of complications related to dissection of the CS during delivery tool and lead manipulation. The dissections are most commonly detected during venography performed to identify the cardiac venous anatomy. Since venography is not routinely performed during standard electrophysiologic studies, the true incidence of dissection for all CS cannulation procedures is unknown. Perforation of the cardiac vein wall resulting in detectable adverse sequelae during or after implantation is rare. The use of soft-tipped delivery sheaths and leads with flexible distal tip designs may contribute to lower dissection and perforation rates.

Phrenic nerve stimulation has emerged as a more common challenge. Hanksy *et al.* reported on phrenic nerve stimulation in 22 of 96 patients with a wide variety of lead types [52]. In general, leads requiring wedging for fixation and those with annular electrodes were associated with greater difficulty in avoiding phrenic nerve stimulation than those with electrodes on the distal tip. A directional electrode has been suggested as a solution, but the technology to achieve reliable placement, in the proper orientation for uniform performance, has not proven feasible at this time. Alternatively, a multitude of electrodes on a single lead body has been proposed but no chronic results are available [53]. Only a few cases describing complications related to cross-chamber stimulation have been reported [54]. Oversensing of the atrial depolarization by the LV lead close to the left atrium has been reported [55,56]. There are no human data on the potential superiority of true bipolar LV leads to prevent such complications.

Pathology of pacing leads in the coronary sinus and cardiac veins

Hozan stated with regard to pacing leads that, 'Although the clinical significance of coronary sinus thrombosis is uncertain, obstruction of coronary sinus blood flow should not be deleterious because of multiple anastamoses between the coronary sinus system and the anterior cardiac veins' [57]. This statement suggests that coronary sinus (CS) thrombosis may not be a significant complication [27,58–62]. Jones *et al.* evaluated 7 hearts (2 at autopsy, 5 post-transplant) with chronically indwelling 6.5 French silicone leads positioned as distally as possible in the CS [63]. The time from implantation to death or cardiac transplantation was 8 ± 6 months (range 1–18 months). They found no venous perforation or injury to the CS or adjacent circumflex artery. There was a scattered thin fibrous membrane on the leads. There was

no CS occlusion, but one lead placed in a small vein showed venous thrombosis distal to the electrode site. Hanksy and coworkers have evaluated a small series of hearts from transplanted patients with biventricular systems implanted from 7 to 15 months [63]. They found minimal fibrosis, with encapsulation of the leads at the CS os and in smaller venous branches. There was no thrombosis or dilatation of the distal veins, nor was there any stenosis or reactions of the associated arteries in the areas where the lead was implanted.

Our own studies on over 100 canines have ranged from 12 weeks to 5 years. Short-term implants (12 weeks) typically reveal about a 0.5– 1-mm-long fibrous collar around the lead at the CS os and a fibrotic capsule at the electrode tip. The remainder of the lead is typically free of thrombus or encapsulation until it enters a cardiac vein branch where encapsulation is more prevalent. This experience is consistent with the reports of human studies of Hansky *et al.* [64]. Lead body encapsulation increases as a function of implantation time in dogs (Plate 10.5, facing p. 84). Within 2 years, the leads are typically completely encapsulated, with the capsule adherent to the lateral, inferior groove of the coronary sinus/great vein (Plate 10.6, facing p. 84). We have not observed significant thrombosis. Venous perforation was seen in 2–3 out of over 100 animals. In those cases where the lead perforated the vein, there was no bleeding or other clinically significant sequelae. Thus, our canine experience supports the belief that chronic cannulation of the CS and cardiac veins is a safe and effective procedure.

Lead extraction

Although methods and specialized tools have been developed to aid in extraction of RV pacing and defibrillation leads, there is limited reported experience describing extraction from the CS and the cardiac vein branches. A small number of reports of successful lead extraction in biventricular systems have been published. Alonso *et al.* reported easy extraction and no complications in 8 patients with implantation times ranging from 1 to 41 months, with 5 of 8 having less than 3 months implantation time [65]. Some workers have observed varying degrees of encapsulation, some only at 'binding sites'. Others reported heavy encapsulation and adhesions in postmortem evaluation of leads in the CV. These observations may become relevant if the population served by CV leads exhibits a longer survival than those without resynchronization therapy [64,66].

Extraction from the proximal CS with countertraction and laser sheaths may be possible based on studies in sheep, but more research is needed [67]. The published animal experience to date has yielded variable results. Some investigators report low extraction forces below 200 g using simple traction to remove the cardiac vein leads from dogs implanted from 42 to 222 days (1.4–7.4 months) [68,69]. Conversely, in dogs implanted for 14–55 months, we found forces of up to 770 g are required to free the distal end of a cardiac vein lead when using a locking stylet and a countertraction sheath advanced to the level of the CS os. Forces of up to 1200 g are required to pull the entire lead into the countertraction sheath [70]. Experience with laser extraction of defibrillation leads with a helical shape for fixation, implanted in the CS and proximal great vein of 9 sheep, has yielded mixed results [71]. Leads were successfully removed from 6 of 9 chronically implanted sheep after 4–12 months' implantation using first- and second-generation extraction equipment (Cook Vascular Inc. lead extraction devices and Spectranetics CVX-300 Excimer Laser System with 12 and/or 14 Fr fiber optic sheaths). Laceration of the great cardiac vein wall, causing cardiac tamponade, was responsible for three deaths. In two of the deaths, the laceration was caused by lasering through the vein wall. Major findings associated with lead extraction in this same study included vascular injury in the form of thrombosis and deposition of fibrin in the coronary sinus and great cardiac vein with hemorrhage into the adjacent epicardium. Thus, it is clear that serious attention needs to be given to the development of safer, easier-to-use tools for extraction of chronic leads from the CS and venous vasculature. As a minimum, many of the curved and shaped leads developed for CV implantation are nearly isodiametric, so that the experience demonstrated on RV lead removal may apply to LV leads in the CV [72].

The ability to recannulate the central lumen of a chronic lead with a locking stylet may be especially important to apply traction to the tip of the lead and make the extraction compatible with currently developed extraction sheaths and tools. A fundamental difference in lead designs exists between currently marketed over-the-wire leads. The Medtronic Model 4193 incorporates a silicone seal at the distal end of the lead to prevent gross leakage of blood into the lumen. This feature is intended to prevent the lumen from becoming obstructed with blood, thus providing the possibility of advancing a locking stylet to the tip of a chronically implanted lead. It will also theoretically decrease the incidence of persistent infection transmitted down the open lead lumen from the pocket. The over-the-wire Guidant Models 4510/4511/4512/4513 employ an open lumen design [73]. The long-term performance of these two fundamentally different designs needs to be established.

Thus, at present, no safe, effective, proven technique exists for routine extraction of old pacing leads implanted deeply within the cardiac vasculature. Early reports are encouraging, but the success rate of attempts to extract leads older than 24 months has not been established. Thus, much remains to be done with future techniques and equipment before extraction of chronic transvenous cardiac vein leads becomes a safe and effective procedure.

Endocardial stimulation of the left ventricle

The placement of chronic endocardial LV leads by transseptal puncture is feasible and requires long-term anticoagulation, but it is highly investigational because of the risk of catastrophic embolic complications [74–77]. Midterm follow-up of endocardial LV leads in a small number of patients has proved to be free of major complications. All the patients had failed transvenous LV implants and had a demonstrated need for biventricular stimulation systems. Autopsy revealed no adherent LV thrombus in one of four patients who have died from intractable heart failure or influenza in this series [78]. The endocardial approach may have potential because it permits LV mapping to institute pacing at a site associated with the best hemodynamic performance, or the optimal cardiac activation pattern or sequence [79].

Thromboembolism from chronically implanted endocardial leads in the LV is a well-known complication requiring long-term anticoagulation therapy [80–83]. Long-term lead interaction with mitral function is unknown. Inadvertent malposition in the LV is often recognized several years after implantation, with or without clinical manifestations. Long-term management with anticoagulation therapy has often been successful [84–88]. This suggests that, with appropriate anticoagulation from the time of implantation, an endocardial LV lead may provide an acceptable alternative, if the clinical benefit of LV stimulation is imperative for managing intractable heart failure, and transvenous or epicardial implant is not feasible.

The adoption of LV endocardial stimulation on a broad scale would require a significant breakthrough in anticoagulation therapy, and a large clinical trial to establish safety. Additionally, this approach, like epicardial and cardiac vein LV stimulation, is likely to require advances in leads and delivery tools. The development of tools to rapidly and safely cross the atrial septum, then negotiate the mitral valve, chordae and papillary structures without adverse interactions, is a substantial challenge. The acceptable implantation site during the procedure would also need to be identified rapidly. While percutaneous extraction of chronic endocardial LV leads has been reported, embolic debris from any extraction procedure poses a significant safety issue [89].

Conclusions

Which surgical approach to achieve LV stimulation will prevail? The transvenous approach is clearly the most widely used procedure today. Reduced implantation times, increased success rates and decreased dislodgement rates have developed rapidly compared to the multidecade evolution of right ventricular transvenous leads [90]. The ability to achieve 100% transvenous success in all patients is unlikely, primarily because of anatomic constraints in up to 10% of the population, and the underlying pathology limiting the acceptable stimulation sites. Epicardial LV stimulation will continue to serve as an alternative to the transvenous approach. The epicardial approach could conceivably become a viable alternative, and even displace a large percentage of transvenous implants. This, however, will require the development of tools and leads to achieve a quick and safe surgical approach under local anesthesia. Growth of the endocardial LV approach seems less likely without a breakthrough

in anticoagulation therapy and the development of special tools and leads for a safe and rapid procedure. It is likely that the favored approach will ultimately be contingent on achieving a fundamental understanding of the mechanism(s) of stimulation to achieve the optimal result in each patient with impaired LV function. Regardless of methodology, the development of highly maneuverable tools, delivery systems and special leads will be needed and will continue to evolve to meet the requirements for a short, predictable, effective and safe implantation procedure.

References

1 Hunter SW, Roth NA, Bernardez D *et al.* A bipolar myocardial electrode for complete heart block. *Lancet* 1959; **79**: 506–8.

2 Jeffrey K. *Machines in our Hearts: the Cardiac Pacemaker, the Implantable Defibrillator, and American Health Care.* Baltimore MD: Johns Hopkins University Press, 2001: 78–81.

3 Bakker P, Sen KCA, de Jonge N *et al.* Biventricular pacing improves functional capacity in patients with end-stage congestive heart failure. *Pacing Clin Electrophysiol* 1995; **18** (4 Pt II): 825.

4 Cazeau S, Ritter P, Lazarus A *et al.* Multisite pacing for end-stage heart failure: early experience. *Pacing Clin Electrophysiol* 1996; **19** (Pt II): 1748–57.

5 Cazeau S, Leclercq C, Lavergne T *et al.* Effects of multisite biventricular pacing in patients with heart failure and intraventricular conduction delay. *N Engl J Med* 2001; **344**: 873–80.

6 Abraham WT, Fisher WG, Smith AL *et al.* Cardiac resynchronization in chronic heart failure. *N Engl J Med* 2002; **346**: 1845–53.

7 Bristow MR, Feldman AM, Saxon LA. Heart failure management using implantable devices for ventricular resynchronization: comparison of medial therapy, pacing, and defibrillation in chronic heart failure (COMPANION) trial. *J Card Fail* 2000; **6**: 276–85.

8 Magilligan DJ Jr, Hakimi M, Davila JC. The sutureless electrode: comparison with transvenous and sutured epicardial electrode placement for permanent pacing. *Ann Thorac Surg* 1976; **22** (1): 80–4.

9 Steinke WE, Thomas FT, Hassan Z *et al.* Subepicardial infarction, myocardial impression, and ventricular penetration by sutureless electrode and leads. *Chest* 1978; **70** (1): 80–1.

10 Ott DA. Epicardial pacemaker implant. In: Gillette PC, Garson A Jr, eds. *Pediatric Arrhythmias: Electrophysiology and Pacing.* Philadelphia: W. B. Saunders, 1990: 575–9.

11 Korhonen U, Karkola P, Takkunen J *et al.* One turn more: threshold superiority of 3-turn versus 2-turn screw in myocardial electrodes. *Pacing Clin Electrophysiol* 1984; **7**: 678–82.

12 Walls JT, Maloney JD, Pluth JR. Clinical evaluation of a sutureless cardiac pacing lead: chronic threshold changes and lead durability. *Ann Thorac Surg* 1983; **36** (3): 328–31.

13 Naclerio EA, Varriale P. The sutureless electrode for cardiac pacing: problems, advantages and surgical technique. *Pacing Clin Electrophysiol* 1980; **3**: 232–5.

14 Zhan C, Furman S. The sutureless myocardial electrode for cardiac pacing. *Chin Med J* 1985; **98** (6): 457–60.

15 Bashore TM, Burks JM, Wagner GS. The epicardial screw-on electrode. *Pacing Clin Electrophysiol* 1982; **5** (1): 59–66.

16 Vecht RJ, Fontaine CJ, Bradfield JWB. Fatal outcome arising from use of a sutureless 'corkscrew' epicardial pacing electrode inserted into apex of left ventricle. *Br Heart J* 1976; **38**: 1359–62.

17 Varriale P, Kwa RP, Niznik J *et al.* Electrical testing in cardiac pacing. In: Varriale P, Naclerio EA, eds. *Cardiac Pacing*. Philadelphia: Lead & Felsbiger, 1979: 247–63.

18 Wolpowitz A. Perforation of the left ventricle using a sutureless screw-in epicardial electrode. *J Cardiovasc Surg* 1981; **22** (6): 585–7.

19 Byrd CL. Pacemaker therapy in cardiac surgery. In: Varriale P, Naclerio EA, eds. *Cardiac Pacing*. Philadelphia: Lead & Felsbiger, 1979: 185–200.

20 DeLeon SY, Ilbawi MN, Koster N *et al.* Comparison of the sutureless and suture-type epicardial electrodes in pediatric cardiac pacing. *Ann Thorac Surg* 1982; **33** (3): 273–6.

21 Hunter SW, Bolduc L, Long V *et al.* New myocardial pacemaker lead (sutureless). *Chest* 1973; **63** (3): 430–3.

22 Lawrie GM, Morris GC Jr, DeBakey ME. An improved introducer for the sutureless myocardial pacemaker lead. *Ann Thorac Surg* 1977; **23** (5): 480–2.

23 Lawrie GM, Seale JP, Morris GC Jr *et al.* Results of epicardial pacing by the left subcostal approach. *Ann Thorac Surg* 1979; **28** (6): 561–7.

24 Ritter P, Mugica J, Lazarus A. Why did we leave the epicardial approach? *Arch Mal Coeur Vaiss* 1998; **91**: 153.

25 Castellanos A Jr, Maytin O, Lemberg L *et al.* Unusual QRS complexes produced by pacemaker stimuli with special reference to myocardial tunneling and coronary sinus stimulation. *Am Heart J* 1969; **77** (6): 732–42.

26 Gordon AJ. Catheter pacing in complete heart block. *JAMA* 1965; **193** (13): 109–14.

27 Gulotta SJ. Transvenous cardiac pacing—techniques for optimal electrode positioning and prevention of coronary sinus placement. *Circulation* 1970; **XLII**: 701–18.

28 Hunt D, Sloman G. Long-term electrode catheter pacing from coronary sinus. *Br Med J* 1968; **4**: 495–6.

29 Kemp A, Johansen KJ, Kjaergaard E. Malplacement of endocardial pacemaker electrodes in the middle cardiac vein. *Acta Med Scand* 1976; **199**: 7–11.

30 Paeprer Von H, Kortmann R, Liebenschutz HW *et al.* Electrocardiographic evidence of malposition of intracardiac pacemaker electrodes, with special regard to the position of the coronary veins. *Dtsch Med J* 1970; **21**: 706.

31 Shettigar UR, Loungani RR, Smith CA. Inadvertent permanent ventricular pacing from the coronary vein: an electrocardiographic, roentgenographic, and echocardiographic assessment. *Clin Cardiol* 1989; **12**: 267–74.

32 Spitzberg JW, Milstoc M, Wertheim AR. An unusual site of ventricular pacing occurring during the use of the transvenous catheter pacemaker. *Am Heart J* 1969; **77** (4): 529–33.

33 Lee ME. Special considerations in ventricular pacing in patients with tricuspid valve disease. *Ann Thorac Surg* 1983; **36** (1): 89–92.

34 Bai Y, Strathmore N, Mond H *et al.* Permanent ventricular pacing via the great cardiac vein. *Pacing Clin Electrophysiol* 1994; **17** (4): 678–83.

35 McVenes R. What tools do we need for multisite stimulation? *Eur J Cardiac Pacing Electrophysiol* 1996; **6** (1): 145.

36 McVenes R, Stokes K. Alternative pacing sites: how the modern technology deals with this new challenge. In: Antonioli GE, ed. *Pacemaker Leads 1997*. Bologna: Monduzzi Editore, 1997: 223–8.

37 Potkin B, Roberts W. Size of coronary sinus at necropsy in subjects without cardiac disease and in patients with various cardiac conditions. *Am J Cardiol* 1987; **60**: 1418–21.

38 Desai AD, Chun SH, Friday KJ *et al.* Analysis of factors influencing successful coronary sinus cannulation during implant of biventricular pacing systems. *Circulation* 2001; **104** (17 Suppl. II): 418.

39 InSync™ Model 8040 with the Medtronic Attain™ LV Leads Model 2187/88 biventricular pacing system. Final Clinical Report, June 27, 2000.

40 VonLudinghausen M. Clinical anatomy of cardiac veins, vv. cardiacae. *Surg Radiol Anat* 1987; **9**: 159–68.

41 Hill MRS, Connors SP, Hassan A. Coronary venous vasculature in congestive heart failure patients: opportunities for left ventricular pacing. *Europace* 2000; **I**: D238.

42 Asirvatham SJ, Talreja DR, Gami AS *et al.* Coronary venous drainage of the lateral left ventricle: implications for biventricular pacing. *Circulation* 2001; **104** (17): II-619.

43 Medtronic Attain™ Side-Wire Lead Model 4191 Study Closure Report 1.1, October 18, 2000.

44 Gurley J, Lamba S, Moulton K *et al.* Does the availability of left-heart lead and delivery system options matter for cardiac resynchronization therapy? *Pacing Clin Electrophysiol* 2002; **24** (Pt II): L597.

45 Neri R, Cesario AS, Palermo P *et al.* Retrograde venography of the coronary sinus in candidates for left ventricular pacing. *Europace* 2000; **1** (Suppl. D): 95.

46 Ritter P, Gras D, Bakdach H *et al.* Material-related complications of multisite pacing in end-stage heart failure. *Arch Mal Coeur Vaiss* 1998; **91**: 143.

47 McVenes R, Stokes K, Christie M, French SN. Technical aspects of simultaneous biventricular stimulation thresholds. *Arch Mal Coeur Vaiss* 1998; **91** (3): 152.

48 Puglisi A, Sgreccia F, Santini M *et al.* InSync Italian registry: Left heart leads performance and optimization of the right ventricular lead choice. *Pacing Clin Electrophysiol* 2000; **23** (Pt II): 581.

49 Kocovic DZ, DeLurgio DB, Daubert JP *et al.* Over the wire lead design: US experience with a new guide wire or stylet delivered left ventricular lead. *Pacing Clin Electrophysiol* 2002; **25** (4 Pt II): 600.

50 Irnich W. The fundamental law of electrostimulation and its application to defibrillation. *Pacing Clin Electrophysiol* 1990; **13** (11 Pt II): 1433–47.

51 Wells CA, Senior AJ. Coronary sinus thrombosis and myocardial infarction secondary to ventriculoatrial shunt insertion. *J Pediatr Surg* 1990; **25** (12): 1214–15.

52 Hansky B, Vogt J, Gueldner H *et al.* Problems of coronary vein leads. In: *Proceedings, 3rd Transmediterranean Congress, 4th Electrical Management of Heart Failure Annual Symposium*. Valletta, Malta, February 8–10, 2001: 50.

53 Aurrichio A, Butter C, Block M *et al.* Left ventricular pacing with a 2nd generation over the wire coronary venous lead. *Pacing Clin Electrophysiol* 2002; **24** (Pt II): 548.

54 Bowman CR, Carter WH. Pacemaker pseudodysfunction with a coronary sinus pacemaker *Am Heart J* 1974; **87** (4): 507–10.

55 Taieb JM, Benchaa T, Foltzer E *et al.* Atrioventricular cross-talk in biventricular pacing: a potential cause of ventricular standstill. *Pacing Clin Electrophysiol* 2002; **6**: 929–35.

56 Lipchenca I, Garrigue S, Glickson, M *et al.* Inhibition of biventricular pacemakers by oversensing of far-field atrial depolarization. *Pacing Clin Electrophysiol* 2002; **25**: 365–7.

57 Hazan MB, Byrnes DA, Elmquist TH *et al.* Angiographic demonstration of coronary sinus thrombosis: a potential consequence of trauma to the coronary sinus. *Catheter Cardiovasc Diagn* 1982; **8**: 405–8.

58 Moss AJ, Rivers RJ, Cooper M. Long-term pervenous atrial pacing from the proximal portion of the coronary vein. *JAMA* 1969; **209** (4): 543–5.

59 Hunt D, Sloman G. Long-term electrode catheter pacing from coronary sinus. *Br Med J* 1968; **4**: 495–6.

60 Castellanos A, Castillo CA, Myerburg RJ. Bipolar coronary sinus lead for left atrial and left ventricular recording. *Fundam Clin Cardiol* 1971; **81**: 832–6.

61 Spitzberg JW, Milstoc M, Wertheim AR. An unusual site of ventricular pacing occurring during the use of the transvenous catheter pacemaker. *Am Heart J* 1969; **77** (4): 529–33.

62 Barold S, Banner R. Unusual electrocardiographic pattern during transvenous pacing from the middle cardiac vein. *Pacing Clin Electrophysiol* 1978; **1**: 31–4.

63 Jones GK, Swerdlow C, Reichenbach DD *et al.* Anatomical findings in patients having had a chronically indwelling coronary sinus defibrillation lead. *Pacing Clin Electrophysiol* 1995; **18**: 2062–7.

64 Hanksy B, Minami K, Vogt J. Changes in coronary vein system due to long-term stimulation with coronary vein leads. *Circulation*; **104** (17 Suppl. II): 418.

65 Alonso C, Leclercq C, Pavin D *et al.* Intravascular extraction of leads chronically implanted into the cardiac veins for permanent left ventricular pacing. *Pacing Clin Electrophysiol* 2000; **23** (Pt II): 561.

66 Rosenthal E, Cook A. Pacing lead adhesions after long-term ventricular pacing via the coronary sinus. *Pacing Clin Electrophysiol* 1999; **22**: 1846–8.

67 Byrd CL, Tacker WA, Schoenlein WE *et al.* Extraction of leads from the coronary sinus and great cardiac vein in sheep. *Pacing Clin Electrophysiol* 1997; **20** (Pt II): 1110.

68 Westlund R, Tockman B, Liu L *et al.* Extraction of coronary vein leads having permanent and resorbable passive fixation mechanisms. *Pacing Clin Electrophysiol* 1999; **22** (4 Pt II): 718.

69 Pianca AM, Bornzin GA, Morgan K *et al.* Evaluation of left ventricular pacing leads. *Pacing Clin Electrophysiol* 1999; **22** (4 Pt II): 874.

70 Hine D, McVenes R. Chronic extraction of coronary sinus/cardiac vein leads in canines. *Europace* 2002; **3** (Suppl. A): 156.

71 Tacker WA, Van Vleet JF, Schoenlein WE *et al.* Postmortem changes after lead extraction from the ovine coronary sinus and great cardiac vein. *Pacing Clin Electrophysiol* 1998; **21** (Pt II): 296–8.

72 Parsonnet V, Harari D. The effect of nonisodiametric design on the ease of extracting chronically implanted pacemaker leads. *Pacing Clin Electrophysiol* 1997; **20** (10 Pt I): 2419–21.

73 Purefellner H, Nesser HJ, Winter S *et al.* Transvenous left ventricular lead implantation with Easytrak® lead system: the European experience. *Am J Cardiol* 2000; **86** (Suppl.): 157K–167K.

74 Garrigue S, Jaïs P, Espil G *et al.* Comparison of chronic biventricular pacing between epicardial and endocardial left ventricular stimulation using Doppler tissue imaging in patients with heart failure. *Am J Cardiol* 2001; **88**: 858–62.

75 Leclercq F, Hager FX, Marcia JC *et al.* Left ventricular lead insertion using a modified transseptal catheterization technique: a totally endocardial approach for permanent biventricular pacing in end-stage heart failure. *Pacing Clin Electrophysiol* 1999; **22**: 1570–5.

76 Gold MR, Rashba EJ. Left ventricular endocardial pacing: don't try this at home. *Pacing Clin Electrophysiol* 1999; **22**: 1567–9.

77 Leclercq F, Kassnasrallah S, Macia JC *et al.* Transcranial Doppler detection of microemboli during endocardial biventricular pacing in end-stage heart failure. *J Am Coll Cardiol* 2000; **35** (Suppl. A): 141–A34.

78 Jais P, Takahashi A, Garrigue S *et al.* Mid-term followup of endocardial biventricular pacing. *Pacing Clin Electrophysiol* 2000; **23**: 1744–7.

79 McVenes R, Christie M. LV endocardial and triple site stimulation—insights to the mechanism of cardiac resync. *Europace* 2002; **3** (Suppl. A): 176.

80 Krein A. Böhler J, Hopp H *et al.* Rare embolic complication after pacemaker lead misplacement in the left ventricle. *Pacing Clin Electrophysiol* 2002; **18** (Pt II): 1760.

81 Lee WL, Kong CW, Chu LS *et al.* Transvenous permanent left ventricular pacing. *Angiology, J Vasc Dis* 1995; **46** (3): 259–64.

82 Liebold A, Aebert H, Muscholl M *et al.* Cerebral embolism due to left ventricular pacemaker lead: removal with cardiopulmonary bypass. *Pacing Clin Electrophysiol* 1994; **17** (1): 2353–5.

83 Sharifi M, Sorkin R, Lakier JB. Left heart pacing and cardioembolic stroke. *Pacing Clin Electrophysiol* 1994; **17** (10): 1691–6.

84 Bauersfeld UK, Thakur RK, Ghani M *et al.* Inadvertent left ventricular placement of pacing lead. *Am J Radiol* 1994; **162**: 290–2.

85 Ghani M, Thakur RK, Boughner D *et al.* Malposition of transvenous pacing lead in the left ventricle. *Pacing Clin Electrophysiol* 1993; **16** (9): 1800–7.

86 Gilon D, Lotan C, Gotsman MS *et al.* Transesophageal echocardiographic imaging of misplaced ventricular pacing electrode. *J Am Soc Echocardiogr* 1995; **8** (1): 103–4.

87 Kusniec J, Mazur A, Hirsch R *et al.* Left ventricular malposition of a transvenous cardioverter defibrillator lead: a 3-year follow-up. *Pacing Clin Electrophysiol* 1998; **21**: 1313–15.

88 Shmuely H, Erdman S, Strasberg B *et al.* Seven years of left ventricular pacing due to malposition of pacing electrode. *Pacing Clin Electrophysiol* 1992; **15**: 369–72.

89 Trohman RG, Wilkoff BL, Byrne T *et al.* Successful percutaneous extraction of a chronic left ventricular pacing lead. *Pacing Clin Electrophysiol* 1991; **14**: 1448–51.

90 Stokes K, Stephenson N. The implantable cardiac pacing lead—just a simple wire? In: Barold S, Mugica J, eds. *The Third Decade of Cardiac Pacing*. Armonk, NY: Futura Publishing, 1982: 365–418.

CHAPTER 11

Permanent and Temporary Single-Lead VDD and DDD Pacing: State of the Art

I. Eli Ovsyshcher and Eugene Crystal

Introduction

A single lead (SL) with non-contact, a floating electrode in the atrium (A) and a standard ventricular part (VDD pacing) was first tested in humans for dual-chamber pacing in 1973 [1]. Several years later permanent SL dual-chamber systems were implanted [2,3]. Clinical results with unipolar atrial sensing were suboptimal, and encouraged the development of SL systems incorporating bipolar atrial sensing [3–12]. SL systems became commercially available in Europe and the US about 12 years ago [5–8].

Detection of atrial signal in SL-VDD systems

There are two groups of factors that influence the detection of atrial (A-) signals. One group includes factors beyond the control of the operator or device, such as the anatomy of the atrium, sequence of atrial activation and atrial arrhythmia. These issues are discussed further in the sections on 'Patient selection for permanent single-lead VDD pacing' and 'Atrial sensing performance and long-term results'. Another group includes factors which depend on the design of the atrial lead, sensing amplifier and technique of implantation; this group includes such factors as the distance between the atrial wall and electrodes, electrode size, interelectrode spacing and dipole orientation. Basic features of those factors will be addressed here.

Although sensing of atrial signal is possible from the ventricular electrodes [13], all modern systems use floating electrodes on the body of the single-pass lead.

Distance between atrial wall and electrode

The greater the distance, the smaller the amplitude of the A-signal.

Electrode size

Small electrodes deliver high-quality signals recorded only from nearby myocardium; larger electrodes can record more distant signals (antenna), but at the expense of recording lower-amplitude signals adjacent to the atrial wall, and increasing the detection of far-field signals. The optimal electrode size will, of necessity, be a compromise between these opposing factors.

Interelectrode spacing

The effects of varying interelectrode spacing are analogous to varying electrode size. A larger interelectrode space records larger cardiac signals (bigger sensing antenna), but at the cost of decreased specificity, e.g. far-field sensing. The larger the interelectrode separation, the more the bipolar lead system behaves like a unipolar system.

Dipole orientation

Two types of electrode dipole orientation in bipolar SL designs have been developed (Figure 11.1a,b):
1 Diagonal atrial bipolar (DAB) leads. Two small split rings are separated by 5 mm. These are available in leads manufactured by Guidant, Inc. (previously by CCS, Inc., and Intermedics). Another version of the half-ring diagonal dipole is now available from Vitatron (Unipass lead).
2 Total ring pair electrode. There are two configurations: a short interelectrode distance of about 10 mm (Biotronik, Guidant, Medtronic and Vitatron);

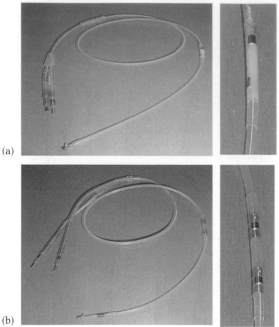

(a)

(b)

Figure 11.1 Two types of electrode dipole orientation in bipolar SL designs. (a) Diagonal atrial bipolar lead consists of two small split rings. On the right, a magnified atrial dipole of half-rings. (b) Typical VDD lead with total ring pair electrode (courtesy of Guidant, Inc.). On the right, a magnified atrial dipole of full rings. The electrodes of similar configuration are manufactured by Biotronic GmbH, Medtronic, Inc., St. Jude, Inc., and Vitatron, Inc. See text for details.

and a long interelectrode distance from 12 mm to 30 mm (St. Jude Medical Company—12 mm, Sorin Biomedica—13 mm and Medico, Italia—30 mm).

Additional details on the SL systems and on differential amplifiers may be found in recent reviews [9–11,14].

Permanent pacing

Atrial sensing performance and long-term results

The clinical significance of intermittent atrial undersensing is limited to a single study, where only inappropriate atrial sensing resulted in > 10% of atrioventricular (AV) asynchrony and was associated with decreased exercise capacity and quality-of-life score in patients with SL devices [15]. With the modern design of the floating sensing electrode, atrial undersensing has been reported in the range of 5–11% [16–22]. Sensing in both SL configura-

tions presently in clinical use (total and splitring systems) is equally efficacious [18–20,22]. The diagonally arranged half-ring dipole showed improved far-field rejection when placed in the high or low right atrium, when compared to the full-ring sensing dipole [20]. Some degree of atrial undersensing was demonstrated by ambulatory ECG monitoring or during physiologic maneuvers and exercise testing. No evidence of atrial oversensing, even at the most sensitive settings, was found with either device. At 6 months postimplantation, the mean A-signal for both systems was 0.8–1.2 mV. As both devices contain amplifiers capable of detecting A-signals as low as 0.10–0.18 mV, these amplitudes still allow for a substantial safety margin before undersensing occurs. A single-center analysis of the Medtronic SL device [7], a multicenter investigation of the same pacing system [21], and direct comparison of two SL systems (Intermedics and Medtronic) [22] showed that they were essentially equivalent [21–23] despite the different sensing strategies of these two devices [9,22]. Importantly, adequate atrial sensing was obtained in 98% of patients with total ring atrial electrodes and was maintained throughout the 2-year follow-up [21]. In 101 consecutive patients with a DAB-SL pacing system the VDD mode survived in 84% for 36 months [24]. For three SL systems, Intermedics, Medtronic and Vitatron, Holter recordings were performed at 1 and 12 months after implantation. AV synchrony with a 2 : 1 programmed safety margin of A-sensitivity was 98.6% ± 2.6%, compared to 99.8% ± 0.4% at highest A-sensitivity ($P = 0.002$), with no difference among the three systems [25]. Similar data were demonstrated with four VDD pacing systems (Biotronik, Intermedics, Medtronic and Medico) implanted in 150 patients [26]. Other studies also demonstrated the similar long-term reliability of bipolar atrial sensing in various SL systems [17,27–37].

The rate of reprogramming to the VVIR mode because of atrial fibrillation (AF) was 2–5% (follow-up 3–63 months), and was similar to that for DDD patients with heart block and predominantly atrial sensing [38]. In another study [39], the incidence of paroxysmal AF was significantly lower in patients with SL systems than in those treated with DDD pacemakers: 4.5% and 8.9% ($P < 0.05$), respectively (10 years' experience, 178 patients). The reliability of diagnosis of intermittent atrial undersensing by various diagnostic features of pacing devices was recently examined [40]. Only the 'P-wave' (atrial signal) amplitude histogram was comparable with Holter monitoring in the detection of atrial undersensing. Atrial sensing reliability in SL systems (180 patients) has been compared with DDD pacing (180 patients): the incidence of atrial undersensing episodes was similar during a mean follow-up of 29 months [41]. The incidence of AF did not differ significantly, and only a trend to a higher reintervention rate in the DDD group was found. The complications related to atrial undersensing (3%) in the VDD group were counterbalanced by complications in the DDD group: atrial lead dislodgment (4%), atrial far-field oversensing (1.4%) and pneumothorax (3%). One recent report [42] demonstrated an inverse relationship between patient age and the amplitude of the A-signal. Intermittent atrial undersensing occurred more frequently in older patients: 6.9% in patients younger than 60 years, 24.1% in patients older than 70 years and 27.6% in patients older than 80 years ($P = 0.02$). However, the percentage of symptomatic atrial undersensing was similar: 1.7% in patients younger than 60 years and 1.7% in patients older than 80 years.

Sensing during activity and body posture

Exercise attenuates the atrial signal of SL VDD pacing systems [7,43–46] compared to the resting upright position. Although values for each individual varied considerably according to maneuver, in all postures, during hyperventilation and maximal exercise, atrial undersensing was rare. When the atrial signal was evaluated by the 'P-wave' amplitude histograms for posture changes, respiration and during exercise, significant variation was shown, with a difference in amplitude of up to 200% in 20% of the patients. During daily activities, 23% of recorded 'P-wave' amplitudes were below 0.5 mV [45].

Cost-effectiveness of SL pacing was evaluated and showed significant estimated cost reduction with the SL pacing versus traditional two-lead systems (Figure 11.2) [47,48].

Patient selection for permanent single-lead VDD pacing

According to the 1998 ACC/AHA guidelines, SL-VDD pacing is indicated for patients with intact sinoatrial (SA) node function and various degrees of all forms of heart block. Such a simple criterion as atrial resting rate ≥ 70 b.p.m. before implantation identified patients with low risk (0.6–0.8%) for subsequent sinus node disease [49]. For diagnosis of SA node disease, Antonioli [11] used criteria of 60 b.p.m. at rest and 85 b.p.m. during exercise. On the basis of retrospective analysis of about 400 VDD implants [14], we employ the following rules of thumb in evaluating patients with complete heart block (before or after temporary VVI pacemaker): the sinus rate should be ≥ 90 b.p.m. at rest; sinus rate < 90 b.p.m. raises the suspicion of SA node dysfunction; in sinus rhythm at rest between 71 and 89 b.p.m. the likelihood of chronotropic incompetence is about 10%; in sinus rhythm ≤ 70 b.p.m. at rest the probability of chronotropic incompetence

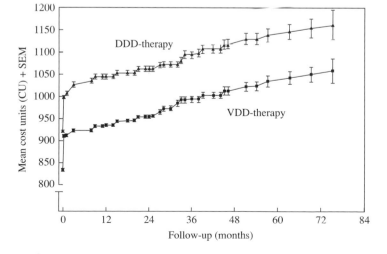

Figure 11.2 Mean and standard deviation of cumulative costs of VDD and DDD pacemaker devices. Costs were significantly lower in VDD pacing therapy ($P < 0.001$) during overall follow-up for about 7 years. Reprinted from [48] by permission of the publisher W. B. Saunders.

is very high (about 30%). Using these criteria, nocturnally and at rest sinus bradycardia < 50 b.p.m. was observed in < 5% of our patients 3 years after implantation. ECG monitoring may be useful at rest and when possible during walking at maximal rate. The preimplant right atrial (RA) volume determined by echocardiography was found to be an accurate predictor of atrial undersensing [50]. It may be expected that in patients with a significantly dilated RA, the probability of SA node disease and atrial arrhythmias is higher than usual.

Selection of suitable criteria for SA node disease is crucial for the appropriate selection of patients for VDD pacing, and should be evaluated in prospective studies. It may also be speculated that the lowest incidence of chronotropic incompetence in patients selected for SL-VDD pacing may prevent the appearance of AF, requiring change of VDD mode to DDD or DDDR.

According to recent publications, paroxysmal AF is not a contraindication in devices with mode switching [11,51,52]. However, it should be mentioned that patients with paroxysmal AF, prior to implantation, had significantly poorer survival rates as a result of VDD pacing over a follow-up of 14 ± 7 months [53].

We do not use any SL systems in patients with paroxysmal AF, or those with frequent premature beats, because we believe that better results are obtainable with DDDR pacing. A recent comparison of VDD and DDD pacing modes in a prospective randomized study of patients with atrial tachyarrhythmia [54] showed no benefit of DDD pacing on the recurrence of atrial arrhythmia. However, in this study no antiarrhythmic therapy was a prerequisite for inclusion, which is not the case in the majority of patients with symptomatic AF.

SL-VDD pacing should also be avoided in patients who may require the administration of antiarrhythmic medication, that may cause drug-induced chronotropic incompetence.

Utilization of VDD

The utilization of reliable VDD technology varies considerably according to centers and geographic regions. One way to estimate the level of utilization of VDD systems is to estimate how many patients with DDD systems and without atrial arrhythmia actually use the VDD mode. In one small survey which used this approach [55], 54% of a total of 165 patients with DDD systems functioned permanently at VDD mode. According to our experience, about 30% of all dual-chamber devices could be VDD systems.

Single leads for dual-chamber systems: SL-DDD pacing

The major limitation of SL systems is their inability to provide A-pacing with the same success as A-sensing. Currently, there are two approaches to using A-pacing clinically with SL systems. The first is to use available SLs and the second is to change the lead shape and thus achieve closer positioning of the stimulation electrode with regard to the atrial wall.

A multicenter study using the Medico Phymos 830-S SL-VDD reported successful atrial stimulation at implantation in 76% of 315 patients with a mean threshold of 3.2 V ± 1.5 V @ 0.5 ms [56]. At 6-month follow-up, only 51% of the patients were responsive to atrial pacing without side-effects, with thresholds of up to 5 V @ 0.5 ms. An interesting approach using a floating atrial dipole for pacing was proposed by Biotronik [23,56–58], by using an overlapping biphasic impulse (OLBI) mode of atrial stimulation. During this mode of pacing, two unipolar rectangular impulses of opposite polarity are delivered simultaneously to each of the floating atrial electrodes. A reduction of atrial stimulation threshold was achieved in comparison to conventional biphasic stimulation (2.5 V ± 1.9 V vs. 5.8 V ± 4.2 V). Atrial capture was reported in 84% of patients at 3 months after implantation [58]. However, in 21% of the patients, phrenic stimulation was observed. Similar results were reported in 125 patients in a multicenter study from 34 centers [58]. The pacing stability was investigated after reprogramming a lower rate of 20% above the resting sinus rate during sitting, left and right decubital positions by Holter ECG monitoring in 32 patients with stable atrial capture when supine. In 83% of patients, loss of atrial capture was observed about 15% of the time. Of note, the initial price of the SL-DDD system, even without OLBI stimulation, is more than the SL-VDD unit and at least equal to the two-lead DDD device [47,48].

Biotronik proposed an SL with three floating atrial rings to improve the results of atrial pacing: VECATS (vena cava atrial stimulation) [59]. The proximal ring is located in the superior vena cava

(SVC), but the medial and distal rings float in the high and midpart of the RA. The pacing stimulus is derived between proximal and medial rings, while sensing occurs between middle and distal rings. In the multicenter European and Canadian clinical study, results of atrial stimulation in 78 patients 3 months after implantation were comparable with those achieved with standard SL and OLBI stimulation [59].

Thus, the results of floating SL-DDD pacing supported the assumption that, for clinically appropriate atrial pacing, the atrial dipole should be positioned as close as possible to the atrial wall, because only the contact lead can provide clinically appropriate pacing [9]. Of note, the best results were achieved in the mid- or lower-atrium position [9,23,57,58,60].

The second approach for SL-DDD pacing is to change the shapes of the lead to favor contact of the atrial part of SL with the atrial wall. Numerous SL-DDD designs are now being studied. Medtronic is currently conducting clinical trials of several DDD single pacing leads [9,61,62] and an ICD lead for DDD pacing [63] which have a preshaped L-curve with a protruding electrically active side-tip designed to lodge in the lower part of the RA. Although sensing in all these leads was appropriate, the mean chronic atrial threshold was $3.4 \text{ V} \pm 0.4 \text{ V}$ @ 0.5 ms [62] and 5 V @ 0.57 ms, and diaphragmatic stimulation was noted in many patients [61].

St. Jude Medical has designed an atrial J-lead with ventricular limb that offshoots 1 cm proximal to the atrial precurved J and can be positioned in the right ventricle apex [64]. This lead was easily placed in dogs and achieved long-term atrial pacing thresholds of less than 1 V. Hirschberg [65], also from St. Jude Medical, have designed an SL for DDD pacing in which the distal tip is an atrial electrode, with an active fixation hooked in the RA, with the body of the lead passing via the tricuspid valve to the ventricle after fixation of the atrial tip. As the authors reported in animals, the implantation of this lead is quite simple [65].

Another type of SL for DDD pacing was designed by CCS, Inc. and has two preformed S-shaped curves: one at the level of the SVC and the other at the level of the mid-to-lower RA [66]. Acute and chronic performance of this version of an SL-DDD has been recently evaluated [66,67]. The mean acute A-signal was 2.5 mV ± 1 mV and mean atrial

stimulation threshold was 1.6 V ± 0.5 V. In a follow-up for 6 months, there was a high rate of atrial part dislocation (3/14) and a relatively high threshold, despite OLBI stimulation, in the remaining patients (mean = 3.1 V ± 1.5 V).

Some modification of regular ventricular lead ICDs was developed by Biotronic [68]. They used a screw-in ventricular ICD lead, as was done in the first models of the Intermedisc SL-VDD lead, with two built-in atrial electrodes in a similar manner as in Biotronic single VDD leads. They proposed placing the atrial part of the lead in contact with the midpart of the lateral wall of the RA because in this position, according to the workers, no far-field signals were observed. Of 30 patients with implanted SL-DDD ICD systems, the system was successfully implanted in 21 (70%); in 5 of these patients (24%), a change of the lead (due to unsuitable distance between the ventricular tip and the atrial part) was necessary to obtain the appropriate atrial signal. The mean atrial signal was 2.7 mV ± 1.1 mV, when the pacing threshold was 2.5 V ± 0.9 V and pacing impedance was $213 \, \Omega \pm 31 \, \Omega$. Thus, pacing parameters in this lead were similar to the standard SL-VDD lead.

Practical aspects of single-lead positioning

SLs are available in several different lengths of atrial to ventricular separation. The decision to choose any AV separation may be made empirically according to the height of the patient. A simple fluoroscopic technique may also be used to predict the best lead size by laying a test electrode over the chest of a supine patient and positioning it under fluoroscopy to approximate the expected intracardiac course of the lead [69].

There is significant controversy regarding placement of atrial electrodes. There are operators who recommend placing an atrial lead in close proximity to the SA node, but not far from the midpart of the RA [11,28,29,41]. Others strongly recommend RA mapping by the atrial part of the SL before selection of the optimal place for the atrial lead [7,10,21,68]. In several reports (about 500 implantations of SL devices) the optimal A-signal was most frequently found in the midlower and lower parts of the RA [7,9,10,21,34,60]. A comparative study of the best position for the two types of leads (total and split rings) was conducted and no significant differences in optimal positioning or achievable atrial signal

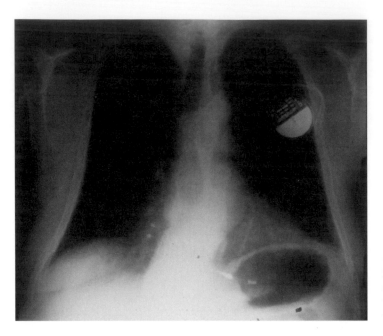

Figure 11.3 Typical location of the atrial part of VDD lead in the lower part of the right atrium, the atrial electrodes far enough from the tricuspid valve and in closest position to the atrial wall. See text for details.

amplitude were found [70]. Non-uniformity of the anatomy in normal and diseased atria leads to multiform atrial depolarization, making individual propagation and sensing of the A-signal via the pacemaker's amplifier unpredictable. This complexity in the anatomoelectrophysiologic substrate could explain the unpredictability of the optimum location for the atrial lead. Therefore, the recommendations of some operators to localize the atrial part of an SL only in the high [28,29,41] or midpart [68] of the RA seem unreliable both practically and theoretically [7,8,14,21]. As expected, the optimum cardiac signal is provided by contact with or at least very close positioning of the electrodes near the endocardium (Figure 11.3). If this is important for atrial sensing by floating electrodes, it is more important if the same leads are to provide atrial pacing. More details regarding the position of the atrial part of an SL and the technique of placing it were discussed in a recently published review [71].

Another important issue during implantation of an SL is the minimum acceptable amplitude of the atrial signal. As was demonstrated for the first time with Medtronic's VDD system [7], and later with the Intermedics device [22–24,27], as well as in the multicenter study using the Biotronik SL-VDD system [33], there is an approximately 50% diminu-

tion in atrial signal amplitude between the values obtained at implantation with a pulse system analyser (PSA) (usually measurements done via a ventricular channel), and the actual atrial sensing threshold detected by the pacemaker immediately after implantation. There are several reasons for this diminution of atrial signal [7,9]. As mentioned above, the A-signal may decrease by up to 200% during exercise or other physiological maneuvers [41–45]. This would suggest that it is necessary to employ a large margin of safety: at least more than twofold according to the above-mentioned data. Therefore, the minimally acceptable A-signal amplitude, during implantation, should be at least twice the desired long-term A-signal and the desired long-term A-signal should be at least 0.5–1 mV (if one assumes amplifiers are capable of detecting A-signals as low as 0.10–0.18 mV; these amplitudes still allow for a substantial margin before undersensing occurs). Accordingly, during implantation of an SL, for appropriate long-term survival of VDD pacing, the minimally acceptable A-signal amplitude measured by the ventricular channel of the PSA should be at least 1–2 mV [7,9]. In follow-up, such diagnostic features as A-signal amplitude histograms (Saphir II, Vitatron; KAPPA 700, Medtronic) can provide further help in adequately programming atrial sensitivity.

Figure 11.4 Temporary VDD lead. Diagrammatic representation of the temporary quadripolar VDD lead from Dr. Osypka GmbH: Grenzach Whylen, Germany. The lead is available in diameters from 4F to 6F. The electrode distances (from distal to proximal) are 10–130–20 mm.

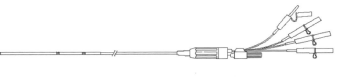

Temporary SL dual-chamber pacing

The idea of giving the advantage of dual-chamber pacing to critically ill patients by means of a temporary SL-VDD system preceded the development of permanent SL-VDD pacing leads but there are only a few pertinent publications on this subject. First attempts to use temporary SL wires were reported three decades ago [1]. The second report from the same group [72] confirmed proposed advantages of such atrial-synchronized SL pacing in patients with compromised hemodynamics. In a more recent report, utilized single modern temporary wire (Mod. TUA, Dr. Osypka GmBH; Grenzach Whylen, Germany), provided the stable atrial sensing in 82% of patients (Figure 11.4) [73].

In our initial experience with using these leads in patients with acute myocardial infarction, high-degree or complete heart block and compromised hemodynamics, the use of SL-VDD pacing as a substitute for single-chamber ventricular pacing has yielded dramatic hemodynamic and clinical improvement. Therefore, over the last few years we have routinely used this lead in patients with acute myocardial infarction, appropriate sinus rhythm, and high-degree or complete heart block, complicated by compromised hemodynamics.

Recently, the success of temporary dual-chamber pacing through a temporary wire using OLBI technology was demonstrated [74]. The report is based on experience in 74 patients, in whom a temporary catheter developed by the authors was inserted under fluoroscopic guidance. Stable dual-chamber pacing was achievable in 95% of patients. In another recent report [75] temporary left ventricle dual-chamber pacing was achieved using an SL temporary wire (VECATS SL, Biotronik, Berlin, Germany), inserted into the coronary sinus. The left ventricle was paced from the distal dipole in the lateral or posterolateral cardiac vein; the left atrium was paced by OLBI technology from the proximal part of the electrode located in the first 2–3 cm of the coronary sinus. Insertion was successful in 13 out of 21 attempts, and changes in the design of the lead were suggested.

Conclusions

1 Single-lead VDD pacing is a reliable, convenient and cost-effective therapeutic alternative for patients with various degrees of AV block and normal sinus node function. A floating single lead may be used for temporary and permanent pacing. To obtain the appropriate long-term results with single-lead systems, it is important to place the atrial lead at a site within the right atrium where it exhibits an optimum A-signal.

2 The performance of various models of a floating single lead with various stimuli configurations does not provide clinically appropriate results for atrial pacing, and cannot currently be used as an alternative to DDD pacing.

3 Proposed models of single-lead DDD pacing, with the atrial part in contact with the atrial wall, are very attractive, but they are still in their early stages of development.

4 There is good reason to hope that in the near future single-lead systems capable of both appropriate atrial sensing and pacing will be available. These systems are particularly suited to electrical therapy of brady- and tachyarrhythmia and to heart resynchronization by future universal antiarrhythmia devices.

References

1 Chamberlain DA, Woollons DJ, White NM *et al.* Synchronous AV pacing with a single pervenous electrode. *Br Heart J* 1973; **35**: 559.
2 Curry PV, Raper DA. Single lead for permanent physiological cardiac pacing. *Lancet* 1978; **2**: 757–9.
3 Antonioli G, Grassi G, Baggioni G *et al.* A single P-sensing ventricle stimulating lead driving a VAT generator. In: Meere C, ed. *Sixth World Symposium on Cardiac Pacing*. Montreal, Canada: 1979: 34–39.

4 Goldreyer BN, Olive AL, Leslie J *et al.* A new orthogonal lead for P synchronous pacing. *Pacing Clin Electrophysiol* 1981; **4**: 638–44.

5 Furman S, Gross J, Andrews C. Single lead VDD pacing. In: Antonioli G, Aubert A, Ector H, eds. *Pacemaker Leads.* Amsterdam, The Netherlands: Elsevier BV, 1991: 183–97.

6 Furman S. Sensing and timing on cardiac electrogram. In: Furman S, Hayes D, Holmes D, eds. *A Practice of Cardiac Pacing.* Mount Kisco, NY: Futura, Inc., 1993: 104–8.

7 Ovsyshcher IE, Katz A, Bondy C. Clinical evaluation of a new single pass lead VDD pacing system. *Pacing Clin Electrophysiol* 1994; **17**: 1859–64.

8 Antonioli GE. Single lead atrial synchronous ventricular pacing: a dream come true. *Pacing Clin Electrophysiol* 1994; **17**: 1531–47.

9 Ovsyshcher I, Wagshal A. Single-lead VDD/DDD pacing. In: Vardas P, ed. *Cardiac Arrhythmias, Pacing and Electrophysiology. The Expert View.* London: Kluwer Academic Publishers, 1998: 389–98.

10 Tse HF, Lau CP. The current status of single lead dual chamber sensing and pacing. *J Interv Card Electrophysiol* 1998; **2**: 255–67.

11 Antonioli G. *Single A-V Lead Cardiac Pacing.* Casalecchio (BO), Italy: Arianna Editrice, 1999.

12 Brownlee RR. Toward optimizing the detection of atrial depolarization with floating bipolar electrodes. *Pacing Clin Electrophysiol* 1989; **12**: 431–42.

13 Greenhut SE, Svinarich JT, Randall NJ *et al.* Detection of atrial activation by intraventricular electrogram morphology analysis: a study to determine the feasibility of P wave synchronous pacing from a standard ventricular lead. *Pacing Clin Electrophysiol* 1993; **16**: 1293–303.

14 Ovsyshcher IE, Crystal E. Single-lead dual chamber pacing: how reliable and effective is it? In: Raviele A, ed. *Cardiac Arrhythmias 2001.* Milan: Springer-Verlag, 2001: 556–65.

15 Van Campen CM, De Cock CC, Huijgens J *et al.* Clinical relevance of loss of atrial sensing in patients with single lead VDD pacemakers. *Pacing Clin Electrophysiol* 2001; **24**: 806–9.

16 Antonioli GE, Ansani L, Barbieri D *et al.* Italian multicenter study on a single lead VDD pacing system using a narrow atrial dipole spacing. *Pacing Clin Electrophysiol* 1992; **15**: 1890–3.

17 Crick JC. European multicenter prospective follow-up study of 1,002 implants of a single lead VDD pacing system. The European Multicenter Study Group. *Pacing Clin Electrophysiol* 1991; **14**: 1742–4.

18 Lau CP, Leung SK, Lee IS. Comparative evaluation of acute and long-term clinical performance of two single lead atrial synchronous ventricular (VDD) pace-

makers: diagonally arranged bipolar versus closely spaced bipolar ring electrodes. *Pacing Clin Electrophysiol* 1996; **19**: 1574–81.

19 Nowak B, Henry S, Knops M. Atrial sensing in VDD stimulation: comparison of full- and half-ring dipole. *Europace* 2001; **2**: B120.

20 Nowak B, Horstick G, Rippin G *et al.* Far-field rejection in single-lead VDD stimulation: are all atrial dipoles the same? *Pacing Clin Electrophysiol* 2001; **24**: 566.

21 Ovsyscher IE, Katz A, Rosenheck S *et al.* Single lead VDD pacing: multicenter study. *Pacing Clin Electrophysiol* 1996; **19**: 1768–71.

22 Wagshal AB, Ovsyshcher IE. Comparing the performance of the Unity VDD and Thera VDD pacing systems. *Pacing Clin Electrophysiol* 1997; **20**: 1888–90.

23 Tse HF, Lau CP, Leung SK *et al.* Single lead DDD system: a comparative evaluation of unipolar, bipolar, and overlapping biphasic stimulation and the effects of right atrial floating electrode location on atrial pacing and sensing thresholds. *Pacing Clin Electrophysiol* 1996; **19**: 1758–63.

24 Palma E, Andrews C, Hanson S *et al.* Atrial arrhythmia and mode survival in single pass VDD pacemakers. *Pacing Clin Electrophysiol* 1997; **20** (II): A1538.

25 Nowak B, Middeldorf T, Voigtlander T *et al.* How reliable is atrial sensing in single-lead VDD pacing: comparison of three systems. *Pacing Clin Electrophysiol* 1998; **21**: 2226–31.

26 Rey JL, Tribouilloy C, Elghelbazouri F *et al.* Single-lead VDD pacing: long-term experience with four different systems. *Am Heart J* 1998; **135**: 1036–9.

27 Naegeli B, Osswald S, Pfisterer M *et al.* VDD(R) pacing: short- and long-term stability of atrial sensing with a single lead system. *Pacing Clin Electrophysiol* 1996; **19**: 455–64.

28 Longo E, Catrini V. Experience and implantation techniques with a new single-pass lead VDD pacing system. *Pacing Clin Electrophysiol* 1990; **13**: 927–36.

29 Ansani L, Percoco GF, Guardigli G *et al.* Long-term reliability of single lead atrial synchronous pacing systems using closely spaced atrial dipoles: five-year experience. *Pacing Clin Electrophysiol* 1994; **17**: 1865–9.

30 Curzio G. A multicenter evaluation of a single-pass lead VDD pacing system. The Multicenter Study Group. *Pacing Clin Electrophysiol* 1991; **14**: 434–42.

31 Lau CP, Tai YT, Li JP *et al.* Initial clinical experience with a single pass VDDR pacing system. *Pacing Clin Electrophysiol* 1992; **15**: 1894–900.

32 Takei Y, Ishibashi H, Tanaka K *et al.* The long-term outcome after VDD pacemaker implantation. *Pacing Clin Electrophysiol* 1997; **20**: A1454.

33 Clinical experience with VDD pacing systems (1995) Review: 6: 1, Biotronik.

34 Gessman L, White M, Ghaly N *et al.* US experience with the AddVent VDD(R) pacing system. AddVent Phase I Investigators. *Pacing Clin Electrophysiol* 1996; **19**: 1764–7.

35 Chamberlain-Webber R, Barnes E, Papouchado M *et al.* Long-term survival of VDD pacing. *Pacing Clin Electrophysiol* 1998; **21**: 2246–8.

36 Sassara M, Achilli A, Guerra R *et al.* [Long-term clinical assessment of single-lead VDD electric stimulation.] *Ital Heart J* 2000; **1**: 777–82.

37 Rosenheck S, Leibowitz D, Sharon Z. Three-year follow-up of atrial sensing efficacy in children and adults with a single lead VDD pacing system. *Pacing Clin Electrophysiol* 2000; **23**: 1226–31.

38 Chamberlain-Webber R, Petersen ME, Ingram A *et al.* Reasons for reprogramming dual chamber pacemakers to VVI mode: a retrospective review using a computer database. *Pacing Clin Electrophysiol* 1994; **17**: 1730–6.

39 Moracchini P, Tesorieri M, Juliani M *et al.* Atrial fibrillation incidence in patients with with VDD single lead and DDD pacing system. *Pacing Clin Electrophysiol* 1997; **20**: A1549.

40 Wiegand UK, Bode F, Schneider R *et al.* Diagnosis of atrial undersensing in dual chamber pacemakers: impact of autodiagnostic features. *Pacing Clin Electrophysiol* 1999; **22**: 894–902.

41 Wiegand UK, Bode F, Schneider R *et al.* Atrial sensing and AV synchrony in single lead VDD pacemakers: a prospective comparison to DDD devices with bipolar atrial leads. *J Cardiovasc Electrophysiol* 1999; **10**: 513–20.

42 Wiegand UK, Potratz J, Bode F *et al.* Age dependency of sensing performance and AV synchrony in single lead VDD pacing. *Pacing Clin Electrophysiol* 2000; **23**: 863–9.

43 Varriale P, Chryssos BE. Atrial sensing performance of the single-lead VDD pacemaker during exercise. *J Am Coll Cardiol* 1993; **22**: 1854–7.

44 Toivonen L, Lommi J. Dependence of atrial sensing function on posture in a single-lead atrial triggered ventricular (VDD) pacemaker. *Pacing Clin Electrophysiol* 1996; **19**: 309–13.

45 Langford EJ, Smith RE, McCrea WA *et al.* Determining optimal atrial sensitivity settings for single lead VDD pacing: the importance of the P wave histogram. *Pacing Clin Electrophysiol* 1997; **20**: 619–23.

46 Ertas F, Karaoguz R, Guldal M *et al.* Atrial sensing performance of a single-lead VDD pacing system during physical activities. *J Electrocardiol* 2000; **33**: 253–60.

47 Lee J, Krahn A, Yee R *et al.* Long-term reliability and cost effectiveness of VDD pacing. *Circulation* 1998; **17**: A427.

48 Wiegand UK, Potratz J, Bode F *et al.* Cost-effectiveness of dual-chamber pacemaker therapy: does single lead VDD pacing reduce treatment costs of atrioventricular block? *Eur Heart J* 2001; **22**: 174–80.

49 Wiegand UK, Bode F, Schneider R *et al.* Development of sinus node disease in patients with AV block: implications for single lead VDD pacing. *Heart* 1999; **81**: 580–5.

50 de Cock CC, Van Campen LC, Huygens J *et al.* Usefulness of echocardiography to predict inappropriate atrial sensing in single-lead VDD pacing. *Pacing Clin Electrophysiol* 1999; **22**: 1344–7.

51 Nowak B, Voigtlander T, Rosocha S *et al.* Paroxysmal atrial fibrillation and high degree AV block: use of single- lead VDDR pacing with mode switching. *Pacing Clin Electrophysiol* 1998; **21**: 1927–33.

52 Buys EM, van Hemel NM, Jessurun ER *et al.* VDDR pacing after His-bundle ablation for paroxysmal atrial fibrillation: a pilot study. *Pacing Clin Electrophysiol* 1998; **21**: 1869–72.

53 Ben Ameur Y, Martin E, Jarwe M *et al.* [VDD mode single electrode cardiac stimulation: indications, results and limitations of the method.] *Ann Cardiol Angeiol (Paris)* 1997; **46**: 585–91.

54 Gillis AM, Connolly SJ, Lacombe P *et al.* Randomized crossover comparison of DDDR versus VDD pacing after atrioventricular junction ablation for prevention of atrial fibrillation. The atrial pacing peri-ablation for paroxysmal atrial fibrillation (PA (3)) study investigators. *Circulation* 2000; **102**: 736–41.

55 Crespo A, Ramella I, Porcile G *et al.* Single lead VDD pacing: is it underutilized? *Europace* 2001; **2**: B119.

56 DiGregorio F, Morra A, Bongiorni M *et al.* A multicenter experience in DDD pacing with single-pass lead. *Pacing Clin Electrophysiol* 1997; **20**: A1210.

57 Del Giudici G, Frabeti L, Cioffi L *et al.* DDD pacing using a single A-V lead with atrial floating dipole and biphasic overlapping stimulation. *Pacing Clin Electrophysiol* 1997; **20**: A1516.

58 Frabetti L, Sassara M, Melissano A *et al.* OLBI pacing— the Italian experience. *Prog Biomed Res* 1997; **2**: 88–94.

59 Res JC, Lau C. First results of the Canadian and European single lead DDD studies. A report of two multicenter studies on vena cava atrial stimulation (VECATS). *Pacing Clin Electrophysiol* 2000; **23**: 1804–8.

60 Calosso E, Verzoni A, Manzo R *et al.* DDD pacing by the floating electrode of a VDD single lead pacemaker. *Pacing Clin Electrophysiol* 1997; **20**: A1516.

61 Israel CW, Kruse IM, Van Mechelen R *et al.* Results from the use of a preshaped lead for single-pass VDD/ DDD stimulation. *Pacing Clin Electrophysiol* 1999; **22**: 1314–20.

62 Naegeli B, Straumann E, Gerber A *et al.* Dual chamber pacing with a single-lead DDD pacing system. *Pacing Clin Electrophysiol* 1999; **22**: 1013–9.

63 Gradaus R, Dorszewski A, Kleeman A *et al.* Acute results with a new single pass, right ventricular defibrillation lead capable for pacing and sensing in right atrium and ventricle. *J Am Coll Cardiol* 1999; **33**: 134A.

64 Morgan K, Bornzin G, Florio J *et al.* A new single pass lead. *Pacing Clin Electrophysiol* 1997; **20**: A1211.

65 Hirschberg J, Ekwall C, Bowald S. DDD pacemaker system with single lead (SLDDD) reduces intravascular hardware. Long-term experimental study. *Rev Esp Cardiol* 1996; **19**: A601.

66 Hazday MS, Mendelson D, Brownlee RR. Acute evaluation of a preformed single-pass VDD/DDD pacing lead. *J Interv Card Electrophysiol* 1998; **2**: 171–3.

67 Antonioli G, Sassara M, Guerra R *et al.* First clinical experience with a new preshaped single AV lead for permanent DDD pacing. *Pacing Clin Electrophysiol* 1999; **22**: A177.

68 Niehaus M, Schuchert A, Thamasett S *et al.* Multicenter experiences with a single lead electrode for dual chamber ICD systems. *Pacing Clin Electrophysiol* 2001; **24**: 1489–93.

69 Nowak B, Voigtlander T, Liebrich A *et al.* A simple method for preoperative assessment of the best fitting electrode length in single lead VDD pacing. *Pacing Clin Electrophysiol* 1996; **19**: 1346–50.

70 Karagouz R, Guldal M, Ertas F *et al.* Comparison of the optimal position of the atrial electrodes in two different single lead VDD pacing systems. *Pacing Clin Electrophysiol* 1997; **20**: A1444.

71 Ovsyshcher IE, Crystal E. Patient selection and lead positioning for single lead dual chamber pacing. In: Ovsyshcher IE, ed. *New Developments in Cardiac Pacing and Electrophysiology.* Armonk, NY: Futura Publishing Company, Inc., 2002: 167–74.

72 Fowler MB, Crick JC, Tayler DI *et al.* Single lead atrial synchronized pacing in patients with cardiogenic shock after acute myocardial infarction. *Br Heart J* 1984; **51**: 622–5.

73 Voigtlander T, Nowak B, Barenfanger P *et al.* Feasibility and sensing thresholds of temporary single-lead VDD pacing in intensive care. *Am J Cardiol* 1997; **79**: 1360–3.

74 Ferguson JD, Lever N, Channon KM *et al.* A simplified approach to temporary DDD pacing using a single lead, balloon-tipped catheter with overlapping biphasic impulse stimulation. *Pacing Clin Electrophysiol* 2001; **24**: 939–44.

75 de Cock CC, van Campen CM, Vos DH *et al.* Left atrial- and left ventricular-based single lead DDD pacing. *Pacing Clin Electrophysiol* 2001; **24**: 486–8.

CHAPTER 12

Pacemaker Memory: Basic Concepts and New Technology

Paul A. Levine, Robert E. Smith Jr., Balakrishnan Shankar, Greg Hauck, Jeffrey Snell, André Walker and Mark Kroll

Introduction

Webster's dictionary [1] has a number of definitions for memory. With respect to individuals, it is 'the power, act or process of recalling to mind facts previously learned or past experiences.' There are two definitions with respect to electronics. The first is 'a device in a computer, guidance system, etc. designed to accept, store and recall information or instructions.' The second is 'storage or storage capacity as of a computer, disk, etc.' Computers are now a routine and virtually essential component in everyone's existence, both at home and in their profession. In this regard, the more memory or storage capacity, the better.

With respect to pacemakers and implantable cardioverter defibrillators (ICDs), memory is needed to maintain the instructions for special algorithms defining how the system behaves as well as capturing and storing system behavior in the form of event counter diagnostics [2–6]. The increased sophistication and diagnostic capabilities of the modern pacemaker and ICD is a direct result of the increasing amounts of memory that can be packaged in these devices and operate at extremely low power. Our ability to incorporate increasing amounts of memory in these small packages is a direct result of technologic advances.

Terminology

In device therapy, we speak of hardware, software and firmware. The *hardware* is the actual physical components that make up the device including, but not limited to, the battery, the integrated circuits (including the microprocessor, memory, etc.) and the physical connections in the device. *Software* is a more nebulous concept comprising the step-by-step instructions that are stored in memory and followed by the microprocessor to execute the algorithms. *Firmware* is software that is permanently stored in a type of memory called read-only memory (ROM).

Software, or the code that controls the behavior of the implanted device, is stored in memory and thus is dependent upon the amount of memory that is available in the device. There are different forms of memory and most devices use a combination of ROM and RAM. The various forms of memory fall into two basic categories—volatile memory and non-volatile memory. While in active use, all types of memory require energy or power to function. If power to the system is lost or falls below a defined minimum, volatile memory will evaporate and be lost, while non-volatile memory will be maintained even when no power is available. This is the same whether it is a personal digital assistant (PDA), a laptop computer or a pacemaker. However, the constraints on a pacemaker are far more severe than my desktop computer or PDA. A computer requires 110 V, while a laptop, which runs best on line power, can run for a short period of time on a battery that is 14.8 V. PDAs have a rechargeable power source. A 2.8 V non-rechargeable lithium iodine battery with a fixed amp-hour capacity powers the pacemaker while an ICD utilizes a 3.5 V lithium vanadium pentoxide cell with similar constraints.

The battery in a laptop computer, if fully charged at the beginning of a session, may allow it to operate for 3–4 h. The significantly smaller battery in an implanted device must not only keep all the software active but also enable the device to function for 5–10 years.

Read-only memory or *ROM* is non-volatile memory. It requires the lowest power and is used primarily for fixed data such as operating programs, look-up tables, etc. ROM is not very flexible and making changes to the firmware contained in ROM is impossible: hence the term 'firm'-ware. All computer-based systems contain some amount of ROM memory. This is used for the 'boot' program, which takes control of the system when power is first applied or when the hardware is reset.

Some ROM memory is manufactured with the programs and data written into the memory during the manufacturing process. This is the classic type of ROM. Other types are manufactured blank and then can be programmed once or programmed, erased and reprogrammed a limited number of times. These are referred to a *programmable ROM (PROM)*. Specific types of PROM are erasable programmable PROM (EPROM), ultraviolet erasable EPROM (UVE-PROM) and electrically erasable PROM (EEPROM), some of which are also called 'flash' memory. All of the PROM memory types require more power to operate than the ROM types.

To make changes or dynamically acquire data, one needs volatile memory, commonly referred to as *random access memory* or *RAM*. *Static random access memory* or *SRAM* is used for code storage that controls the special algorithms in the pacemaker and for event counter data storage. SRAM is progressively increasing in devices. SRAM requires more energy to operate than ROM and is susceptible to loss if the power level drops.

Dynamic RAM (DRAM) has the highest density among memories that can be written to but has the disadvantage of even higher power consumption, limiting its utility in implanted devices with fixed relatively small batteries. All desktop and laptop computers use predominantly DRAM with a small amount of ROM. The DRAM provides a high-density, high-speed memory for the programs and data while the programs are executing. When not executing, the programs and data are stored on a different type of memory device, the disk drive.

Most low-power hand-held devices such as a PDA use a combination of SRAM and flash but their batteries can either be replaced or are rechargeable. In addition, flash memory is not used for firmware storage as it has a limit on the number of cycles and also is more complicated to use.

Most current generation pacemakers use a combination of ROM and SRAM.

The unit of memory that allows a device to store information is a *bit*. A bit has a value of either 1 or 0. Bits are stored and accessed in electronic memory in 'packets of eight bits' or a *byte*. Bytes can be used to store data in the form of numbers or encoded symbols. A byte can store 256 unique values, or combinations of 0 and 1, for each of the 8 bits.

When information (or data) is read or stored in electronic memory, it is done by selecting a specific byte using an address. Like data, the address is also composed of bits. Since the memory can become very large, the standard unit of memory is the *kilobyte (K)*. This is actually 1024 bytes, the number of unique data addresses that can be created using 10 bits.

St. Jude Medical's Synchrony® pacemaker introduced in 1989 had 8 K of random access memory or 8192 bytes. A little over half of this was used for diagnostic event counter storage while the remainder operated the special algorithms such as rate modulation. The memory availability in Trilogy® increased to 16 K while Affinity® had 36 K and the recently released Identity® has 64 K, virtually all of which is SRAM. In the next generation of pacemaker currently under development, 64 K of memory will be used for code and data while an additional 256 K will be available but only used for data storage. ICDs have a higher-voltage battery and a physically larger size than pacemakers and have always had more memory. St. Jude Medical's Photon® has 32 K of ROM and 128 K of SRAM while ICDs presently under development will have 256 K of ROM and 512 K of SRAM. Even greater memory capacity will be the norm in the next decade.

Costs associated with memory

Ideally, more memory is better. If there were no constraints, the increased memory capacity would allow the implanted device to have protracted periods of beat-by-beat monitoring such as an implanted Holter monitor [2]. There is a commercially available external multichannel Holter monitor that can record 7 days of continuous rhythm with a digital 90-MB flash card. The data is downloaded from this flash card by way of a line-powered computer. Increased memory would allow implanted devices to be mini-Holter monitors. At present, these devices can store only brief snapshots of specific rhythm that activate a specific, often programmable, trigger. Stored electrograms in current devices allow a cumulative maximum of 128–150 s of rhythm (single or dual channel). In addition, the diagnostic event counter can graphically display data that is sequentially collected over time to provide a trend for virtually every possible variable (battery and lead status, heart rates, atrial and ventricular ectopic beats, etc). Additional memory would enable the development of even more sophisticated algorithms and increasing storage of diagnostic information. However, there are a number of issues with respect to cost or constraints imposed by increasing memory. One is the power required to operate the memory. Another is the space that is available in the device to place the memory chip and the third is the financial cost. Most important and a key limiting factor is the telemetry or the speed with which the data can be downloaded out of the implanted device to the programmer.

The financial cost of adding a couple more megabytes of RAM memory to the home computer is relatively minimal but the hardware socket that is the receptacle for this memory is larger than the current implantable devices. However, the size of the chips is steadily decreasing while technology is improving. Additional increases in memory will be very feasible in the not too distant future. Ideally, memory would not require any battery current. In reality, it costs energy to store, retrieve and maintain the data. Commercially available chips are not particularly efficient since they assume the availability of line power or sizable and easily replaced batteries. Implanted devices are constrained by very low supply voltages which need to be able to function even at the Elective Replacement Indicator voltages (2.2–2.8 V). In addition, when memory is being accessed, an extremely low current drain is required or devices would last only a few months before battery depletion occurred. Low power consumption is also required during active download. If the current consumption were very high, this might drive a system with a partially depleted battery to an end-of-life or even no output state.

There are two levels of power consumption with respect to memory. *Static current consumption* is the current required to maintain the memory when it is not otherwise being used. This can be under 0.5 microamperes (μA) and will have a minimal effect on overall device longevity. *Dynamic current consumption* can be quite high. This is the current required when the memory is being actively accessed to perform an algorithm, adjust a parameter or acquire data for storage. Commercial 'off the shelf' memory is not very efficient but when it has access to either line power or rechargeable energy sources, one can sacrifice efficiency. That is not the case with an implanted device. Consequently, most manufacturers use their own custom-designed memories for frequent usage while commercially available memory is used for less frequent applications such as storage but not acquisition of data.

One of the challenges of increasing memory and the ability of devices to acquire more data such as stored electrograms is the telemetry system, allowing the pacemaker to communicate with the programmer and transfer these data. Active communication causes a huge current consumption penalty and increases the requirements on the battery. Just as a lithium iodine cell cannot be used in a high voltage system such as an ICD, the speed of telemetry is limited with the lithium iodine cell. Hence, other power sources need to be investigated and developed as future devices increase their ability to store electrograms and increasing amounts of data over protracted periods of time.

The current telemetry schemes transmit 8 kilobauds (8 kBd) (approximately 8000 bits per second or 1000 bytes per second). This is assuming 100% utilization of the bandwidth. More rapid communication is feasible with optical fibers or coaxial cables but this is not feasible in an implanted device. Hence, there needs to be cross-checking and validation that the data being transmitted are not corrupted. The result is overhead associated with the telemetry protocols that lowers the average data transfer rates to 700–800 bytes per second, if not lower. The earlier generation pacemakers were even slower. It can take several minutes to transfer a sizable series of stored electrograms and their associated markers. Sixty-four kilobytes of RAM now require 80 s to download while 256 kilobytes would require 320 s or more than 5 min to download. Future devices will have even more memory but to make this practical, industry must find ways of significantly increasing the communication speed. If one were to increase the memory capacity to 128 megabytes, the amount currently available in a flash card for digital cameras, downloading all the data at the current telemetry speed and assuming that the memory was full, would require 4.4 h. This is simply not practical. Hence, in order to incorporate additional memory in future pacemakers, particularly that which is dedicated to capturing diagnostic information, concomitant advances in low-voltage telemetry communication will be required.

One way to speed up communication is data compression [4] where this is opened up and expanded by the programmer. Compression algorithms identify redundant pieces of information and code them so that every item of information need not be transmitted. This requires that the implanted device actively process the data. For example, the implanted system could maintain a running sum or average of lead impedance, battery impedance and signal amplitudes over periods of time, and then transfer the averages rather than transmit all the raw data in order that the programmer then processes the data. Once the compressed file is received, it can be expanded so that it appears, to the clinician, to contain all the original information. This requires that the device compress the incoming information to reduce the size of the packets that need to be transmitted. The complexity of the data compression may increase the duty cycle of the microprocessor in the pacemaker. This, in turn, may increase the housekeeping current and result in higher energy costs with a negative impact on battery consumption and projected longevity.

Summary

Memory is a wonderful thing. As technology advances, increasing amounts of memory can be compressed into smaller and smaller packages and operate at lower voltages. Increasing memory will allow future pacemakers to increase their diagnostic and therapeutic capabilities. The rate with which advances are occurring is so rapid that capabilities of devices available in 2002 were not available 10 years ago. The sophisticated algorithms such as ventricular AutoCapture, tachycardia recognition and dynamic preventive algorithms, automatic adjustments in paced and sensed atrioventricular delays depending on the status of the native conduction system that are standard in many pacemakers today are all made possible by increasing amounts of memory. At the same time, there are increased diagnostic capabilities in current pacemakers providing broad overviews of pacing system behavior, algorithm specific event counters, time-based event counters and stored electrograms from one or both channels, complete with event markers along with documentation of the events immediately preceding the trigger.

However, memory is associated with additional 'costs'. Even if the financial and spatial considerations were trivial, the telemetry download time will be a rate-limiting step. This chapter has reviewed some of the technologic concepts associated with device memory and the constraints that must be considered when increasing the memory content of the next generation of implantable device.

References

1 Neufeldt V, Guralnik DB, eds. *Webster's New World Dictionary*, 3rd College edn. New York: Simon and Shuster Publishers, 1988.

2 Levine PA. Holter and pacemaker diagnostics. In: Aubert AE, Ector H, Stroobandt R, eds. *Cardiac Pacing, a Bridge to the 21st Century*. Dordrecht, The Netherlands: Kluwer Academic Publishers, 1994: 309–24.

3 Levine PA, Markowitz T, Sanders R. Diagnostic features of the modern pacemaker. In: Ellenbogen K, Wilkoff B, Kay N, eds. *Cardiac Pacing*. Philadelphia: W. B. Saunders, 1995: 639–55.

4 Barold SS, Bornzin G, Levine P. Development of a true pacemaker Holter. In: Vardas PE, ed. *Cardiac Arrhythmias, Pacing and Electrophysiology*. Dordrecht, The Netherlands: Kluwer Academic Publishers, 1988: 421–6.

5 Sermasi S, Marconi M, Monti M, Temporin S. Temporary RAM programming of pacemaker diagnostics: tachyarrhythmias. *Pacing Clin Electrophysiol* 1997; **20**: 1173 [abstract].

6 Sermasi S, Marconi M. Temporary RAM programming of pacemaker capabilities. In: Santini M, ed. *Progress in Clinical Pacing 1996*. Armonk, NY: Futura Media Services, 1997: 85–91.

CHAPTER 13

Future Trends in Pacemaker Technology

Michael R. Gold and David A. Casavant

Introduction

While the task of attempting to predict the future of cardiac pacing is replete with possibilities given the rapid evolution of technologic advances in recent times, our challenge is to speculate on those advances that are most likely to be realized in the relative near term. In this chapter we will make some perhaps obvious and other more esoteric predictions in this field. The discussion will focus on recent developments in cardiac pacing and their potential implications for future pursuits.

Possible future trends can be considered according to whether they are therapy driven or technology driven. The former are addressed in the first part of this chapter and are relatively straightforward to discuss, given the active investigation in the field. Technology-driven trends, on the other hand, are endless in their possibilities and, if allowed to expand without clinician input, ultimately provide a disservice. Paradoxically, devices are now capable of providing so much information that the opportunity for confusion has become greater than ever. Possible solutions to the challenge of data overload include artificial intelligence for discriminating real problems from diagnostic 'noise', with possible sharing of limited information with patients to empower them to participate in the management of their diseases within physician-prescribed guidelines. Regardless of the strategy employed, it will be critically important that technologically driven advances simplify patient management and outcomes, otherwise, devices are likely to become so complex their follow-up will fall solely within the domain of electrophysiologists.

Therapeutic trends

Temporal versus spatial cardiac stimulation

For more than 30 years, pacemakers were used primarily to correct problems in the temporal domain (i.e. the timing of atrial and ventricular activation). During the past decade, however, the same technologies have been increasingly applied to the spatial domain (i.e. the activation pattern of myocardium) to prevent atrial fibrillation and effect favorable hemodynamic changes in subjects with dilated cardiomyopathy and pathophysiologic ventricular activation (Table 13.1).

Atrial fibrillation prevention in sinus node dysfunction
Device strategies aimed at reducing atrial fibrillation (AF) have been temporal as well as spatial in nature. Substantial evidence now exists that atrial pacing using conventional DDDR (or AAIR) pacing decreases the incidence of AF in the paced population [1], and delays progression to chronic AF [2]. It is noteworthy that these studies only compared atrial-based pacing with ventricular pacing. There is no evidence that such pacing reduces the incidence of AF compared with no pacing in subjects without symptomatic bradycardia and a standard pacemaker indication.

Newly implemented pacemaker timing algorithms can dynamically adapt the atrial pacing rate in order to overdrive the sinus mechanism consistently. These algorithms maintain the circadian and other physiologic changes in heart rate normally observed, while minimizing the symptoms (insomnia, palpitations, etc.) associated with persistent rapid rates. The initial studies of these algorithms

Table 13.1 Temporal versus spatial pacing strategies.

	Temporal			Spatial			
	Maximum atrial pacing strategies	Minimum ventricular pacing strategies	Rhythm control strategies	Preferred conduction system pacing	Septal pacing	Bi-(L/R) chamber pacing	Dual-site (DS) same chamber pacing
AF prevention in sinus node dysfunction (SND)	Atrial overdrive, rate stabilization pacing (P,M,R,B,+S;P,M,R,B,N)	AAIR, AV hysteresis, AAIR-DDDR (P,R,B,+S;P,M,R,B,O)		Bachmann's bundle pacing (P,M,R,B,+S)	Septal pacing (P,M,R,B,N), triangle of Koch pacing (P,R,+S)	Biatrial pacing (P,+S)	Combined high RA, CS os pacing (P,R,B,+S;P,M,R,B,O)
Chronic AF w/DCM			Ventricular rate regularization (P,M,R,B,O)	Permanent His bundle pacing, post-AVN ablation (P,+S)	RVOT pacing, post-AVN ablation (P,M,R,B,N)	Biventricular pacing, post-AVN ablation (P,M,R,B,O)	Combined RVOT, RVA pacing (P,M,R,B,N)
Wide QRS DCM				His bundle pacing, if proximal AV block with wide, paced QRS (proposed)		Biventricular pacing (P,M,R,B,+S)	Combined RVOT, RVA pacing (P,R,+S)
Narrow QRS DCM		AAIR, AV hysteresis, AAIR-DDDR (P,M,R,B,P)		Permanent His bundle pacing, if delayed AV conduction (proposed)		Biventricular pacing, if long PR interval (proposed)	

Trial type: P, prospective; R, retrospective; M, multicenter; R, randomized; B, blinded.

Trial results: +S, positive significance; (+), positive trend; N, neutral; O, ongoing.

AF, atrial fibrillation; AVN, atrioventricular node; CS, coronary sinus; DCM, dilated cardiomyopathy; RVA, right ventricular apex; RVOT, right ventricular outflow tract.

showed early promise in reducing AF episodes and AF triggers such as premature atrial contractions [3]. However, results from prospective, multicenter trials sponsored by two different manufacturers have been contradictory. The ADOPT-A (St. Jude Medical, Inc.) trial showed a significant reduction in patient-reported symptomatic atrial tachyarrhythmia (AT) burden with dynamic overdrive pacing [4], whereas similar trials using the AT500 pacemaker (Medtronic, Inc.), incorporating a comparable overdrive pacing algorithm, failed to show reduction in electrogram-documented AT/AF burden [5,6]. These discrepancies may be due to differences in endpoints (symptomatic episodes vs. total AF burden), the proportion of atrial pacing or the patient population evaluated.

In addition to conventional atrial pacing from the high right atrium, pacing from alternate sites to influence spatial atrial activation patterns and thereby reduce AF propensity is also being investigated. Early studies of strategic atrial pacing, including pacing at the posterior triangle of Koch [7] and from the intratrial septum (e.g. Bachmann's bundle) [8], as well as dual-site right atrial [9] and biatrial pacing [10], have all demonstrated AF reduction. However, recent results from the large, multicenter, randomized atrial septal pacing efficacy trial (ASPECT) failed to show a reduction in AT/AF frequency or burden, even when combined with atrial overdrive pacing [11]. Studies of dual-site pacing within the right atrium (RA) have provided inconsistent results in the ability to decrease AF further compared with single-site RA pacing [9,12]. Early results from the multicenter, randomized, crossover study of dual- versus single-site atrial pacing for prevention for AF (DAPPAF) have been positive [13]. Whether the combination of temporal and spatial strategies imparts additive benefit remains to be seen, but this is a promising strategy that may address several of the abnormalities associated with the induction of AF. By suppressing both triggers and anisotropic conduction patterns, a more effective therapy may be available. In this regard, the combination of dual-site right atrial pacing with atrial overdrive pacing has shown early promise in preventing AF in patients lacking a pacemaker indication [14]. One of the limitations of the dual site technology is the need for multiple leads with the inherent increased complication rate associated with such a strategy. Combining intra-atrial septal lead placement with advanced pacing algorithms should be evaluated as this can be achieved without the need for additional hardware.

A final approach aimed at possibly reducing AF in paced patients with sinus node dysfunction (SND) can be referred to as a whole as minimal ventricular pacing strategies. The hypothesis that the ventricular pacing associated with DDDR mode also causes pathophysiologic effects in the atrium was recently shown to have some basis. In fact, investigators in Denmark recently reported results from a 3-year, randomized, 177-patient study showing that DDDR pacing, even with a long atrioventricular (AV) delay, causes left atrial dilatation [15] and a greater AF propensity as compared to AAIR pacing [16]. Moreover, compared with ventricular pacing, a greater benefit is noted with atrial pacing than with dual-chamber pacing. In Europe and Canada, AAIR pacing continues to be advocated by some as the preferred mode for SND with a low (i.e. < 2%) reported incidence of required upgrade to DDDR and decreased costs [17]. In the US, however, AAIR is considered an obsolete mode, probably owing to the fact that physicians are concerned that heart block can occasionally have drastic consequences in an overly litigious society. A direct comparison of AAIR and DDDR pacing in patients with sick sinus syndrome is presently being performed in Scandinavia and should help clarify this issue.

Recent studies in large paced populations including the Canadian Trial of Physiologic Pacing (CTOPP) [1] and the Mode Selection Trial (MOST) (not yet published) have not demonstrated a survival benefit or reduction in non-fatal stroke in DDDR over VVIR pacing. The combined observed benefits included a decreased incidence of AF, less pacemaker syndrome, and a mild reduction of heart failure symptoms and marginally improved quality of life (QOL), causing some speculation that asynchronous ventricular activation is disadvantageous with DDDR and not just VVIR pacing. Minimal ventricular pacing strategies are more actively being employed in the paced population with sinus node dysfunction. Pacemaker manufacturers have implemented a number of timing strategies to encourage AV conduction including adaptive search AV hysteresis [18,19] and automatic AAIR–DDDR mode switching [20].

Dilated cardiomyopathy

There has been tremendous interest and research in the field of pacing for hemodynamic improvement in subjects with dilated cardiomyopathy (DCM) and congestive heart failure. Initial reports suggested that standard right ventricular pacing with a short AV delay could improve functional status. However, subsequent controlled studies failed to confirm these benefits. Pacing from either the right ventricular apex (RVA) and outflow tract (RVOT) was evaluated. A more novel approach that is being investigated in DCM patients involves pacing from two RV sites (i.e. RVA and RVOT). Preliminarily, dual-site RV pacing has been shown to improve cardiac function and QOL as compared to RVA pacing [21]. However, a larger multicenter study (i.e. the right outflow versus apical, ROVA, trial) failed to confirm any benefit of dual-site right ventricular pacing in DCM. In contrast to the disappointing results obtained with short AV delay VDD/DDD pacing [22,23], accumulating data have shown the ability to improve cardiac function by resynchronizing ventricular systole in heart failure patients with intra- and interventricular conduction delay (i.e. wide QRS), usually in the form of left bundle branch block activation. Pacing strategies aimed at restoring spatial (i.e. left–right) ventricular synchrony are categorized as cardiac resynchronizaton therapies (CRTs). Acute hemodynamic studies have demonstrated that biventricular or left ventricular pacing alone could improve cardiac systolic performance. Results from prospective, randomized multicenter trials including PATH-CHF [24], MUSTIC [25] and MIRACLE (not yet published) have extended these observations to demonstrate long-term functional improvement with CRT therapy.

Today, left ventricular (LV) pacing is most commonly accomplished using specially adapted, transcoronary sinus LV venous leads. Other possibly viable methods for LV lead placement include placement of epimyocardial leads via a limited thoracotomy or thorascopic approach. Transatrial septum deployment of endocardial LV pacing leads is also being explored. Although early investigation has suggested that there may be an added benefit [26] of this approach, its acceptance remains controversial because of the need for chronic anticoagulation and the risk of embolic events. Despite the recent enthusiasm for CRT therapy, there is still much to be learned which will likely affect this pacing approach. The ability to measure hemodynamic parameters in real time will allow for the optimization of AV and VV timing. Also, there is a clear need to predict responders to avoid unnecessary pacing and to identify those subjects without classic wide left bundle branch block who will respond.

In DCM patients with narrow QRS (i.e. ≤ 120 ms) who ultimately receive a dual-chamber pacemaker or implantable cardioverter defibrillator (ICD) for a sinus brady- or tachyarrhythmia indication, pacing-imposed ventricular dysynchrony often results. Obligatory DDDR programming constraints due to maximum atrial tracking requirements, mode-switching and other features frequently disallow programming of sufficiently long AV intervals to permit normal ventricular activation. As a moderately prolonged PR interval is common in this population and is often exacerbated by negative dromotropic agents such as beta-blockers, ventricular pacing is often the norm. Whether this results in the same degree of dysynchrony as a native left bundle branch block that would improve with left ventricular-based pacing is unknown. Another potential option in this setting is permanent His bundle pacing to optimize AV timing while maintaining normal ventricular activation. Minimal ventricular pacing strategies may also be useful in this patient subgroup in order to provide atrial rate responsiveness while maintaining the 'idioventricular kick' that results during normal ventricular activation.

Chronic atrial fibrillation and dilated cardiomyopathy

Several investigators have demonstrated that permanent His bundle pacing using a transvenous approach is feasible in DCM patients with chronic AF [27–29]. Septal pacing within the right ventricular outflow tract (RVOT), while easier to achieve than His bundle pacing, has been largely abandoned as long-term results have been equivocal [30]. Most recently, the multicenter, ROVA trial failed to demonstrate a long-term advantage of RVOT [31] or dual-site (i.e. RVA and RVOT) [32] pacing over RVA pacing using a rigorous crossover study design involving 103 patients. Biventricular pacing post AV node ablation in this subgroup is being investigated in an ongoing multicenter trial (i.e. PAVE, St.Jude, Inc.). An alternate, less aggressive pacing strategy involves ventricular rate regularization (VRR) without AV node ablation

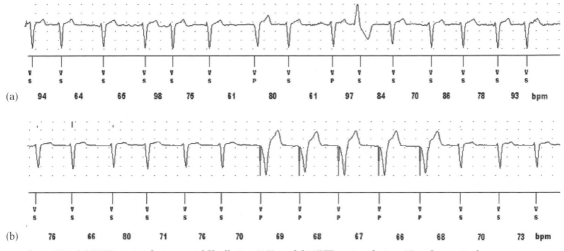

Figure 13.1 (a) VVIR pacing during atrial fibrillation (AF), and (b) VVIR pacing during AF with ventricular rate regularization (VRR). Both ECGs were collected from the same patient during separate applications of a specialized Holter monitor capable of simultaneous recording of ECG and Marker Channel™ information (with permission from Medtronic, Inc.).

[33–36]. The supposed advantage of this approach is the maintenance of a significant amount of normally activated ventricular contractions with ventricular pacing occurring only as necessary. The variability of RR intervals is minimized which results in more consistent ventricular filling and ejection periods (Figure 13.1). Moreover, potentiated beats following pauses are eliminated, thereby ameliorating symptoms and perhaps the progression of structural disease. Early investigation has shown that VRR may be well suited as a compliment to biventricular pacing [37].

Technology trends

There are a number of principal areas of accelerated technologic innovation and development that will lead to improved management of patients having implanted pacemakers and other devices. These are: multitasking devices; unattended pacemaker self-evaluation for remote follow-up; wireless technologies; and internet connectivity to centralized data servers. Each of these topics is described in the context of pacemaker technology.

Multitasking devices

The concept that devices can treat more than one problem, or can use multiple modalities to treat an arrhythmia, is already well established. For instance, atrial defibrillators incorporate pacing strategies,

atrial defibrillation and ventricular defibrillation modalities. Similarly CRT devices have been combined with ICDs to improve functional status and treat life-threatening arrhythmias in the heart failure population. Other areas under investigation include combining invasive hemodynamic monitoring with pacing technology and the use of drug pumps with hemodynamic or cardiac rhythm devices. For instance, when a device detects AF, a local infusion of an antiarrhythmic drug can be given in an attempt to terminate the arrhythmia or facilitate pace termination before cardioversion is performed. Similarly, intravenous vasodilator therapy can be triggered by hemodynamic parameters such as increasing filling pressures.

Unattended pacemaker self-evaluation

The notion that pacemakers will one day automatically check themselves is not far from being a reality. In fact, the one outstanding element required for achieving this goal has remained somewhat elusive: that is, atrial capture determination. Although ventricular capture detection has been implemented in pacemakers and has been shown to work reliably [38,39], atrial capture detection is complicated by the fact that evoked P waves are of an order of magnitude smaller than evoked R waves. Despite this, manufacturers have made important strides in this area using direct methods to improve atrial capture visualization [40,41], and through deduction using indirect clues including the presence of AV conduction [42] and atrial chamber reset [43]. First-generation atrial capture detection capabilities will soon be incorporated into pacemakers. While one can argue that the addition of more electrodes in future treatment approaches including atrial fibrillation prevention and cardiac resynchronization will result in more complicated, attended follow-up, on the other hand, multiple electrodes will allow verification of same- or opposite-chamber capture and may actually facilitate automated follow-up.

Remote pacemaker follow-up

Transtelephonic, remote interrogation of implantable devices is today a reality using specialized clinic or home-based monitors (Figure 13.2: Medtronic CareLink™ Receiver). As this technology is nearly mature, the widespread acceptance of unattended, remote pacemaker follow-up therefore becomes more a question of whether clinicians, insurers and patients will develop a trust, and 'buy in' to this completely different paradigm for pacemaker follow-up. The addition of pacemaker accessories for patients, such as a hand-held device having audio and/or visual cues to indicate presence of AF, may further help patients to become more independent and active in the management of their disease using adjunctive treatments (i.e. medicines) within physician-prescribed limits. The ability of devices to empower patients in their care is relatively new in arrhythmia management, but is now standard for glycemic control with home glucose monitoring, hypertension control with automated blood pressure cuffs, and heart failure management with daily weighings.

Wireless technologies

The most important near-term opportunities in this area include wireless (i.e. leadless) electrocardiography (ECG), long-range pacemaker telemetry, and in-hospital wireless local area networks (WLANs).

Wireless ECG

In the future, the potential to rid follow-up of programmer ECG wires may be achieved by using electrodes residing on the pacemaker can [44,45]. In fact, this concept has been employed in the implantable loop recorder (ILR) with maintained signal quality after pocket maturation [46]. The immediate value of leadless ECG will be realized during attended follow-up in terms of increased efficiency, as patients will not have to disrobe for clinicians to apply ECG electrodes. Ultimately, the potential implications for leadless ECG are even greater if one considers the possibilities for improved remote diagnosis and disease management by storing patient-triggered, leadless ECG recordings in pacemaker memory. Patient trigger devices that exist today include hand-held magnets and telemetry units. In the future, leadless ECGs may contain

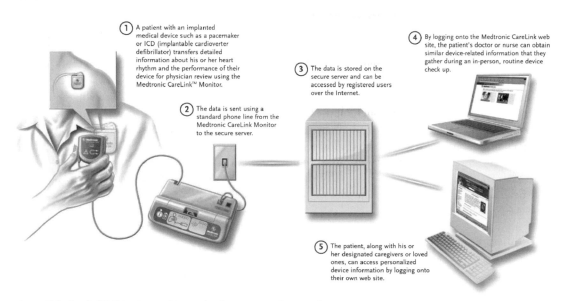

1. A patient with an implanted medical device such as a pacemaker or ICD (implantable cardioverter defibrillator) transfers detailed information about his or her heart rhythm and the performance of their device for physician review using the Medtronic CareLink™ Monitor.

2. The data is sent using a standard phone line from the Medtronic CareLink Monitor to the secure server.

3. The data is stored on the secure server and can be accessed by registered users over the Internet.

4. By logging onto the Medtronic CareLink web site, the patient's doctor or nurse can obtain similar device-related information that they gather during an in-person, routine device check up.

5. The patient, along with his or her designated caregivers or loved ones, can access personalized device information by logging onto their own web site.

Figure 13.2 Carelink™ Monitoring System (with permission from Medtronic, Inc.).

important information not currently available in stored EGMs including confirmation of pacemaker capture [45], P-wave morphology, and T-wave changes indicative of ischemia or infarct.

Long-range pacemaker telemetry

The development of pacemaker telemetry to allow bidirectional communication to transmitter/receivers such as programmers over greater distances will be an important enhancement. An immediate, albeit subtle, benefit will allow attended follow-up without a programmer head but rather via an antenna located within the nearby programmer. Eventually, when pacemakers are able to perform complete self-evaluation, the concepts of home-based, bedside receivers capable of 'while you were sleeping' interrogation may become a reality. Combined with wireless phone technology, real-time monitoring of ambulatory patients becomes possible. Long-range telemetry (e.g. ≥ 10 m) is not inconceivable, yet probably would require more significant engineering trade-offs such as increased pacemaker size. However, it perhaps would further enhance patient management by allowing improved real-time monitoring of patients in the hospital and at home.

Wireless local area networks (WLANs)

The use of wireless technology within hospitals has been restricted due to concerns related to interference with patient monitors, particularly in telemetry units. To overcome this, the prospect of an in-hospital wireless network operating on non-interfering frequency bands and capable of interfacing with a wide variety of equipment has been described [17]. Although many pacemaker programmers are frequently stationary within hospital electrophysiology labs, clinics, etc., many are nomadic in that they are used throughout the hospital. WLANs enable the concept of programmers being continuously linked to technical support, to remote programmers at off-site clinics, to patient databases outside of the hospital, etc., all through a central in-hospital server.

Internet

The possibilities enabled by the worldwide web are already becoming evident. For instance, a system already exists for ICD patients whereby patient information is uploaded from an ICD via telephone to a remote server using a specialized in-home

device interrogation unit as previously described and shown in Figure 13.2. The advantage of uploading to a central server managed either by a pacemaker manufacturer or by an independent third-party service provider will lie in the clinician's subsequent ability to access the patient information using a secure access application from any computer connected to the internet. A secondary benefit of this approach is that limited information can also be made available back to the patient via internet and perhaps allow some degree of self-management of their disease using adjunctive medical therapy, such as medicines, within prescribed limits. As devices become more sophisticated and begin to incorporate improved diagnostics from hemodynamic sensors including those capable of trending absolute right ventricular pressure [47], remote patient management via the internet will become even more attractive.

Conclusions

The results from current investigations will help define future trends in cardiac pacing therapy. Preliminary data are now available to justify the further pursuit of multisite atrial pacing for AF prevention. Biventricular pacing for cardiac resynchronization has gained widespread acceptance and is swaying clinician sentiment towards minimizing ventricular pacing in patients with SND and narrow QRS. Future pacing strategies for SND using conventional two-lead pacing systems will emphasize maximal atrial, *but* minimal ventricular pacing. It remains to be seen whether technologic advances will allow the 'holy grail' of ventricular stimulation, i.e. permanent His bundle pacing, to be readily achieved in order that it be accepted on a widespread basis.

With respect to patient management, although the prospect of automated, wireless, remote follow-up via the internet is exciting, the overabundance of information that will result from the technologies described herein, however, will require large data repositories having automatic, rule-based artificial intelligence in order to sort through the data and report only clinically relevant information. Reimbursement is a prerequisite in order for the concept to succeed. Moreover, freedom from liability for data that are collected and screened by a computer but not directly reviewed by a clinician is a concern that will need to be addressed. Overcoming these challenges is essential, however, in order to allow more efficient and effective delivery of pacemaker therapies to a greater number of patients.

References

1 Connolly SJ, Kerr CR, Gent M *et al.* Effects of physiologic pacing versus ventricular pacing on the risk of stroke and death due to cardiovascular causes. Canadian Trial of Physiologic Pacing Investigators. *N Engl J Med* 2000; **342** (19): 1385–91.

2 Skanes AC, Krahn AD, Yee R *et al.* Progression to chronic atrial fibrillation after pacing: the Canadian Trial of Physiologic Pacing. CTOPP Investigators. *J Am Coll Cardiol* 2001; **38** (1): 167–72.

3 Ricci R, Santini M, Puglisi A *et al.* Impact of consistent atrial pacing algorithm on premature atrial complex number and paroxysmal atrial fibrillation recurrences in brady–tachy syndrome: a randomized prospective cross over study. *J Interv Card Electrophysiol* 2001; **5** (1): 33–44.

4 Carlson M, Gold M, Messenger J *et al.* Dynamic atrial overdrive pacing decreases symptomatic atrial arrhythmia burden in patients with sinus node dysfunction [abstract]. *Circulation* 2001; **104** (17): 1825.

5 Israel CW, Hugl B, Unterberg C *et al.* Pace-termination and pacing for prevention of atrial tachyarrhythmias: results from a multicenter study with an implantable device for atrial therapy. *J Cardiovasc Electrophysiol* 2001; **12** (10): 1121–8.

6 Lee M, Weachter R, Pollak S, Kremers MS *et al.* Can preventive and antitachycardia pacing reduce the frequency and burden of atrial tachyarrhythmias? The ATTEST Study Results [abstract]. *Pacing Clin Electrophysiol* 2002; **25** (4 Pt II): 541.

7 Padeletti L, Pieragnoli P, Ciapetti C *et al.* Randomized crossover comparison of right atrial appendage pacing versus interatrial septum pacing for prevention of paroxysmal atrial fibrillation in patients with sinus bradycardia. *Am Heart J* 2001; **142** (6): 1047–55.

8 Bailin SJ, Adler S, Giudici M. Prevention of chronic atrial fibrillation by pacing in the region of Bachmann's bundle: results of a multicenter randomized trial. *J Cardiovasc Electrophysiol* 2001; **12** (8): 912–17.

9 Delfaut P, Saksena S, Prakash A *et al.* Long-term outcome of patients with drug-refractory atrial flutter and fibrillation after single- and dual-site right atrial pacing for arrhythmia prevention. *J Am Coll Cardiol* 1998; **32** (7): 1900–8.

10 Witte J, Reibis R, Bondke HJ *et al.* [Biatrial pacing as an effective therapy method of paroxysmal atrial fibrillation.] *Wien Med Wochenschr* 2000; **150** (19–21): 419–23.

11 Padeletti L, Purerfellner H, Adler S *et al.* Atrial septal lead placement and atrial pacing algorithms for prevention of paroxysmal atrial fibrillation: ASPECT Study Results [abstract]. *Pacing Clin Electrophysiol* 2002; **25** (4 Pt II): 687.

12 Levy T, Walker S, Rex S *et al.* No incremental benefit of multisite atrial pacing compared with right atrial pacing in patients with drug refractory paroxysmal atrial fibrillation. *Heart* 2001; **85** (1): 48–52.

13 Saksena SPA, Fitts S, Ziegler P, Hettrick D, for the DAPPAF Investigators. Dual Site Atrial Pacing for Prevention of Atrial Fibrillation (DAPPAF) Trial: substudy on device-based detection of recurrent atrial fibrillation [abstract]. *Pacing Clin Electrophysiol* 2001; **24** (4 Pt II): 616.

14 Lau CP, Tse HF, Yu CM *et al.* Dual-site atrial pacing for atrial fibrillation in patients without bradycardia. *Am J Cardiol* 2001; **88** (4): 371–5.

15 Nielsen J, Kristensen L, Pedersen A *et al.* Changes in left atrial size and left ventricular size and function during follow-up of 177 patients with sick sinus syndrome randomized to atrial or dual chamber pacing [abstract]. *Pacing Clin Electrophysiol* 2001; **24** (4 Pt II): 697.

16 Andersen H, Kristensen L, Nielsen J *et al.* Atrial versus dual chamber pacing in patients with sick sinus syndrome. atrial fibrillation, congestive heart failure and mortality during follow-up in a randomized trial of 177 consecutive patients [abstract]. *Pacing Clin Electrophysiol* 2001; **24** (4 Pt II): 575.

17 Kristensen L, Nielsen JC, Pedersen AK *et al.* AV block and changes in pacing mode during long-term follow-up of 399 consecutive patients with sick sinus syndrome treated with an AAI/AAIR pacemaker. *Pacing Clin Electrophysiol* 2001; **24** (3): 358–65.

18 Silverman RCD, Loucks S, Lundstrum R, Lynn T. Atrioventricular interval search: a dual-chamber pacemaker feature to promote intrinsic A-V conduction [abstract]. *Pacing Clin Electrophysiol* 1999; **22** (4 Pt II): 837.

19 Stierle U, Kruger D, Vincent AM *et al.* An optimized AV delay algorithm for patients with intermittent atrioventricular conduction. *Pacing Clin Electrophysiol* 1998; **21** (5): 1035–43.

20 Himmrich E, Kramer LI, Fischer W *et al.* [Support of spontaneous atrioventricular conduction in patients with DDR(R) pacemakers: effectiveness and safety.] *Herz* 2001; **26** (1): 69–74.

21 Pachon JC, Pachon EI, Albornoz RN *et al.* Ventricular endocardial right bifocal stimulation in the treatment of severe dilated cardiomyopathy heart failure with wide QRS. *Pacing Clin Electrophysiol* 2001; **24** (9 Pt 1): 1369–76.

22 Gold MR, Feliciano Z, Gottlieb SS *et al.* Dual-chamber pacing with a short atrioventricular delay in congestive

heart failure: a randomized study. *J Am Coll Cardiol* 1995; **26** (4): 967–73.

23 Linde C, Gadler F, Edner M *et al*. Results of atrioventricular synchronous pacing with optimized delay in patients with severe congestive heart failure. *Am J Cardiol* 1995; **75** (14): 919–23.

24 Huth C, Friedl A, Klein H *et al*. [Pacing therapies for congestive heart failure considering the results of the PATH-CHF study.] *Z Kardiol* 2001; **90** (Suppl. 1): 10–5.

25 Cazeau S, Leclercq C, Lavergne T *et al*. Effects of multisite biventricular pacing in patients with heart failure and intraventricular conduction delay. *N Engl J Med* 2001; **344** (12): 873–80.

26 Garrigue S, Jais P, Espil G *et al*. Comparison of chronic biventricular pacing between epicardial and endocardial left ventricular stimulation using Doppler tissue imaging in patients with heart failure. *Am J Cardiol* 2001; **88** (8): 858–62.

27 Deshmukh P, Casavant DA, Romanyshyn M *et al*. Permanent, direct His-bundle pacing: a novel approach to cardiac pacing in patients with normal His–Purkinje activation. *Circulation* 2000; **101** (8): 869–77.

28 Padeletti L, Colella A, Porciani M *et al*. Permanent His bundle pacing in man: a comparison with right ventricular apical pacing [abstract]. *Pacing Clin Electrophysiol* 2000; **23** (4 Pt II): 679.

29 Yamuauchi YAK, Hachiya J, Harada J *et al*. Significant reduction of mitral regurgitation by direct His-bundle pacing in comparison with right ventricular apical pacing in patients with chronic atrial fibrillation and mitral regurgitation [abstract]. *Pacing Clin Electrophysiol* 2001; **24** (4 Pt II): 583.

30 Victor F, Leclercq C, Mabo P *et al*. Optimal right ventricular pacing site in chronically implanted patients: a prospective randomized crossover comparison of apical and outflow tract pacing. *J Am Coll Cardiol* 1999; **33** (2): 311–16.

31 Stambler B, Ellenbogen K, Zhang X *et al*. Right ventricular outflow tract versus apical pacing (ROVA): results of a randomized, single-blind, crossover trial in pacemaker recipients with congestive heart failure [abstract]. *Pacing Clin Electrophysiol* 2002; **25** (4 Pt II): 557.

32 Stambler B, Ellenbogen K, Zhang X *et al*. Is dual site superior to single site right ventricular pacing in patients with heart failure? [abstract]. *Pacing Clin Electrophysiol* 2002; **25** (4 Pt II): 554.

33 Buhr T, Yee R, Hayes D *et al*. Novel pacemaker algorithm diminishes short-coupled ventricular beats in atrial fibrillation [abstract]. *Pacing Clin Electrophysiol* 2001; **24** (4 Pt II): 729.

34 Muno E, Neuzner J, Kramer A *et al*. Ventricular pacing during atrial fibrillation reduces rate and hemodynamic variability [abstract]. *Pacing Clin Electrophysiol* 2001; **24** (4 Pt II): 576.

35 Lau CP, Jiang ZY, Tang MO. Efficacy of ventricular rate stabilization by right ventricular pacing during atrial fibrillation. *Pacing Clin Electrophysiol* 1998; **21** (3): 542–8.

36 Wittkampf FH, De Jongste MJ. Rate stabilization by right ventricular pacing in patients with atrial fibrillation. *Pacing Clin Electrophysiol* 1986; **9** (6 Pt 2): 1147–53.

37 Muno E, Neuzner J, Kramer A *et al*. New algorithm for continuous heart failure resynchronization therapy and reduced heart rate variability in presence of atrial fibrillation [abstract]. *Pacing Clin Electrophysiol* 2001; **24** (4 Pt II): 729.

38 Lundstrom R, Dinneen J, Vlach K *et al*. Automatic capture detection: success with multiple lead types. *Pacing Clin Electrophysiol* 1999; **22** (4 Pt II): 873.

39 Verma PK, Sharma JK, Khan IA *et al*. A cardiac evoked response algorithm providing automatic threshold tracking for continuous capture verification: a single-center prospective study. *Indian Heart J* 2001; **53** (4): 467–76.

40 Vonk BF, Van Oort G. New method of atrial and ventricular capture detection. *Pacing Clin Electrophysiol* 1998; **21** (1 Pt II): 217–22.

41 Butter C, Hartung WM, Kay GN *et al*. Clinical validation of new pacing-sensing configurations for atrial automatic capture verification in pacemakers. *J Cardiovasc Electrophysiol* 2001; **12** (10): 1104–8.

42 Rueter J, Heynen H, Meisel E *et al*. Automatic measurement of atrial pacing thresholds by AV conduction [abstract]. *Pacing Clin Electrophysiol* 2000; **23** (4 Pt II): 659.

43 Sheldon T, Nelson L, Vatterott P *et al*. Atrial threshold measurement using atrial chamber reset method [abstract]. *Pacing Clin Electrophysiol* 2000; **23** (4 Pt II): 634.

44 Mazur A, Wang L, Anderson ME *et al*. Functional similarity between electrograms recorded from an implantable cardioverter defibrillator emulator and the surface electrocardiogram. *Pacing Clin Electrophysiol* 2001; **24** (1): 34–40.

45 Theres H, Combs W, Fotuhi P *et al*. Electrogram signals recorded from acute and chronic pacemaker implantation sites in pacemaker patients. *Pacing Clin Electrophysiol* 1998; **21** (1 Pt I): 11–17.

46 Krahn AD, Klein GJ, Yee R *et al*. Maturation of the sensed electrogram amplitude over time in a new subcutaneous implantable loop recorder. *Pacing Clin Electrophysiol* 1997; **20** (6): 1686–90.

47 Steinhaus D, Reynolds D, Gadler F *et al*. Chronicle implantable hemodynamic monitor: implant experience in the multi-center trial in heart failure patients. *Pacing Clin Electrophysiol* 2001; **24** (4 Pt II): 567.

PART IV
Pacemaker Follow-Up

CHAPTER 14

Diagnosis of Supraventricular Tachyarrhythmias by Automatic Mode-Switching Algorithms of Dual-Chamber Pacemakers

S. Serge Barold, Carsten W. Israel, Roland X. Stroobandt, Stéphane Garrigue, Chu-Pak Lau and Ignacio Gallardo

Most contemporary dual-chamber pacemakers come equipped with automatic mode-switching (AMS) algorithms to control the paced ventricular rate if supraventricular tachyarrhythmias (SVTs) are detected by the devices [1–12]. Beyond this, AMS episodes may be stored by the device to provide information about the incidence and type of SVT in the individual patient. This chapter focuses on the fundamental principles of SVT detection by dual-chamber pacemakers because correct device SVT diagnosis is the key to reliable AMS performance. Optimal SVT detection calls for a high atrial sensitivity and short atrial blanking periods [2–5,10,13, 14]. Very high atrial sensitivity carries the risk of sensing noise generated within the pacing system itself.

Basic concepts

AMS requires fundamental changes in the operation of pacemaker timing cycles to maximize SVT detection above the programmed upper rate (Figure 14.1). The atrial channel must be insensitive during certain parts of the pacing cycle to avoid two potential problems:

1 near-field double sensing of atrial activity; and
2 far-field R-wave sensing or ventriculoatrial crosstalk.

Near-field double sensing of atrial activity

The duration of the atrial blanking period initiated by a paced or sensed atrial event is designed to prevent undesirable near-field atrial sensing or double counting of atrial events. Double atrial counting (double sensing of P waves and possible detection of polarization after atrial pacing) may occur if the atrial blanking period is too short [15–17] (Figure 14.2). This problem is especially important with dual-site atrial pacing for the prevention of atrial fibrillation. In this setting, double counting of atrial activity will occur when the atrial blanking period is shorter than atrial conduction time between the two atrial pacing sites, particularly in the presence of severe intra- and interatrial conduction delay or block.

Far-field R-wave sensing or ventriculoatrial crosstalk

Far-field R-wave sensing by the atrial channel generally occurs because a high atrial sensitivity is needed to detect atrial fibrillation which generates atrial signals substantially smaller than those in normal sinus rhythm [4,7,18–20]. Indeed, for proper AMS function, a device should be programmed at maximal atrial sensitivity or with a sensing safety margin of 300–350% (for a P-wave amplitude of 2.0 mV, atrial sensitivity should be programmed to 0.5 mV or higher, i.e. < 0.5 mV) to avoid atrial

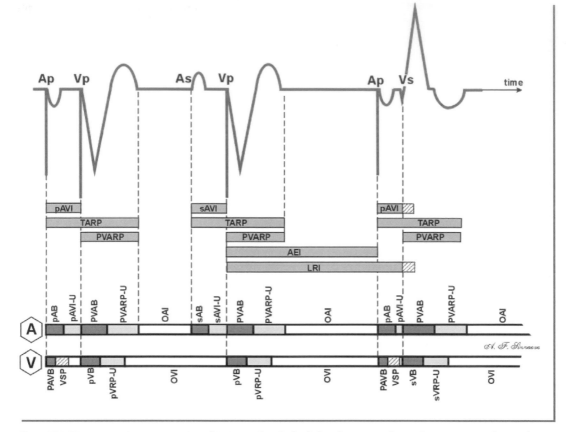

Figure 14.1 Diagrammatic representation of timing cycles of a dual-chamber pacemaker with automatic mode-switching capability.

Atrial events and intervals. Ap, atrial paced event; As, atrial sensed event; Ar, atrial refractory sensed event; AVI, atrioventricular interval, the interval between an atrial event (either sensed or paced) and the scheduled delivery of a ventricular stimulus; pAVI, paced atrioventricular interval, the time from a paced atrial event to the succeeding ventricular paced event; sAVI, sensed atrioventricular interval, the time from a sensed atrial event to the succeeding ventricular paced event; AB, atrial blanking period, first portion of the AVI during which the detection of all signals is blocked. A paced event initiates the pAB and a sensed event initiates the sAB. An atrial event sensed in the refractory period (Ar) usually initiates the same sAB. AVI-U, unblanked second part of the AVI after AB when P waves can be sensed and used in the mode-switching algorithm, although they are unable to trigger a new ventricular stimulus; PVAB, postventricular atrial blanking, first part of the PVARP initiated by a ventricular event during which the atrial sensing amplifier is turned off (PVAB < PVARP); PVARP, postventricular atrial refractory period, interval after a ventricular paced or sensed event during which the atrial channel is refractory. It consists of PVAB + PVARP-U (defined below). In some pacemakers the duration of the PVARP (but not the PVAB) may vary according to sensor input or the atrial rate. In some AMS algorithms the PVARP duration is mandated by the programmed settings. The DDIR destination mode during AMS may not have the same PVARP as the DDDR mode before AMS. PVARP-U, unblanked postventricular atrial refractory period, second part of the PVARP during which the atrial channel can sense but cannot initiate an AV delay; TAB, total atrial blanking period (AB + PVAB). For sensing regular SVT, the functional TAB, AVI + PVAB if AVI < atrial cycle when the AVI is partially blanked. TARP, total atrial refractory period; TARP = AVI + PVARP. The AVI may be pAVI, sAVI or AVE where E indicates extended by upper rate limitation. OAI, open atrial interval, a sensing interval during which a sensed atrial event will trigger a ventricular stimulus according to the programmed AV delay. During the OAI, a pacemaker with atrial-based lower rate timing will reset the lower rate interval upon atrial sensing or pacing. The OAI starts at the end of PVARP and ends with the next paced or sensed atrial event unless interrupted by a ventricular sensed event that starts the PVARP. OAI = lower rate interval – PVARP.

Ventricular events and intervals. Vp, ventricular paced event; Vs, ventricular sensed event; PAVB, postatrial ventricular blanking interval, a brief interval initiated by an atrial output pulse when the ventricular sensing amplifier is switched off. It prevents AV crosstalk or sensing of the atrial stimulus by the ventricular channel. VB, ventricular blanking period, free-standing or first portion of the ventricular refractory period initiated by a ventricular paced or sensed event during which the detection of all signals is blocked; VRP, ventricular refractory period (= VB + VRP-U); VRP-U, unblanked ventricular refractory period; OVI, open ventricular interval during which a sensed ventricular event initiates the lower rate or atrial escape interval in devices with ventricular-based lower rate timing. (Reproduced from [3] with permission.)

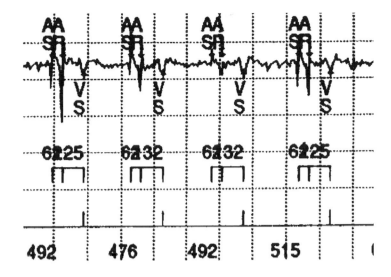

Figure 14.2 Double sensing of the P wave (stored atrial electrogram of supraventricular tachyarrhythmia episode) by Medtronic Kappa 700 pacemaker programmed to nominal settings. The markers are on top, and the atrial electrogram is at the bottom. Abbreviations as in Figure 14.1.

undersensing during atrial fibrillation [18]. Therefore, the elimination of ventriculoatrial (VA) crosstalk by reducing atrial sensitivity carries the risk of atrial undersensing during SVT. There are two forms of VA or reverse crosstalk according to their timing in the pacemaker cycle.

1 *VA crosstalk in the postventricular atrial refractory period (PVARP)*. Atrial sensing of ventricular signals (usually from a paced ventricular beat) occurs in the unblanked portion of the PVARP beyond

the initial postventricular atrial blanking period (PVAB) [19–28] (Figure 14.3). Far-field sensing within the PVARP can be corrected by decreasing atrial sensitivity, provided the atrial signals during SVT can be sensed at the lower sensitivity, or by programming the PVAB to a longer value. A long PVAB predisposes to atrial undersensing, especially of atrial flutter.

2 *VA crosstalk in the atrioventricular (AV) delay*. The atrial channel may sense the spontaneous QRS

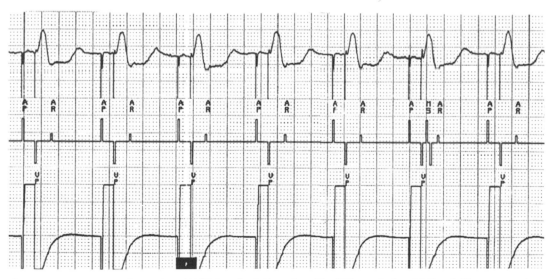

Figure 14.3 Automatic mode switching (AMS) from far-field sensing of the QRS complex by a Medtronic Thera pacemaker. The ECG is on top, the annotated markers in the middle and the ventricular electrogram at the bottom. The AMS algorithm uses the mean atrial rate (MAR) so that alternation of short intervals (shorter than the tachycardia detection interval) and long intervals (longer than the tachycardia detection interval) eventually activates AMS. Abbreviations as in Figure 14.1. (Reprinted from [2], with permission from Elsevier.)

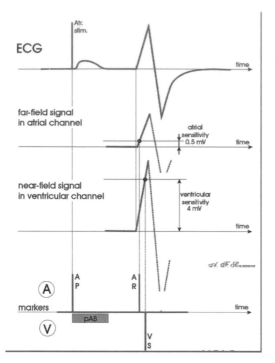

ECG

Atr.
stim.

time

far-field signal
in atrial channel

atrial
sensitivity
0.5 mV

time

near-field signal
in ventricular channel

ventricular
sensitivity
4 mV

time

A. F. Sinners

(A)

A
P

A
R

markers

time

pAB

(V)

V
S

Figure 14.4 Diagrammatic representation of the mechanism of far-field sensing by the atrial channel during the AVI. The spontaneous QRS complex generates an intracardiac electrogram capable of being sensed by the ventricular channel as a near-field signal and the atrial channel as a far-field event. Because of its high sensitivity (0.5 mV), the atrial channel senses the smaller far-field signal before the ventricular channel programmed with a lower sensitivity (4 mV) can sense the near-field signal. Abbreviations as in Figure 14.1; stim, stimulus. (Reproduced from [3] with permission.)

complex within the unblanked terminal portion of the AV delay [2,3,26]. Partial blanking of the AV delay was designed to enhance sensing of atrial fibrillation during the pacing cycle. At high atrial sensitivity, the atrial channel can sense the deflection of spontaneous ventricular depolarization because it registers sufficient voltage for detection in the atrial before the ventricular channel (programmed at a lower sensitivity than the atrial channel). Sequential sensing by the two channels creates an atrial sensed–ventricular sensed (As–Vs) AV interval close to zero (Figures 14.4 & 14.5). If this form of far-field R-wave sensing cannot be eliminated by reprogramming atrial sensitivity, the paced AV delay can be shortened to ensure continual ventricular pacing. Shortening the paced AV delay cannot prevent far-field R-wave sensing from

ventricular premature complexes (VPCs) but counting these signals should not interfere with AMS function unless ventricular premature complexes develop into ventricular tachycardia. Alternatively, ventricular sensitivity can be increased to permit earlier near-field ventricular sensing before far-field R-wave sensing by the atrial channel. In this respect the Frontier (St. Jude) biventricular pacemaker, presently under clinical investigation in the US, is designed with a special timing cycle to prevent VA crosstalk within the AV interval [5]. This interval is called the 'preventricular atrial blanking period' though it is a timing cycle and not really a true blanking period (Figure 14.6). The preventricular atrial blanking is programmable between 0 and 62 ms. The algorithm cancels (for the purpose of AMS) counting of far-field R waves detected by the atrial channel. The preventricular blanking is initiated whenever a P-wave or sensed atrial signal (such as a far-field R wave) is detected either inside or outside the unblanked refractory period of the atrial channel. If a ventricular depolarization is detected by the ventricular channel within the preventricular atrial blanking period, the P-wave or atrial signal that initiated the preventricular atrial blanking will be invalidated for counting purposes. The atrial event sensed in the AV delay (which cannot trigger an atrial output pulse) will not be included in the calculation of the atrial rate for the purpose of AMS. Thus the algorithm cancels the preventricular atrial blanking period as soon as the ventricular channel senses the ventricular electrogram as a near-field event after a sensed atrial event.

Testing for VA crosstalk

The propensity for VA crosstalk during the unblanked PVARP should be tested during ventricular pacing and sensing. For VA crosstalk after ventricular pacing, the sensed AV delay is shortened to permit continual ventricular capture. The pacemaker is then programmed to the highest atrial sensitivity and the largest ventricular output (voltage and pulse duration). These settings should be evaluated at several pacing rates to at least 110–120 p.p.m. because faster ventricular pacing rates impair dissipation of the afterpotential or polarization voltage at the electrode–myocardial interface. Such parameters enhance the afterpotential and therefore generate a voltage superimposed on the tail end of the paced QRS complex. The combined

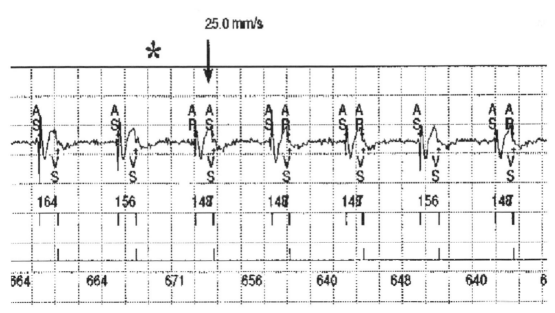

Figure 14.5 Stored atrial electrogram of supraventricular tachyarrhythmia by Medtronic Kappa 700 pacemaker. The markers are on top and the atrial electrogram at the bottom. There is far-field R-wave oversensing in the terminal part of the AV delay provoked by automatic atrial sensitivity adjustment which was programmed to 0.18 mV. Abbreviations as in Figure 14.1.

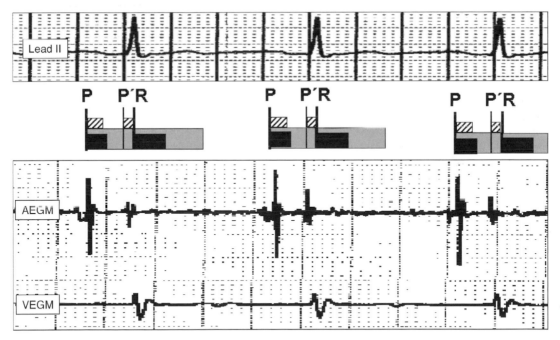

Figure 14.6 Diagrammatic representation of the Pre-Ventricular Atrial Blanking™ (VAB) algorithm. This algorithm is designed to avoid atrial oversensing of the far-field R wave of spontaneous ventricular beats by the atrial channel before the ventricular channel detects the R wave as a near-field signal. The problem can only occur in devices with a partially blanked AV delay. A sensed atrial signal (either inside or outside the atrial refractory period) initiates a pre-VAB shown as a box with black and white stripes. A far-field R wave detected by the atrial channel also initiates a pre-VAB interval at P[1]. However, the far-field signal P[1] is not counted as an atrial event if the ventricular channel senses the near-field R wave before the pre-VAB has terminated. Top: Surface lead II electrocardiogram. Middle: Diagram of blanking periods (black boxes) and refractory periods (gray boxes). Bottom: Atrial electrogram (AEGM) and ventricular electrogram (VEGM). The AEGM shows a P wave (large signal) and a sensed far-field R wave (smaller signal). The simultaneously recorded VEGM shows that the R wave is sensed later by the ventricular channel than the atrial channel. The pre-VAB algorithm avoids inappropriate atrial tachyarrhythmia detection in this situation (algorithm implemented in St. Jude Medical Frontier™ pacemaker systems).

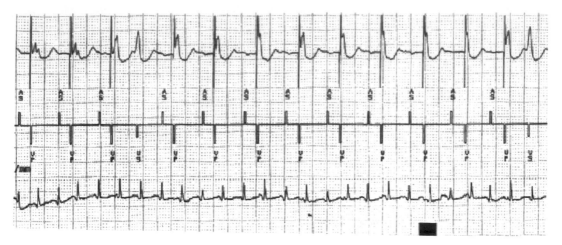

Figure 14.7 Failure of automatic mode switching (AMS) in a Medtronic Kappa 700 DDDR pacemaker due to the 2 : 1 lock-in response in atrial flutter. The recording (25 mm/s) shows, from top to bottom, the electrocardiogram, marker channel and atrial electrogram. Lower rate = 60 p.p.m., upper rate = 120 p.p.m., AV delay = 160 ms, PVARP = 310 ms, PVAB = 150 ms, tachycardia detection rate = 175 p.p.m. The atrial cycle measures about 280–300 ms. Every second atrial signal falls in the PVAB and is undetected. The sum of the AV delay and the PVAB is equal to 310 ms, longer than the atrial cycle. Restoration of AMS requires reprogramming of the pacemaker and/or use of the blanked flutter search algorithm shown in Figure 14.9. Abbreviations as in Figure 14.1. (Reproduced from [3] with permission.)

voltage from these two sources may be sensed as a far-field signal by the atrial channel.

In devices with a programmable PVAB, if the testing procedure is positive for VA crosstalk it can be performed at various durations of the PVAB until VA crosstalk is eliminated. VA crosstalk related to the tail end of the spontaneous QRS complex should be tested in devices where by design the PVAB after sensing is shorter than after ventricular pacing. VA crosstalk within the AV delay is evaluated by programming the highest atrial sensitivity and a slow lower rate with a long AV delay to promote spontaneous sinus rhythm and AV conduction.

Extraneous signals sensed by the atrial channel can also activate AMS. These include myopotentials in unipolar systems, loose electrode in the connector block, etc [29].

Atrial flutter: 2 : 1 lock-in response and special algorithms

The duration of the atrial blanking periods may prevent detection of atrial flutter. If AV interval + PVAB > atrial cycle length, the pacemaker will exhibit 2 : 1 atrial sensing if unblanked AV interval < atrial flutter cycle [2,3,5,30]. Sensing of alternate atrial signals is also called the 2 : 1 lock-in response (Figure 14.7). For example, if AV interval = 140 ms

and PVAB = 120 ms, the pacemaker cannot sense atrial flutter at a rate of 280/min (cycle length = 214 ms) on a 1 : 1 basis because 140 + 120, or 260, > 214 ms (concealed or blanked atrial flutter). If PVAB is non-programmable, restoration of 1 : 1 atrial sensing would require programming the AV interval to 90 ms. Now, the sum of the AV interval + PVAB, 90 + 120 or 210, becomes shorter than the atrial flutter cycle length of 214 ms. The pacemaker will now sense atrial flutter on a 1 : 1 basis and activate AMS. Restoration of AMS function by shortening the AV delay to circumvent a fixed PVAB produces unfavorable hemodynamics for long-term pacing if the AV interval remains permanently short in the absence of SVT. For this reason, a design that allows substantial shortening of the sensed AV interval only with increasing sensed atrial rates (so-called 'rate-adaptive AV delay'), optimizes sensing of atrial flutter, and yet preserves a physiologic AV interval at rest and low levels of exercise [2]. During SVT when sensed AV interval + PVAB = 30 + 120 = 150 ms, this combination allows sensing of atrial flutter with short cycle lengths (Figure 14.8).

Dedicated algorithms for atrial flutter detection
Supplemental or parallel algorithms for the detection of atrial flutter unrecognized by the primary

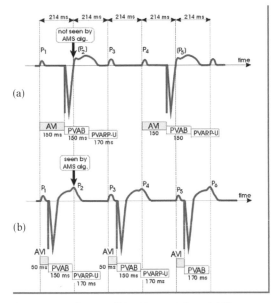

Figure 14.8 Influence of blanking periods and AVI on atrial sensing during atrial tachycardia. (a) The second and fifth P waves fall in the PVAB and are unsensed; sAVI + PVAB > P–P interval. A shorter PVARP would have caused 2 : 1 atrial sensing if sAVI + PVARP < two atrial cycles. (b) All the P waves are detected when the sAVI is shortened to 50 ms so that sAVI + PVAB < P–P interval. Abbreviations as in Figure 14.1. (Reproduced from [3] with permission.)

AMS algorithm have been designed to circumvent the 2 : 1 lock-in response. No data have yet been published on the sensitivity and specificity of these special atrial flutter detection algorithms. In the Medtronic Kappa 700 and 900 series of pacemakers, the Blanked Flutter Search™ algorithm is automatically activated whenever the device senses a high atrial rate consistent with atrial flutter and a possible 2 : 1 lock-in situation, i.e. if 8 consecutive atrial cycles are shorter than twice (AV interval + PVAB) and shorter than twice the tachycardia detection interval [2,5,31]. The algorithm 'shifts' all atrial blanking times by prolonging one PVARP cycle only (Figure 14.9). This disrupts synchronization of every second atrial flutter wave with the atrial blanking times. If the Blanked Flutter Search™ algorithm does not disclose atrial flutter, it is automatically deactivated for 90 s. The algorithm may rarely be active during exercise-induced sinus tachycardia in young patients with unusual programmed parameters when it may cause pauses

related to undetected sinus P waves falling in the intermittently extended PVARP for the flutter search mechanism [32].

The Pulsar max™ system (Guidant) offers an 'atrial flutter response'. This algorithm starts another atrial refractory period ('AFR window') of 260 ms (equivalent to an atrial rate of 230 b.p.m.) if atrial events are sensed within the PVARP beyond the PVAB [33]. Any atrial signal sensed within the PVARP triggers another 260-ms atrial refractory period (concept of retriggerable atrial refractory periods). As long as the pacemaker senses an atrial rate > 230 b.p.m., successive AFR windows are continually initiated and ventricular pacing becomes independent of atrial sensing, thereby establishing AMS. The atrial flutter response therefore provides instantaneous AMS. However, if every second atrial flutter potential occurs during the blanked portion of the PVARP, the atrial flutter response cannot detect the SVT and 2 : 1 tracking will persist.

Basic algorithms for the detection of atrial tachyarrhythmias

SVT detection should be highly sensitive in order to prevent rapid tracking of SVT and highly specific to prevent loss of AV synchronous pacing from inappropriate AMS during sinus rhythm. Manufacturers have designed a variety of AMS algorithms based on the following concepts [4–6,10,34].

Calculation of a matching or mean atrial rate

The 'running average' of the atrial rate or mean atrial rate (MAR) was developed to provide AMS with high specificity (Figure 14.10) and to prevent frequent mode oscillations back and forth in the presence of intermittent atrial undersensing [2,4–7]. The device continuously calculates the MAR interval and compares it with the actual sensed atrial interval. If the MAR interval exceeds the sensed atrial interval, it shortens by a fixed value (e.g. 39 ms). If the MAR interval is shorter than the sensed atrial cycle, it lengthens by either the same (unbiased MAR calculation) or a different value (biased MAR calculation). Thus the MAR represents an artificial atrial rate and a moving value that bears a constantly changing relationship to the true or sensed atrial rate. AMS will occur when the MAR reaches the programmed tachycardia detection interval (TDR). This algorithm is used in the

ATRIAL MARKERS
1
2
3
4
5
AS
time
ECG
NOT SEEN
sAB
PVAB
sAVI
PVARP
6
7
8
AR
MODE SWITCH
SEEN BY AMS ALG.
PVARP extension
AVI
A.F. Sinnaeve

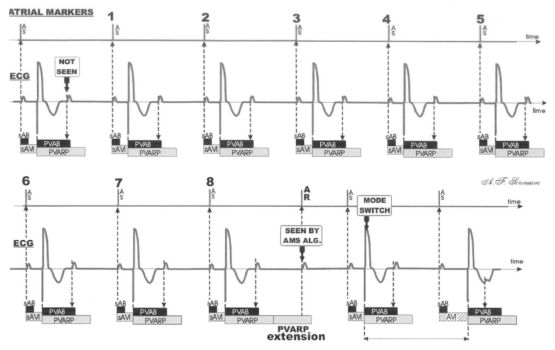

Figure 14.9 Medtronic® blanked atrial flutter search algorithm (Kappa 700 and 900 series). The algorithm prolongs the PVARP for one beat (arrow) after 8 cycles whenever twice the P–P interval is less than twice (sAVI + PVAB) and less than twice the tachycardia detection interval. PVARP prolongation allows a P wave to occur within the unblanked part of the PVARP. This detected P wave in the PVARP-U, together with the succeeding and sensed P wave (outside the atrial refractory period), reveals the *true* P–P interval of the tachycardia whereupon AMS occurs. AVI bottom right refers to the AVI during DDI pacing but it is not initiated by As. Abbreviations as in Figure 14.1; see text for details. (Reproduced from [3] with permission.)

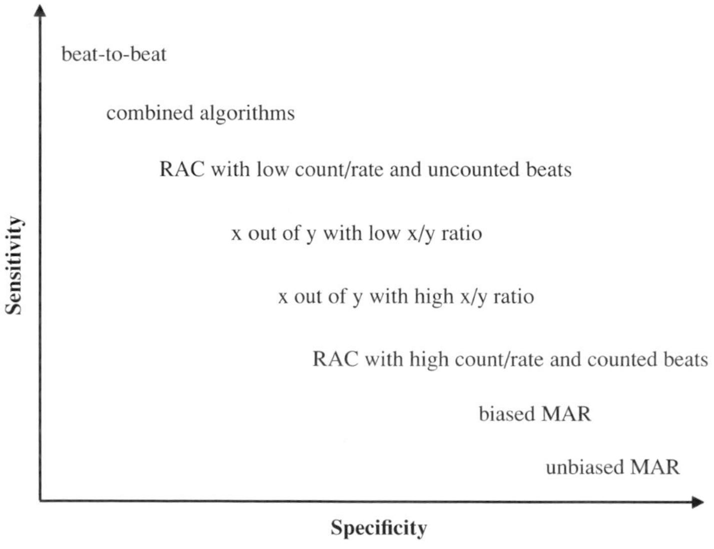

beat-to-beat
combined algorithms
RAC with low count/rate and uncounted beats
x out of y with low x/y ratio
x out of y with high x/y ratio
RAC with high count/rate and counted beats
biased MAR
unbiased MAR
Sensitivity
Specificity

Figure 14.10 Sensitivity vs. specificity of the various mode-switching algorithms. See text for details.

Medtronic Thera DR and Kappa 400 pacemakers (also in the Gem I and II ICDs) and the St. Jude Trilogy DR+/Affinity/Integrity and Identity devices [2,3,5,7,35].

In the biased concept used clinically, undersensing of occasional atrial signals related to blanking periods or intermittent signal drop-out does not prevent or significantly delay SVT detection. Such algorithms are resistant to sudden changes in atrial rate, making them effective against intermittent atrial undersensing. Several detected long As–As intervals secondary to undersensing can be compensated with just one short As–As interval, enabling SVT detection even if as much as 50% of atrial signals are unsensed. MAR-calculating algorithms are highly specific for SVT. They do not trigger inappropriate AMS in response to occasional far-field R-wave oversensing, short runs of SVTs or atrial premature beats. Because the process is gradual, the rapidity of AMS will depend on the pre-existing sinus rate, the SVT rate itself, and the programmed TDR. It is easier for the MAR to reach the TDR when SVT occurs in the setting of a higher resting sinus rate than starting from a sinus bradycardia. This is because the MAR interval starts from a shorter baseline duration on its gradual way to reach the TDR interval. MAR algorithms achieve AMS slowly so that patients may become symptomatic during the delay phase from SVT onset to AMS. Depending on the sinus rate before SVT, there is a minimum delay between SVT onset and AMS of 2.5–10 s when the SVT is tracked at the upper rate limit. Intermittent atrial undersensing may further delay AMS.

Three types of atrial events are available to the Medtronic AMS algorithm for monitoring the interval between two consecutive atrial events: an atrial paced event (Ap); an atrial sensed event (As); and an atrial sensed event in the refractory period (Ar). There are therefore nine possible ways to form a measured atrial interval. The pacemaker utilizes all these intervals (including the Ap–Ap) to calculate the MAR, except for the As–Ap and Ar–Ap intervals. As indicated above, the MAR interval shortens by 24 ms when it is equal to or longer than the measured atrial cycle, and increases by 8 ms when it is shorter than the measured atrial cycle.

In the Trilogy Pacemaker (St. Jude) the microprocessor only begins to sense in the unblanked part of the PVARP when there is a rapid sensed atrial rate that initiates Wenckebach upper rate behavior. This can be a single cycle with an early P wave resulting in prolongation of the sensed AV interval in accord with normal upper rate behavior. At that point the microprocessor 'wakes up' and begins to look in the unblanked PVARP for additional P waves. If the rhythm abruptly jumps from 1 : 1 tracking to abrupt 2 : 1 tracking and it never

passes through even a brief period of Wenckebach behavior, the microprocessor remains quiescent with respect to the AMS algorithm. Subsequent generations of St. Jude pacemakers do not have this limitation.

Long–short cycles. If alternating sensed atrial cycle lengths are shorter and longer than the TDR interval (e.g. far-field R-wave oversensing (Figure 14.3), supraventricular bigeminy), inappropriate SVT detection may result in biased MAR calculating systems [2]. The algorithm of the Medtronic Thera and Kappa 400 devices subtracts 24 ms from the MAR interval with shorter atrial cycles and adds only 8 ms to the MAR interval with longer atrial cycles. This process eventually allows the MAR interval to reach the TDR interval and AMS becomes established. The AMS algorithm was designed to weather intermittent undersensing and is resistant to sudden changes in atrial rate by virtue of its biased character with the 24 ms–8 ms relationship. Thus, although this algorithm is helpful in detecting an irregular tachycardia with detection gaps (atrial beats undetected in the blanking period or one associated with intermittent undersensing), it may also induce AMS in circumstances without SVT (e.g. frequent atrial premature beats, atrial bigeminy or runs).

Repetitive non-reentrant ventriculoatrial synchrony
Repetitive VA synchrony can occur in the absence of endless loop tachycardia when retrograde P waves are not sensed (i.e. they cannot initiate an AV delay) because they fall within the postventricular atrial refractory period (PVARP) of a dual-chamber pacemaker [36]. In this situation, an atrial stimulus (Ap) following the P wave (Ar: detected by the pacemaker in the PVARP) will be ineffectual as it falls within the absolute atrial myocardial refractory period generated by the preceding retrograde atrial depolarization. This self-perpetuating process is often called repetitive non-reentrant VA synchrony (RNRVAS) because the pacemaker does not sense the retrograde P wave (beyond the PVARP) and the potential macroreentrant circuit of endless loop tachycardia is never completed. This non-reentrant process has also been called AV dysynchronization arrhythmia or pseudoatrial exit block, and creates a sequence of Vp–Ar–Ap–Vp–Ar–Ap (Ar is detected in the unblanked part of the PVARP and Ap is ineffectual). Sweeney [37] recently described the occurrence of AMS during this process with Medtronic

Kappa 401 DDDR pacemakers. As indicated above, the pacemaker uses an MAR algorithm and counts all atrial intervals except As–Ap or Ar–Ap (obviously barring Ap–Ap intervals), i.e. all atrial intervals initiated by atrial sensing and terminated by atrial pacing. The sequence in repetitive non-reentrant VA synchrony consists of Ap–Ar–Ap–Ar atrial events. Consequently, the pacemaker ignores Ar–Ap cycles but deducts 24 ms from the MAR interval upon detection of an Ap–Ar cycle shorter than the tachycardia detection interval. This process continues until the MAR interval reaches the tachycardia detection interval whereupon AMS occurs.

Behavior of the AV delay according to the mean (matched) atrial rate

When AMS of the Thera/Kappa 400 devices (as well as GEM DR I and II ICDs) is programmed, the obligatory SAV algorithm (S, sensed) shortens the As–Vp interval according to the sensed atrial rate to a minimum of 30 ms to enhance sensing of SVT, especially atrial flutter. Shortening of the As–Vp interval is rate-adaptive and controlled by the atrial rate via the prevailing MAR interval. Consequently, after the onset of SVT, As–Vp shortening like the MAR interval, occurs gradually from beat to beat. If the sinus rate increases quickly, or jumps to a tachycardia level, the MAR interval will follow and shorten by 24 ms per beat, and As–Vp intervals will shorten, eventually (within a few seconds) reaching the rate-adaptive value appropriate for that sensed atrial rate. If SVT terminates before AMS activation (MAR interval > tachycardia detection interval), the MAR interval will have already shortened the As–Vp interval to some extent. Without SVT recurrence the shortened As–Vp interval will then gradually lengthen to its programmed value in the setting of sinus rhythm as the MAR interval gradually returns to baseline in the presence of the measured normal sinus rhythm interval or rate. A similar response occurs with St. Jude's devices. This behavior of the As–Vp interval outside of SVT may cause difficulty in electrocardiographic interpretation of pacemaker function. Of note, the programming interlock while facilitating atrial tachyarrhythmia detection may severely limit pacemaker performance. In first-degree AV block or only intermittent AV block, permanent ventricular pacing is forced by a shorter rate-adaptive AV delay.

Number of beats above a tachycardia detection rate ('rate and count')

The pacemaker detects SVT by counting sensed atrial signals occurring at a rate above the programmed TDR [5]. Every short atrial cycle increases the counter by 1 until the required number of short cycles triggers AMS. Rate and count algorithms designed to count only consecutive short cycles reset the counter to 0 if an atrial cycle lengthens beyond the TDR interval before the number of short cycles required for SVT detection is reached. In rate and count algorithms that utilize non-consecutive short atrial cycles for SVT detection, an atrial cycle greater than TDR interval only decreases the counter by 1 without resetting it to baseline or 0. AMS performance in rate and count algorithms is highly dependent on atrial sensing and device programming. Every short atrial cycle increases the counter by 1 until the required number of short cycles is reached, triggering AMS. The sensitivity and specificity of rate and count algorithms for SVT detection depend primarily on the inclusion or exclusion of non-consecutive short atrial cycles into the algorithm (Figure 14.10). Algorithms using only consecutive sensed atrial cycles less than TDR interval are highly immune to VA crosstalk because the alternation of short and normal atrial cycles prevents inappropriate SVT detection. Intermittent atrial undersensing may severely delay or prevent AMS by continually resetting the counter to 0. In contrast, rate and count algorithms using non-consecutive atrial intervals are better suited in an environment of intermittent atrial undersensing, but intermittent oversensing may more easily cause inappropriate AMS. AMS may be rapid if the required number of short cycles less than TDR interval is low (e.g. 5 beats), but delayed if the programmed number of short cycles is high. However, inappropriate AMS is frequent with sensitive rate and count criteria, and mode oscillations secondary to intermittent atrial undersensing (with marked variation of the ventricular cycles) are more frequent than with other SVT detection algorithms. Inappropriate reaction of 'rate and count' algorithms may be prevented if a preliminary detection criterion (e.g. 8 non-consecutive short atrial cycles) is combined with another criterion which confirms that the atrial tachyarrhythmia is sustained (e.g. another 8 non-consecutive short atrial cycles). During this confirmation phase, the ventricular

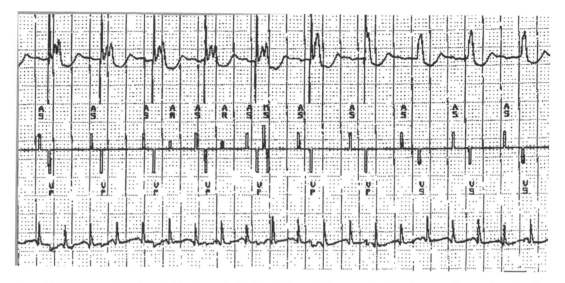

Figure 14.11 Automatic mode switching (AMS) by Medtronic Kappa 700 pacemaker. The electrocardiogram is on top, the annotated markers in the middle and the atrial electrogram at the bottom. There is 2 : 1 sensing of atrial flutter, probably because the atrial electrogram falls very close to the termination of the PVAB. As soon as 1 : 1 sensing returns, probably from slight fluctuations in the timing of the atrial signal, AMS occurs rapidly after 4 out of 7 short intervals. Abbreviations as in Figure 14.1.

response is already limited and a Wenckebach upper rate response is applied until AMS is initiated.

The 'x out of y' concept

The 'x out of y' concept was introduced to reduce the consequences of intermittent atrial undersensing on the delay to achieve AMS [31,38,39]. The algorithm resembles some rate and count algorithms that depend on sensing non-consecutive short cycles for AMS activation (Figures 14.11 & 14.12). Consecutive and non-consecutive 'run and count' algorithms as well as 'x out of y' algorithms basically use a number of beats above a certain rate for activation. However, a 'rate and run' algorithm using non-consecutive short cycles cannot go below a ratio of 0.5, i.e. a minimum of > 50% of atrial

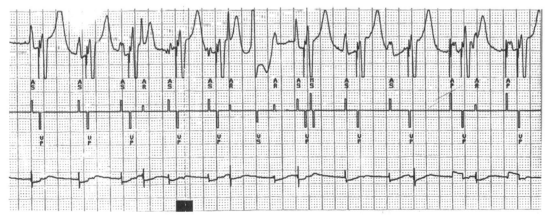

Figure 14.12 Automatic mode switching (AMS) of Medtronic Kappa 700 pacemaker triggered by multifocal atrial premature complexes. The electrocardiogram is on top, the annotated markers in the middle and the atrial electrogram at the bottom. Three premature atrial events produce 4 short intervals out of 7, thereby activating AMS (MS). AS, AR and VS abbreviations are listed in the legend to Figure 14.1.

cycles must be short. If every second atrial cycle is short, there will be no SVT detection (counter always +1 and then −1). In contrast, 'x out of y' algorithms can be programmed to a ratio < 0.5 (e.g. programmable x out of 8 in the Biotronik Logos pacemaker). In addition, two criteria can be used, one rather stringent for relatively small y values (e.g. 28 out of 32 = 87.5%, 'strong criterion' in the ELA Talent pacemaker) and one less stringent for relatively large y values (e.g. 36 out of 64 = 56%, 'weak criterion' in the ELA Talent) to avoid inappropriate AMS for short periods of fast atrial rates while maintaining high sensitivity for longer periods of fast atrial rates. 'x out of y' algorithms are commonly used in implantable cardioverter defibrillators (ICDs) to ensure detection of ventricular fibrillation even if some fibrillation potentials are too small to be sensed. Most designs favor a small value for 'y'. 'x' and 'y' values are usually non-programmable and come as fixed ratios such as 4/7, 5/8, 28/32 and 36/64 for SVT detection (Figure 14.4). Rapidity of SVT detection depends on 'x' and 'y' values and can be as fast as 2.3 s for a 4/7 criterion. The combination of fast reactivity with good performance even in the setting of a high degree of atrial undersensing represents a major advantage of the 'x out of y' concept. Their sensitivity seems higher than

that of MAR algorithms and comparable to 'rate and count' algorithms (including non-consecutive short cycles). The specificity of 'x out of y' algorithms appears reduced compared to MAR algorithms, depending on the 'x and y' values (Figure 14.10).

Beat-to-beat

AMS in response to one single short atrial cycle is the most sensitive and fast-reacting response, but the least specific AMS concept (Figure 14.10). The first AMS algorithm (Telectronics Meta DDDR 1250) was highly unspecific in that a single sensed event within the unblanked PVARP triggered AMS [1].

The Biotronik Actros and Kairos family of DDDR pacemakers use a 'retriggerable' atrial refractory period algorithm for AMS. This algorithm is simple and responds rapidly to the onset and termination of SVT [40,41]. In such a relatively simple system, an atrial signal detected in the PVARP beyond the initial postventricular blanking period does not start an AV interval but reinitiates a new total atrial refractory period (TARP) or the sum of AV interval and PVARP (Figure 14.13). This process repeats itself so that SVT faster than the programmed upper rate (i.e. P–P interval < TARP) automatically converts the atrial channel to the asynchronous mode and the pacemaker to the DVI mode at the lower

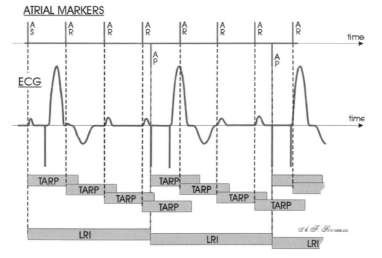

Figure 14.13 Diagrammatic representation of retriggerable atrial refractory periods. All the atrial events are detected by the atrial channel outside the blanking periods which are not shown. There is an atrial tachycardia and the first atrial event is sensed (As). The next atrial signal (Ar) falls in the unblanked portion of the PVARP and is sensed. This signal does not start an AVI but it initiates a new total atrial refractory period (TARP). Continual retriggering of the TARP by the rapid atrial rate causes operation of the pacemaker in the DVI mode at the lower rate interval (LRI). Note that the emission of an atrial stimulus also reinitiates the TARP. Abbreviations as in Figure 14.1. (Reproduced from [3] with permission.)

rate, or the DVIR mode according to design and programmability. The function of dual-demand anti-tachycardia pacemakers is based on this concept. The atrial stimulus emitted at the end of the atrial escape interval also initiates another TARP. The TARPs will continue to be reinitiated and overlap until the P–P interval lengthens beyond the duration of the TARP whereupon the pacemaker will regain normal AV synchrony. Instantaneous resynchronization occurs when an atrial event occurs outside the TARP, or an atrial paced event is initiated at the termination of the atrial escape interval. Rapid oscillations of the paced ventricular rate may occur with intermittent atrial undersensing.

Competitive (asynchronous) atrial pacing occurs during SVT. Upper rate control with fixed-ratio AV block obviously cannot occur in designs with a retriggerable atrial refractory period, but a Wenckebach upper rate response is possible only if the upper rate interval is greater than the TARP.

The Vitatron Diamond and Clarity DDDR pacemakers employ a physiologic band to define normal vs. pathologic atrial rate [42,43]. A physiologic atrial rate is calculated from the running average of the actual sensed or paced atrial beats and the rate change in this moving average is limited to 2 b.p.m. The physiologic band is defined by an upper boundary equal to the physiologic rate plus 15 b.p.m. (minimum value of 100 b.p.m.) and the lower boundary by the physiologic rate minus 15 b.p.m. (or the sensor-indicated rate if it is higher). As the physiologic rate during sensor driven pacing will be determined by the sensor, it follows that SVT detection is sensor based when the sensor is active. If an atrial event occurs above the upper boundary of the physiologic band, it is not tracked and AMS to DDIR mode will occur. The paced ventricular rate is the sensor-indicated rate or lower boundary of the physiologic band, whichever is higher. It seems inappropriate to activate AMS after a single atrial premature beat. For this reason, after every atrial sensed event that is not tracked secondary to AMS, the pacemaker tries to pace the atrium with an atrial 'resynchronization' beat that is delivered with a safety delay after the atrial sensed beat. The mode switch feature can be programmed as either 'auto' or 'fixed'. If the automatic mode is programmed, the SVT detection rate varies with the upper boundary of the physiologic band and allows AMS to occur below the upper rate. When programmed to the fixed mode, the SVT detection rate is equal to the upper rate and AMS is allowed only when the atrial rate exceeds the upper rate.

The Vitatron Diamond II DDDR pacemaker can respond to atrial flutter by generating ventricular paced cycles varying by about 40 ms during automatic mode switching to the DDIR mode [44]. The device activates mode switching on a beat-to-beat basis and exhibits 'ventricular hysteresis' in the DDIR mode when an atrial sensed event is detected during the period corresponding with the (implied) AV delay prior to emission of the ventricular stimulus (Figure 14.14). Such unusual behavior must not be interpreted as pacemaker malfunction.

New mode-switching algorithms

New concepts have been developed to accelerate appropriate AMS activation and prevent inappropriate AMS due to VA crosstalk or short atrial runs. The Medtronic AT500 pacemaker uses the PR Logic algorithm found in Medtronic dual-chamber defibrillators (Jewel AF, Gem series, Marquis DR) to control mode-switching operation [45,46]. The device evaluates two criteria: the atrial cycle length, and evidence of atrial tachycardia based on the pattern of atrial and ventricular events (evidence counter). The median of the most recent 12 atrial intervals (PP median equivalent to the longest of the two middle values) must be shorter than the programmed AT detection zone (the zone the device can be programmed to treat with antitachycardia pacing). If the PP median is less than this programmed value, the device then evaluates the 'AT/AF Evidence Counter'. The AT/AF Evidence Counter increases by 1 when there are two or more intrinsic atrial events between ventricular events and there is no evidence of far-field R-wave sensing (discussed below). The counter decreases by 1 if, for two beats, the criteria to increase the counter are not met—namely if atrial pacing occurs or if there is only one atrial sensed event within the next ventricular cycle. When the counter reaches 3, and the PP median is less than the programmed AT detection interval, the device mode switches to the DDIR mode.

The dedicated algorithm for ventricular far-field detection (e.g. PR Logic™) is a promising system for optimal AT detection with improved discrimination between far-field R-wave oversensing and AT. It

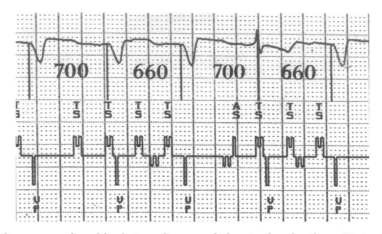

Figure 14.14 Simultaneous recording of the electrocardiogram and telemetered markers from a Vitatron Diamond II DDDR pacemaker during 'slow' atrial flutter (atrial rate about 220 b.p.m.) producing automatic mode switching to the DDIR mode. The prevailing paced rate is sensor controlled and faster than the programmed lower rate. The ventricular pacing cycles (VP–VP) alternate between 660 and 700 ms. Atrial signals in the postventricular atrial blanking period are unsensed. AS is an atrial sensed event that falls in the physiologic band (proprietary) and is classified as a normal atrial sensed event. TS is an atrial sensed event labeled as a tachycardia event because it occurs outside the physiologic band. A physiologic atrial rate (proprietary) is calculated from the running average of the actual sensed or paced atrial beats. The physiologic band is defined by an upper boundary equal to the physiologic rate plus 15 b.p.m. (minimum value of 100 b.p.m.), and the lower boundary by the physiologic rate minus 15 b.p.m. (or the sensor-indicated rate if it is higher). Atrial tachycardia sensed events (TS) detected just before completion of the ventricular lower rate interval induce slightly longer VP–VP intervals (700 ms). The short double marker pointing down represents T-wave sensing for input into the QT sensor. Note that cycle alternation is more evident in the marker channel recording because of the greater delay in the emission of VP when it is closely preceded by a TS event (Reproduced from [44] with permission.)

takes into account atrial rate/cycle length, AV association, AV, AA and VA intervals, and the number of atrial events between ventricular signals. The AT 500 pacemaker has a PVAB of 0 after ventricular sensing and 30 ms after ventricular pacing. The minimal blanking times provide a very large atrial sensing window to activate the AMS algorithm. The AMS algorithm of the AT 500 device therefore relies on data that must be appropriately interpreted by the PR logic of the system. A dedicated algorithm identifies ventricular far-field oversensing if a short–long pattern of atrial intervals is detected together with a short PR interval (< 60 ms) or a short RP interval (< 160 ms) in the preceding 12 ventricular cycles. If ventricular far-field oversensing is detected, the respective cycles will not be used for atrial tachyarrhythmia detection. This complex AMS algorithm is combined with an atrial sensitivity adjustment algorithm which in effect replaces long atrial blanking periods after ventricular pacing by very short ones combined with a period of reduced atrial sensitivity after a ventricular stimulus (e.g. 1.2 mV for 100 ms). These features have virtually eliminated the problem of VA crosstalk with atrial

leads implanted at conventional sites. The increased accuracy of atrial arrhythmia detection is of particular importance in this device which can deliver antitachycardia pacing to sustained atrial tachyarrhythmias.

Towards more meaningful SVT detection and storage

Devices with fast-reacting mode-switching algorithms can store many relatively unimportant unsustained AT episodes that quickly fill up the memory capacity. Thus, the number of recorded mode-switching episodes may be misleading in assessing the presence and frequency of intermittent atrial fibrillation. In some systems, there is a fast AT detection algorithm to allow rapid mode switching followed by confirmation of sustained AT (during which AMS is already operating) that ensures storage for only sustained AT episodes, thereby discarding clinically irrelevant shorter AT episodes. Thus, storage of an AT episode (including its onset) occurs according to the tachycardia detection criteria of the AMS algorithm only if the

AT persists beyond this confirmation period. For example in the Medtronic AT 500 device, atrial detection is totally independent of mode switching. The AT diagnostics system and the AMS algorithm share the same counter which is incremented to trigger mode switching and atrial diagnostics, and they both use the same detection interval. The nominal 24 beats for diagnostic logging of SVT episodes is programmable from 12 to 128 beats. Event markers and electrograms (EGMs) from the time of arrhythmia onset and mode switch are frozen in device memory and only stored if the subsequent confirmation of the episode occurs.

Some devices provide another monitor to count the number of 'atrial high-rate episodes'. These may be programmed to detection criteria different from those of mode switching. For example, high atrial rate detection may occur if a rate above 200 b.p.m. is sensed for 10 s, and its termination may require 10 consecutive beats below this value. These more stringent criteria are generally not useful for effective mode switching function because of the high risk of AT underdetection and patient symptoms associated with maintaining the DDD pacing mode during this confirmation period. For example, the Medtronic Kappa 900 pacemaker permits the selection of either mode-switching diagnostics or high atrial rate diagnostics. If the mode-switch diagnostic function is selected, the AT rate that triggers memory storage of the episode is the same as the one that causes mode switching. If atrial high-rate diagnostics is selected, the rate that triggers data collection may be different from the mode-switching trigger rate (and mode-switching episodes will not be stored).

Special considerations and future directions

1 *Signal morphology.* Optimal discrimination between small atrial fibrillation potentials and far-field R-wave oversensing will be achieved if signal morphology criteria beyond mere amplitude are incorporated for atrial detection.

2 *Automatic adjustment of atrial sensitivity.* Intermittent atrial undersensing during atrial fibrillation is a common cause of AMS failure. While this can be partially offset by the use of a running average (MAR) algorithm, this necessarily slows the onset of AMS. A fixed atrial sensitivity setting for atrial fibrillation sensing is not optimal for AMS function because there is substantial variability of the atrial

electrogram amplitude during atrial fibrillation [47, 48]. Thus atrial sensitivity should vary throughout the atrial cycle, being high at the time when an atrial signal is expected and low at the time when a ventricular far-field signal is expected.

3 *Detection of termination of atrial tachyarrhythmia.* Similar to detection of SVT onset, the reliable detection of its termination also determines AMS performance. If premature sinus rhythm redetection occurs from intermittent undersensing of atrial fibrillation, inappropriately high and irregular ventricular pacing may result and lead to 'mode oscillations' (permanent alternation between detection of SVT and sinus rhythm redetection). On the other hand, if criteria for switching back to the tracking mode are very stringent, atrial premature beats may significantly delay return to the DDD pacing mode and prolong ventricular pacing in the DDI or DDIR mode during sinus rhythm. Therefore, criteria for sinus rhythm redetection should be programmable (e.g. 'x out of y' with the 'x' value programmable independently from onset detection criteria).

4 *Sophisticated algorithms.* Algorithms developed for ICDs will also be used in pacemakers for the improved diagnosis of arrhythmias and elimination of false-positive AMS. The PR Logic of the Medtronic AT 500 pacemaker is an example of such an intelligent algorithm.

5 *Memory.* Pacemaker memory functions should provide insights into AMS performance [49,50]. For optimal interpretation, stored EGMs require the following:

(a) Separate channels for atrial and ventricular EGMs of sufficient resolution and duration. The summated (superimposed) atrial and ventricular EGMs in a single channel are not able to distinguish atrial premature beats or atrial flutter from far-field R-wave sensing.

(b) An EGM scale should be available to quantify signal amplitude.

(c) Onset data. Stored EGMs should include a programmable number of cardiac cycles before arrhythmia onset ('pretrigger EGM').

(d) Annotations. To facilitate understanding of why and how the pacemaker detected and classified an event, stored EGMs need to be annotated with markers and intervals. An additional marker annotation (e.g. arrow, line) should indicate the exact moment when arrhythmia detection criteria were fulfilled.

(e) Selective EGM storage.

To avoid consumption of device memory by unimportant information (short atrial tachyarrhythmia episodes of few seconds, short episodes of ventricular far-field oversensing), different criteria should be available for AMS that should be performed rapidly to avoid fast tracking, and episode storage that should only consider sustained atrial tachyarrhythmias.

6 *Manual readjustment.* This needs to be available if memory functions demonstrate that automatic parameter adjustment fails or needs to be optimized.

7 *Device intelligence and learning capability.* The pacemaker should 'learn' the patient's most likely rhythms and optimize SVT detection parameters and pacing responses to individual conditions.

References

1 Mond HG, Barold SS. Dual chamber rate adaptive pacing in patients with paroxysmal supraventricular tachyarrhythmias. Protective measures for rate control. *Pacing Clin Electrophysiol* 1993; **16**: 2168–84.

2 Barold SS. Timing cycles and operational characteristics of pacemakers. In: Ellenbogen K, Kay GN, Wilkoff B, eds. *Clinical Cardiac Pacing and Defibrillation*, 2nd edn. Philadelphia, PA: W. B. Saunders, 2000: 727–825.

3 Stroobandt RX, Barold SS, Vandenbulcke FD *et al.* A reappraisal of pacemaker timing cycles pertaining to automatic mode switching. *J Interv Card Electrophysiol* 2001; **5**: 417–29.

4 Lau CP, Leung SK, Tse HF *et al.* Automatic mode switching of implanted pacemakers: I. Principles of instrumentation, clinical, and hemodynamic considerations. *Pacing Clin Electrophysiol* 2002; **25**: 967–83.

5 Lau CP, Leung SK, Tse HF *et al.* Automatic mode switching of implantable pacemakers. II. Clinical performance of current algorithms and their programming. *Pacing Clin Electrophysiol* 2002; **25**: 1094–113.

6 Israel CW, Barold SS. Automatic mode switching. Basic concepts and overview. In: Israel CW, Barold SS, eds. *Advances in the Treatment of Atrial Tachycardias: Pacing, Cardioversion and Defibrillation*. Armonk, NY: Futura, 2002: 193–218.

7 Kay GN, Bubien RS. Algorithms for management of atrial fibrillation in patients with dual chamber pacing systems. In: Rosenqvist M, ed. *Cardiac Pacing. New Advances*. London: W. B. Saunders, 1997: 61–82.

8 Ellenbogen KA, Wood MA, Mond HG *et al.* Clinical applications of mode switching for dual-chamber pacemakers. In: Singer I, Barold SS, Camm AJ, eds. *Nonpharmacological Therapy of Arrhythmias for the 21st Century. The State of the Art.* Armonk, NY: Futura, 1998: 819–44.

9 Sutton R, Stack Z, Heaven D *et al.* Mode switching for atrial tachyarrhythmias. *Am J Cardiol* 1999; **83**: 202D–210D.

10 Israel CW. Analysis of mode switching algorithms in dual chamber pacemakers. *Pacing Clin Electrophysiol* 2002; **25**: 380–93.

11 Wood MA, Swerdlow C, Olson WH. Sensing and arrhythmia detection in implantable devices. In: Ellenbogen K, Kay N, Wilkoff B, eds. *Clinical Cardiac Pacing and Defibrillation*, 2nd edn. Philadelphia, PA: W. B. Saunders, 2000: 68–126.

12 Fu EY, Ellenbogen KA. Management of atrial tachyarrhythmias in patients with implantable devices. *Cardiol Clin* 2000; **18**: 37–53.

13 Wiegand UK, Bode F, Peters W *et al.* Efficacy and safety of bipolar sensing with high atrial sensitivity in dual chamber pacemakers. *Pacing Clin Electrophysiol* 2000; **23**: 427–33.

14 Nowak B, Kraker S, Rippin G *et al.* Effect of the atrial blanking time on the detection of atrial fibrillation in dual chamber pacing. *Pacing Clin Electrophysiol* 2001; **24**: 496–9.

15 Johnson WB, Bailin SJ, Solinger B *et al.* Frequency of inappropriate automatic pacemaker mode switching as assessed 6–8 weeks post implantation [abstract]. *Pacing Clin Electrophysiol* 1996; **19**: 720.

16 Fröhlig G, Kindermann M, Heisel A *et al.* Mode switch without atrial tachyarrhythmias [abstract]. *Pacing Clin Electrophysiol* 1996; **19**: 592.

17 Fitts SM, Hill MR, Mehra R *et al.* High rate atrial tachycardia detections in implantable pulse generators: low incidence of false-positive detections. The PA Clinical Trial Investigators. *Pacing Clin Electrophysiol* 2000; **23**: 1080–6.

18 Leung SK, Lau CP, Lam CT-F *et al.* Programmed atrial sensitivity: a critical determinant in atrial fibrillation detection and optimal automatic mode switching *Pacing Clin Electrophysiol* 1998; **21**: 2214–19.

19 Wood MA, Moskovljevic P, Stambler BS *et al.* Comparison of bipolar atrial electrogram amplitude in sinus rhythm, atrial fibrillation, and atrial flutter. *Pacing Clin Electrophysiol* 1996; **19**: 150–6.

20 Walfridsson H, Aunes M, Capocci M *et al.* Sensing of atrial fibrillation by a dual chamber pacemaker: how should atrial sensing be programmed to ensure adequate mode shift? *Pacing Clin Electrophysiol* 2000; **23**: 1089–93.

21 Brandt J, Fåhraeus T, Schüller H. Far-field QRS complex sensing via the atrial pacemaker lead. II. Prevalence, clinical significance and possibility of intraoperative prediction in DDD pacing. *Pacing Clin Electrophysiol* 1988; **11**: 1540–4.

22 Brouwer J, Nagelkerke D, den Heijer P *et al.* Analysis of atrial sensed far-field ventricular signals: a reassessment. *Pacing Clin Electrophysiol* 1997; **20**: 916–22.

23 Nowak B, Kramm B, Schwaier H *et al.* Is atrial sensing of ventricular far-field signals important in single-lead VDD pacing? *Pacing Clin Electrophysiol* 1998; **21**: 2236–9.

24 Fröhlig G, Helwani Z, Kusch O *et al.* Bipolar ventricular far-field signals in the atrium. *Pacing Clin Electrophysiol* 1999; **22**: 1604–14.

25 Brandt J, Worzewski W. Far-field QRS complex sensing: prevalence and timing with bipolar atrial leads. *Pacing Clin Electrophysiol* 2000; **23**: 315–20.

26 Theres H, Sun W, Combs W *et al.* P wave and far-field R wave detection in pacemaker patient atrial electrogram. *Pacing Clin Electrophysiol* 2000; **23**: 434–40.

27 Maury P, Schlaepfer J, Arbane M *et al.* Incessant atrioventricular dissociation due to far-field oversensing and recurrent mode switch in a dual chamber pacemaker. *Europace* 2002; **4**: 149–53.

28 Weretka S, Becker R, Hilbel T *et al.* Far-field R wave oversensing in a dual chamber arrhythmia management device: predisposing factors and practical implications. *Pacing Clin Electrophysiol* 2001; **24**: 1240–6.

29 Kuruvilla C, Voigt L, Kachmar K *et al.* Inappropriate mode switching in a dual chamber pacemaker due to oversensing of a high frequency signal from conductor/ring discontinuity (loose set screw). *Pacing Clin Electrophysiol* 2002; **25**: 115–17.

30 Ellenbogen KA, Mond HG, Wood MA *et al.* Failure of automatic mode switching: recognition and management. *Pacing Clin Electrophysiol* 1997; **20**: 268–75.

31 Israel CW. Automatic mode switching based on a '4 out of 7' algorithm in Medtronic Kappa 700 dual chamber pacemaker systems. *Herzschr Elektrophys* 1999; **10** (Suppl. 1): I/32–I/45.

32 Dodinot B. Effondrement de la fréquence de stimulation à l'effort. *Stimucoeur* 2000; **28**: 89–92.

33 Sutton R, Stack Z, Bruls A. Tiered management of atrial arrhythmias: the Pulsar Max™ family of pacemakers. *Herzschr Elektrophys* 1999; **10** (Suppl. 1): I/8–I/14.

34 Leung SK, Lau CP, Lam CT *et al.* A comparative study on the behavior of three different automatic mode switching dual chamber pacemakers to intracardiac recordings of clinical atrial fibrillation. *Pacing Clin Electrophysiol* 2000; **23**: 2086–96.

35 Levine PA, Bornzin GA, Hauck G *et al.* Implementation of automatic mode switching in Pacesetter's Trilogy DR+ and Affinity DR pulse generators. *Herzschr Elektrophys* 1999; **10** (Suppl. 1): I/46–I/57.

36 Barold SS, Levine PA. Pacemaker repetitive nonreentrant ventriculoatrial synchronous rhythm. A review. *J Interv Card Electrophysiol* 2001; **5**: 45–58.

37 Sweeney MO. Novel cause of spurious mode switching in dual chamber pacemakers: atrioventricular desynchronization arrhythmia. *J Cardiovasc Electrophysiol* 2002; **13**: 616–19.

38 Gencel L, Géroux L, Clementy J *et al.* Ventricular protection against atrial arrhythmias in DDD pacing based on a statistical approach: clinical results. *Pacing Clin Electrophysiol* 1996; **19**: 1729–33.

39 Géroux L, Limousin M, Cazeau S. Clinical performance of a new mode switch function based on a statistical analysis of the atrial rhythm. *Herzschr Elektrophys* 1999; **10** (Suppl. 1): I/15–I/21.

40 Barold SS, Byrd CL. Automatic mode switching variants: dual demand pacing, retriggerable atrial refractory periods, automatic mode adaptation, and pseudomode switching. Enlightenment or obfuscation? *Pacing Clin Electrophysiol* 2000; **23**: 1065–7.

41 Jayaprakash S, Sparks PB, Kalman JM *et al.* Dual demand pacing using retriggerable refractory periods for ventricular rate control during paroxysmal supraventricular tachyarrhythmias in patients with dual chamber pacemakers. *Pacing Clin Electrophysiol* 2000; **23**: 1156–63.

42 Israel CW. Automatic 'beat-to-beat' mode-switch: Advantages, possible problems and recommendations to optimize programming. *Herzschrittmacher* 1999; **19**: 88–108.

43 Boute W. Beat-to-beat mode switching for effective ventricular rate control in the presence of atrial tachyarrhythmias—how to maintain a stable ventricular rhythm. *Herzschr Elektrophys* 1999; **10** (Suppl. 1): I/22–I/31.

44 Barold SS, Sayad D, Gallardo I. Alternating duration of ventricular paced cycles during automatic mode switching of a DDDR pacemaker. *J Interv Card Electrophysiol* 2002; **7**: 185–7.

45 Barold SS, Cantens F. Characterization of the 16 blanking periods of the GEM DR dual chamber defibrillators. *J Interv Card Electrophysiol* 2001; **5**: 319–25.

46 Israel CW, Gronefeld G, Elrlich JR *et al.* Suppression of atrial tachyarrhythmias by pacing. *J Cardiovasc Electrophysiol* 2002; **13** (1 Suppl.): S31–S39.

47 Lam CTF, Lau CP, Leung SK *et al.* Improved efficacy of mode switching during atrial fibrillation using automatic atrial sensitivity adjustment. *Pacing Clin Electrophysiol* 1999; **22**: 17–25.

48 Wood MA, Ellenbogen KA, Dinsmoor D *et al.* Influence of autothreshold sensing and sinus rate on mode switching algorithm behavior. *Pacing Clin Electrophysiol* 2000; **23**: 1473–8.

49 Israel CW, Barold SS. Pacemaker systems as implantable cardiac rhythm monitors. *Am J Cardiol* 2001; **88**: 442–5.

50 Nowak B. Pacemaker stored electrogram: teaching us what is really going on in our patients. *Pacing Clin Electrophysiol* 2002; **25**: 838–49.

CHAPTER 15

Pacemaker Memory: Diagnosis of Atrial Tachyarrhythmias

Carsten W. Israel and S. Serge Barold

Introduction

The diagnosis of atrial tachyarrhythmias (ATs) in pacemakers enhances clinical care in the following situations:

1 detection of atrial flutter for which curative ablative therapy (cavotricuspid isthmus ablation) is available;

2 correlation of symptoms (e.g. palpitations, perception of a fast heart beat or presyncope) with registered data;

3 evaluation of pharmacologic treatment such as rhythm or rate control in patients with paroxysmal atrial fibrillation;

4 optimal pacemaker programming, e.g. automatic mode-switching function;

5 need for anticoagulation in patients with paroxysmal atrial fibrillation; and

6 detection of progression of underlying cardiac disease.

In certain forms of ATs (atrioventricular (AV) nodal reentry tachycardia, AV reentry tachycardia) only the surface electrocardiogram (ECG) may provide the diagnosis. In these ATs, the pacemaker is only a bystander and usually unable to detect these arrhythmias or to store the episodes in its memory because the atrial signal typically occurs simultaneously with or shortly after the ventricular signal and thus coincides with the postventricular atrial blanking period. However, these ATs are rare in pacemaker patients. Therefore, this chapter focuses on the diagnosis of atrial fibrillation, different forms of atrial flutter, and ectopic atrial tachycardia in patients with implanted dualchamber pacemakers.

Diagnosis of atrial tachyarrhythmias in pacemaker patients

Many ATs remain undetected, partly because of the paroxysmal, self-terminating nature of most episodes. In a patient with a single 2-h episode of atrial fibrillation every 2 months, it is very unlikely that the arrhythmia will be detected by a resting ECG during pacemaker follow-up or with a 24-h Holter recording. Furthermore the interpretation of the pacemaker ECG during AT can be difficult because the rather tiny deflections of atrial fibrillation may be missed, especially during continuous pacing [1]. In the presence of high-grade atrial undersensing of atrial fibrillation, the emission of atrial stimuli may even be misinterpreted as successful atrial capture. Similarly, during regular VVI pacing it may be difficult to distinguish fine atrial fibrillation from sinus rhythm with retrograde P waves obscured by the T wave.

Although telemetric recording of marker annotations and intracardiac electrograms (EGMs) aid the detection of otherwise inapparent atrial fibrillation or atrial flutter occurring during a follow-up visit (Figure 15.1), the memory function of devices offers much higher accuracy by virtue of continuous monitoring and recording of abnormal atrial rates.

Counter functions

The most basic memory function in pacemakers consists of simple counting of detected ATs and presenting the result as a number at the time of device interrogation. Systems report detection of a certain number of AT episodes, commonly in the form of a

Figure 15.1 Atrial flutter with 2 : 1 atrioventricular conduction in a Kappa 700™ DDDR pacemaker (Medtronic). From the surface ECG (lead I on top), atrial flutter is difficult to detect because every second atrial flutter wave is obscured by the T wave. The marker recordings (shown in the middle) depict only every second flutter potential. However, the simultaneously recorded atrial electrogram (bottom) documents that every second atrial flutter potential is not sensed (arrow) because it falls into the postventricular atrial blanking period. This causes 2 : 1 tracking of atrial flutter. Paper speed 25 mm/s. AS, atrial sense; AR, refractory atrial sense; VP, ventricular pace.

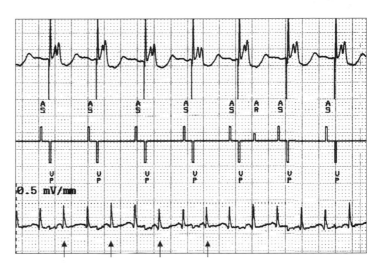

number of automatic mode-switching episodes as a surrogate for the ATs. However, if the mode-switching function is programmed to a very sensitive setting (e.g. beat-to-beat mode switching), the counter may report many such events based upon the quick conversion to a non-tracking mode in response to short atrial runs or far-field R-wave oversensing (Figure 15.2). Intermittent atrial undersensing is common during atrial fibrillation and can result in incorrect detection of AT termination. In this situation, the device soon redetects atrial fibrillation and activates another mode switch which again ends prematurely due to atrial undersensing. Apart from disadvantageous effects on pacing performance, these pacing mode oscillations register a high number of mode switches and quickly increase the counter for mode-switching episodes (Figure 15.3). Thus, a counter report of many recorded AT episodes does not prove that the patient experienced intermittent spontaneous conversion to sinus rhythm (and presumably cardioversion not being necessary) since a single AT episode may be cut into numerous short pieces by the mode-switching algorithm in the presence of intermittent undersensing of the AT. Similarly, a patient with many recorded mode-switching episodes may be falsely considered to spend a high percentage of time in AT when, in fact, only frequent short atrial runs have occurred.

Some devices offer different criteria for mode switching and AT detection. The combination of a rapid and very sensitive mode-switching algorithm and a stringent and very specific AT detection algorithm, both with separate counters, improves the reliability of AT diagnosis by counter data. For instance, in Kappa 700™ dual-chamber systems (Medtronic, Inc.) mode switching occurs if the duration of 4 out of 7 atrial cycles is sensed below a programmable mode-switching cycle length (e.g. 343 ms for a mode-switching rate at 175 b.p.m.) or if the Blanked Flutter Search™ finds a single short interval [2]. Switch back to tracking mode occurs as soon as 5 consecutive beats are paced or 7 consecutive beats are sensed at a normal rate. This mode-switching algorithm reacts very fast and can even be triggered by single atrial premature beats or ventricular far-field signals [3] (Figure 15.4). Thus, the number of mode-switching episodes may be misleading in assessing the presence and frequency of intermittent atrial fibrillation. Therefore, another monitor counts the number of 'atrial high-rate episodes'. These may be programmed to detection criteria different from those of mode switching; for example, high atrial rate detection may occur if a rate above 200 b.p.m. is sensed for 10 s, and its termination may require 10 consecutive beats below this value. These more stringent criteria are generally not useful for effective mode-switching function because of the high risk of AT underdetection and consequent rapid and irregular tracking of AT.

In conclusion, counter data may be useful in the diagnosis of ATs in pacemaker patients but they

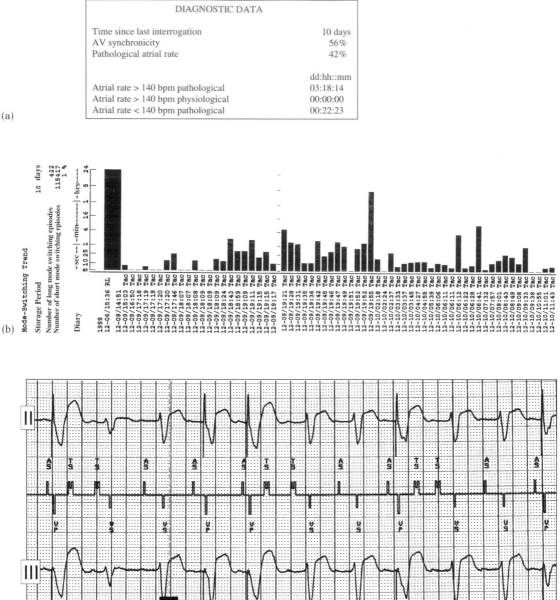

Figure 15.2 Counter report of numerous false-positive mode-switching episodes in a Vitatron Diamond™ 3 DDDR pacemaker (Vitatron). At a follow-up visit 10 days after DDDR pacemaker implantation, the counter reported pacing in the AV synchronous mode for only 56% of the time, and a fast pathologic atrial rate for 42% of the time (a). The 'Mode-Switching Trend' histogram confirms that during the preceding 10 days, 422 long and 115 417 short mode-switching episodes occurred, typically lasting less than 4 min (b). However, telemetry (leads II and III, in the middle marker annotation channel, paper speed 25 mm/s) demonstrates that these mode-switching episodes were most likely caused by periodic far-field T-wave oversensing (c). After an AV synchronous paced ventricular complex (VP, ventricular pace), the T wave is sensed in the atrium (TS, tachy sense) causing a short interval also to the next regular P wave. This P wave is no longer tracked because the beat-to-beat mode-switching algorithm changed the pacing mode to DDIR. However, the P wave is conducted and the intrinsic ventricular complex (VS, ventricular sense) does not exhibit T-wave oversensing by the atrial channel. Therefore, detecting the second normal atrial interval, the pacemaker switches back to the DDDR mode. The second ventricular paced beat is a fusion beat and is not associated with T-wave oversensing by the atrial channel. All subsequent ventricular paced beats cause T-wave oversensing by the atrial channel and mode switching again ('mode oscillation'). This behavior may explain the very high number of short mode-switching episodes in this patient.

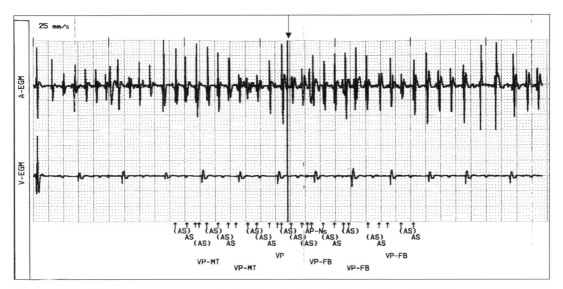

Figure 15.3 Stored electrogram in a patient with multiple atrial tachyarrhythmia (AT) episodes (Pulsar max™ II DR, Guidant). In this patient, the counter reported that 6432 AT episodes had occurred within the preceding 30 days, each lasting only few minutes. However, the electrogram (A-EGM, atrial electrogram; V-EGM, ventricular electrogram) stored at the moment of detection of AT by the device (black line, highlighted by an arrow) shows an AT episode already in progress. It is likely that this patient with persistent atrial fibrillation for several months had only one sustained AT episode which was cut into 6432 short pieces secondary to intermittent atrial undersensing of small fibrillation potentials (note changes in A-EGM amplitude) resulting in repeated premature mode-switching termination and AT redetection. AS, atrial sense; (AS), atrial sense in the refractory period, AP-Ns, noise; VP, ventricular pace; VP-MT, VP at maximum tracking rate; VP-FB, VP during fallback; paper speed 25 mm/s.

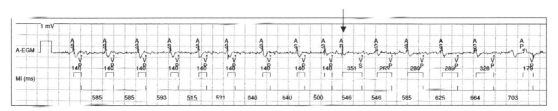

Figure 15.4 Inappropriate mode switching triggered by a single atrial premature beat in a Kappa 700™ DDD pacemaker (Medtronic). This atrial electrogram (A-EGM) stored upon the start of mode switching shows regular sinus rhythm with a single atrial premature beat (arrow). This beat occurred fortuitously in the period dedicated to detection of blanked atrial flutter so that it immediately triggered mode switching to the DDIR mode (note the successive prolongation of the AV delay to 328 ms). Such mode-switching episodes are not useful as a surrogate for ATs in this patient. Paper speed 25 mm/s; MI, marker intervals in ms.

always require confirmation with stored EGMs. AT diagnosis by counter data alone is not feasible and potentially misleading when signals such as myopotentials or far-field R waves are interpreted as AT.

Other numerical memory data

Several numerical data for AT diagnosis are available in modern dual-chamber pacemakers. Some systems report the exact time (date, hour, min, s) of

AT detection, the duration of an AT episode, and its maximum or mean rate. These data may be useful for assessing the maximum AT duration in an individual patient and the need for anticoagulation. The dosage or timing of antiarrhythmic drugs can be optimized using these data, and information about the arrhythmia mechanism may be derived, e.g. if it starts only at night. However, these data alone are of little value if they cannot be verified by stored AT episodes. Apart from limitations of counter data of

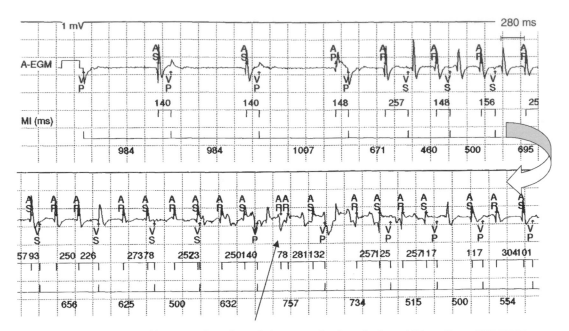

Figure 15.5 Double counting of fractionated atrial signals during atrial tachyarrhythmia (AT) in a Kappa 700™ DDD pacemaker (Medtronic). In this atrial electrogram (A-EGM) stored upon mode switching, there is a very regular AT with a cycle length of 280 ms. However, one interval as short as 78 ms is sensed (arrow), presumably due to double counting of a split potential (beyond the blanking period of about 50 ms). Thus, the counter characterizes this episode erroneously as having a maximum atrial rate > 400 b.p.m. suggestive of atrial fibrillation. Paper speed 25 mm/s; for marker annotations see Figure 15.4.

the number and duration of AT episodes outlined above, the maximum atrial rate during AT (tempting to use for discrimination of atrial flutter and fibrillation) may be misleading in the presence of atrial oversensing or double counting of atrial potentials during AT (Figure 15.5).

Some newer devices report the cumulative time or 'AT burden' during which the patient experienced AT, usually expressed as a percentage of the follow-up period or in hours per week. This parameter may be more useful than others (such as the number of AT episodes or the time to first recurrence) for assessing the success of treatment. In this respect the number of AT episodes may not reflect the severity of disease because, during a period of 6 months, one patient may experience 300 episodes of 3 s each (AT burden < 1%) while another may have only a single sustained episode (AT burden 100%). The AT burden is also less vulnerable than the data on the number of AT episodes in the setting of intermittent atrial undersensing during atrial fibrillation. In a patient with a single sustained episode of atrial fibrillation, the device may report about 500 AT episodes secondary to intermittent atrial undersensing. However, as the periods of atrial fibrillation undersensing are usually short, the AT burden may still be above 90% in this situation. Device-derived AT burden also requires confirmation by stored AT episodes. In the case of severe atrial undersensing, the true AT burden would be much higher, while it may be significantly lower if predominantly atrial oversensing activated AT detection.

Histograms

Several forms of graphic representations of stored data aid the assessment of frequency and duration of ATs. The most common form is an atrial rate histogram (Figure 15.6). This may display the percentage of atrial beats sensed at a high rate during follow-up. However, during a monitoring period of 6 months, approximately 20 million atrial beats will occur. Even an AT episode of 200 000 beats (> 16 h) sensed at a rate > 180 b.p.m. will only represent 1% of atrial beats and will be invisible in a

Follow-up period: Dec 30, 1998 to Apr 13, 1999 (104 days)

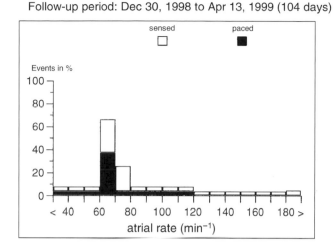

Initial Interrogation
Mode   DDI
Lower rate   60 bpm

Total Atrial Beats   10 215 214
Atrial Runs   121 158

(a)

Follow-up period: Apr 08, 1999 to Apr 13, 1999 (5 days)

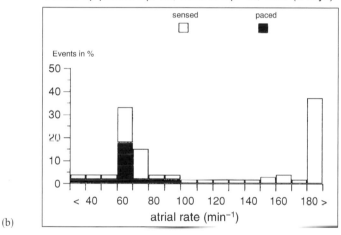

Initial Interrogation
Mode   DDI
Lower rate   60 bpm

Total Atrial Beats   759 315
Atrial Runs   > 65 534

(b)

Figure 15.6 Atrial rate histograms in a Kappa 700™ DDD pacemaker (Medtronic). In this example, the device offers short- and long-term atrial rate histograms for the preceding follow-up period. (a) The long-term histogram covers a time period of 104 days during which 10 215 214 atrial beats were sensed. The percentage of atrial beats sensed at a rate > 180 b.p.m. seems rather low and not suggestive of AT. (b) The short-term histogram of the same pacemaker interrogation summarizes the sensed atrial rates for 5 days before pacemaker interrogation. Now the percentage of atrial rates > 180 b.p.m. of more than 35% may indicate the occurrence of AT.

long-term atrial rate histogram (Figure 15.6a). This problem can be avoided if an additional short-term rate histogram displays the sensed atrial rate during some days before interrogation (Figure 15.6b). However, the interpretation of atrial rate histograms for AT diagnosis presents two fundamental problems: (i) inability to distinguish sustained AT from frequent atrial premature beats in the case of a high percentage of fast (short cycle length) atrial beats (50% of fast atrial beats may represent either an ongoing AT or supraventricular bigeminy); and

(ii) inability to exclude oversensing of far-field R-wave potentials when atrial events are sensed at a high rate.

Histograms displaying the distribution of the maximum rate and the duration of ATs are used to characterize the type of AT (Figure 15.7). Sensed fast atrial rates in a single rate bin may indicate far-field R-wave oversensing with a constant and short ventriculoatrial (VA) interval. However, atrial flutter with a constant cycle length or premature atrial beats with a constant coupling interval may

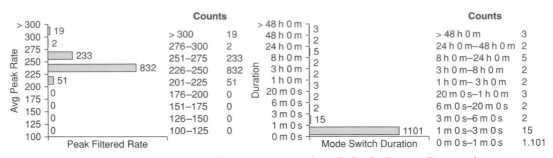

Figure 15.7 Mode-switching histogram in an Affinity™ DDDR (St. Jude Medical). This diagram illustrates the maximum sensed rate during atrial tachyarrhythmia (AT) episodes (left panel) as a discriminator between atrial fibrillation or flutter, and the device-based AT duration (right panel). However, the AT duration may be misleading if intermittent atrial undersensing is registered as premature AT termination.

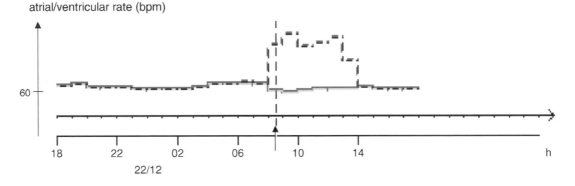

Figure 15.8 Atrial and ventricular rate diagram during 24 h (Talent™ DDDR pacemaker, Ela Medical). The diagram provides the mean atrial (dotted line) and ventricular (solid line) rate during 24 h. At 8 AM, the two lines separate, indicating the onset of an AT which terminated at approximately 2 PM. This monitor provides a useful overview for detection of AV asynchronous pacing at a glance. Arrow/dashed line, mode-switching operation.

also produce the same recording. Like counter data, registration of AT episode duration in histograms is misleading if a single episode is cut into many short fragments because of intermittent atrial undersensing. Similarly, the bar graph for the maximum atrial rate detected during AT may be misleading in the presence of oversensing or double counting (cf. Figure 15.5).

A graphic representation of the atrial and ventricular rate in a single diagram provides a useful overview about the time that the patient was paced in an AV synchronous mode or an asynchronous DDIR/VDIR mode due to AT and mode switching (Figure 15.8). Again, short periods of AT may not be detected depending on the time resolution of this diagram, and AV asynchronous pacing may be due to causes other than AT, particularly ventricular far-field oversensing. Both criticisms also apply to 24-h atrial rate histograms that display the mean

atrial rate for every 20–60 min during the day preceding interrogation.

AT episode storage

AT diagnosis based on memory data requires accurate retrieval of stored AT episodes. AT onset and termination should be displayed. Graphic representations of marker annotations should indicate whether detection of AT onset and termination is reliable or whether atrial undersensing (premature AT termination detection) or oversensing (inappropriate AT detection) is present (Figures 15.9–15.12). Episode storage can be implemented as soon as the patient perceives symptoms, by applying either a magnet or a special activator to permit correlation of symptoms with an atrial arrhythmia or its absence. In a recent study, pacemakers capable of memorizing AT automatically and upon application

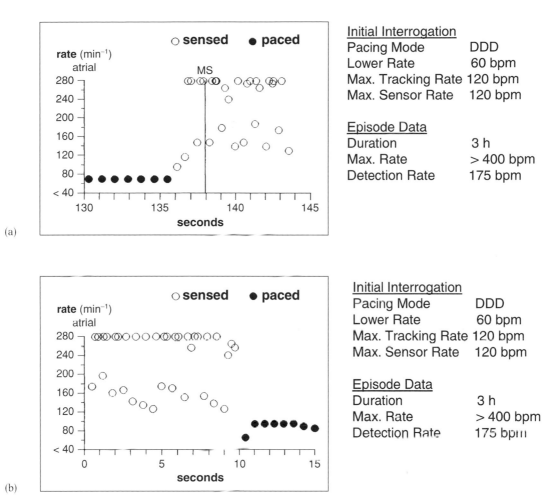

Figure 15.9 Diagram of atrial events at the onset and termination of an atrial tachyarrhythmia (AT) episode (Medtronic Kappa™ 700 DDDR). (a) At AT onset, atrial pacing is present before 2 intrinsic atrial beats are sensed according to a rate of 100 and 120 b.p.m. (atrial premature beats?) which are followed by a sensed fast atrial rate. Mode switching is maintained despite significant atrial undersensing (intermittent atrial sensed events at 120 to 170 b.p.m.: AT signals in the blanking period or with an amplitude not sufficient for detection). (b) At detection of AT termination, spontaneous atrial activity sensed at a high rate (intermittent atrial cycles sensed at a lower rate due to signal drop-out—small amplitude, blanking periods) is followed by atrial pacing at the lower rate limit. The clear cut between continuous atrial sensing and pacing indicates correct AT termination detection; in the case of inappropriate detection of AT termination, intermittent atrial sensed events are to be expected after atrial pacing started again.

of a magnet during symptoms were used in 122 patients [4]. In 45 patients (37%), asymptomatic arrhythmias were stored automatically by the device. Of 36 patients who applied a magnet over the device during symptoms, only 11 revealed EGMs that documented an arrhythmia (Figure 15.13).

In addition to atrial and ventricular marker annotations, stored AT episodes should also display atrial and ventricular cycle lengths and the moment of detection of the onset and termination of AT by a special marker. These functions do not consume much memory capacity. However, without stored atrial EGM, stored marker diagrams of detected AT episodes still lack the definitive differentiation between AT and an atrial sensing artifact (Figure 15.14).

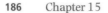

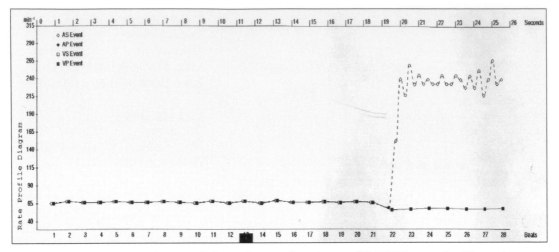

Figure 15.10 Marker diagram at the onset of a detected AT episode in a Diamond™ 3 DDDR pacemaker (Vitatron). Marker annotations indicate that after 21 cycles of AV synchronous pacing (atrial tracked ventricular pacing) at 65 b.p.m., the atrial rate drops to the lower rate limit and AV sequential pacing ensues. Immediately after an atrial paced cycle, the device senses an atrial premature beat with a coupling interval corresponding to a rate of approximately 150 b.p.m. The atrial premature beat triggers an AT with a rate constantly sensed at 240 ± 30 b.p.m., most probably atrial flutter.

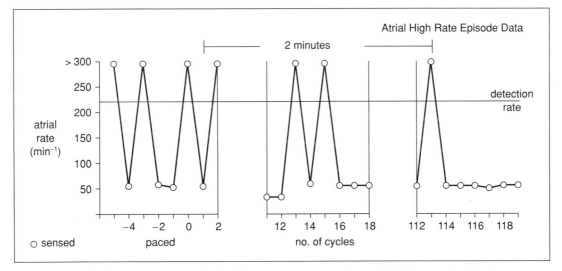

Figure 15.11 Marker diagram suggestive of far-field R-wave oversensing in a Thera™ DDDR pacemaker (Medtronic, Inc.). In this stored episode, a mean atrial rate above a detection rate of 225 b.p.m. was sensed by the device (system programmed to a lower rate limit of 45 b.p.m.). However, the sensed atrial rate alternates between 50 b.p.m. and > 300 b.p.m. This pattern is highly suggestive of far-field R-wave oversensing, most likely in the unblanked terminal portion of the AV delay because the sum of the programmed AV interval (120 ms) and the postventricular atrial blanking period (180 ms) prevents the pacemaker from sensing far-field R waves occurring less than 300 ms after an atrial event.

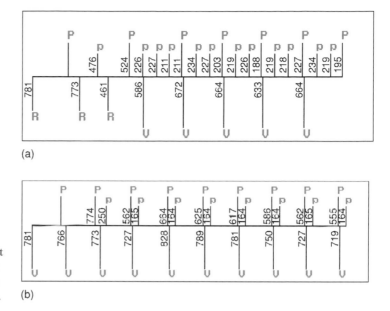

(a)

(b)

Figure 15.12 Marker and cycle length annotations during an atrial tachyarrhythmia (AT) episode in a Talent™ DDDR pacemaker (Ela Medical). (a) Example of an episode where marker annotations show a stable fast sensed atrial rate highly suggestive of correct AT detection. (b) Example of an episode where cycles depicted by marker annotations alternate from very short to near-normal intervals, suggesting that ventricular far-field oversensing triggered inappropriate AT detection.

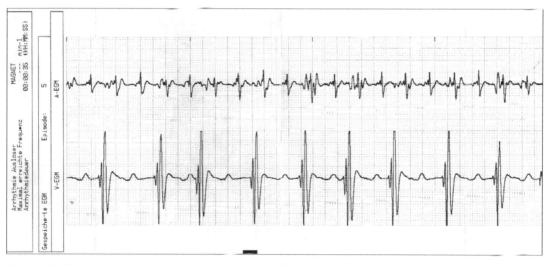

Figure 15.13 Electrogram stored upon application of a magnet (Discovery™ II DDDR pacemaker, Guidant). This recording was obtained by a patient who perceived palpitations and applied a magnet over his pacemaker thereby storing data during a symptomatic episode. The stored electrogram shows an AT with appropriate automatic mode switching. A-EGM, atrial electrogram; V-EGM, ventricular electrogram. Paper speed: 50 mm/s.

Stored electrograms

The diagnostic value of stored atrial EGMs to document AT depends on quality (low baseline noise, adequate amplitude of the atrial signal) and duration of recording (e.g. 3 s). 'Hybrid' EGMs (e.g. ventricular tip to atrial ring) are less useful because they do not distinguish between ventricular far-field oversensing and true atrial potentials

(Figure 15.15). Also, atrial EGMs without annotations are difficult to interpret (Figure 15.16). Annotated high-quality atrial EGMs allow reliable assessment of stored episodes in practically 100% of cases (Figures 15.17–15.20). This combination of recordings is especially useful in the differentiation of far-field R-wave oversensing from supraventricular premature beats [5] (Figures 15.21–15.23).

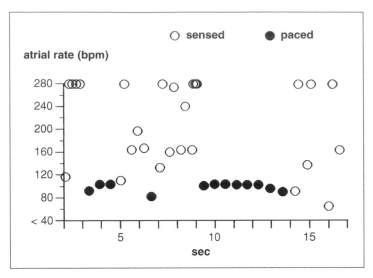

Figure 15.14 Uncertain validity of AT termination detection by a Kappa 700™ DDD pacemaker (Medtronic, Inc.). This marker diagram was stored upon detection of AT termination by the device (criterion: 5 consecutive paced beats). However, after only 8 paced cycles, another AT appears to start. There are also 3 consecutive paced atrial cycles before device detection of AT termination. In the context of a sensed P-wave amplitude of only 0.7–1.2 mV determined at follow-up, this pattern is suspicious of intermittent undersensing during AT. It cannot be determined on the basis of this diagram whether the device detected correctly the moment of AT termination: was it earlier (see 3 consecutive paced cycles) but failed to meet AT termination criteria because of multiple atrial premature beats, or was it a single sustained AT episode with intermittent atrial undersensing (see also Figure 15.24).

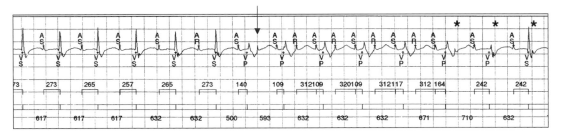

Figure 15.15 'Hybrid' atrioventricular electrogram (EGM) in a Kappa 700™ DDD pacemaker (Medtronic, Inc.). This summated atrioventricular electrogram (AV-EGM) was stored upon mode switching. At the beginning of the tracing, there are ventricular annotations (VS, ventricular sensed; VP, ventricular paced) and atrial marker annotations (AS, atrial sensed) corresponding with small signals, presumably atrial potentials. An atrial tachyarrhythmia (AT) starts at the arrow, but during mode switching alternate atrial signals fall into the postventricular atrial blanking period and are not sensed by the device (*). The tracing illustrates the limitation of hybrid or summated EGM recordings. The atrial signals are difficult to discern from the AV-EGM, so that the sequence could be misinterpreted as showing AT termination.

Stored atrial EGMs provide a unique tool for investigating AT in terms of onset mechanisms, such as the frequency of atrial premature beats with an identical coupling interval before AT, a situation suggesting a focal trigger [6]. Similarly, stored atrial EGMs reliably detect the immediate reinitiation of AT (IRAT), a phenomenon observed after electrical cardioversion [7–12] and after spontaneous AT termination [13]. Such observations may have important implications for the identification of the underlying AT mechanism (e.g. unifocal or multi-focal), the risk of progression from paroxysmal to persistent AT, and the optimization of pacing for AT prevention. In this respect, the differentiation of

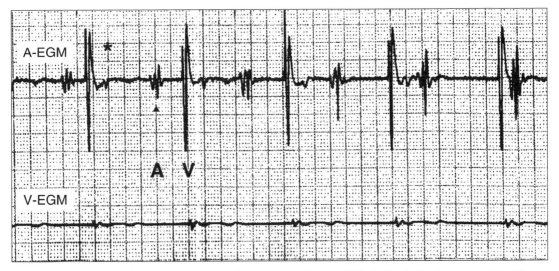

Figure 15.16 Stored atrial electrogram without marker annotation (Pulsar DDDR, Guidant). The device reports that this electrogram (A-EGM, bipolar atrial electrogram; V-EGM, unipolar ventricular electrogram) was stored upon detection of an atrial tachyarrhythmia (AT) followed by mode switching. However, no AT can be seen in the stored A-EGM but mode switching produces prolongation of the AV delay (A, atrial signal; V, far-field paced R-wave signal falling into the postventricular atrial blanking period) causing AV dissociation during mode switching. The small ventricular far-field signals (T wave, *) may have caused this inappropriate AT detection. Marker annotations (available in newer generations of this device) are required to interpret the stored A-EGM.

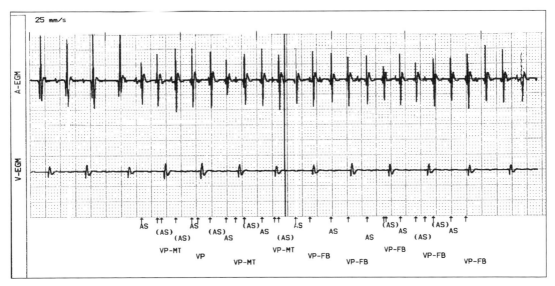

Figure 15.17 Correct detection of atrial tachyarrhythmia (AT) onset during sinus tachycardia (Pulsar max II™, Guidant). In this AT episode stored upon detection, the atrial electrogram (A-EGM) starts with an atrial cycle length of approximately 360 ms (167 b.p.m.). The morphology and cycle length of the A-EGM then changes to an AT of 240 ms. Marker annotations: AS, atrial sensed; (AS), atrial refractory sensed; VP, ventricular paced; VP-MT, ventricular pacing at the maximum tracking rate; VP-FB, ventricular pacing during fallback mode. The black line indicates the moment of AT detection by the device.

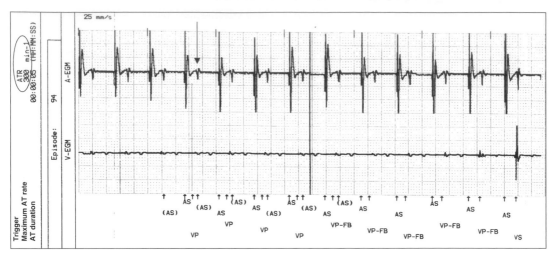

Figure 15.18 False-positive atrial tachyarrhythmia (AT) detection due to ventricular far-field oversensing in the atrium (Pulsar max II™, Guidant). This episode, stored upon 'atrial tachy reaction' (ATR), shows sinus rhythm with a cycle length of approximately 520 ms. However, slightly more than 200 ms after each large atrial signal and 80 ms after a ventricular paced event (first VP annotation), a smaller signal representing a ventricular far-field signal (arrow) is sensed by the atrial channel beyond the postventricular atrial blanking period of 80 ms. Note the misleading maximum sensed atrial rate (circle) and the AT duration of only 5 s.

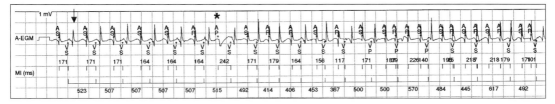

Figure 15.19 Inappropriate atrial tachyarrhythmia (AT) detection due to P-wave double sensing (Kappa 700™ DDD pacemaker, Medtronic). In this device with an unblanked second part of the AV delay, a local conduction delay or block (double potentials) causes double counting of the P wave resulting in inappropriate mode switching. Note the interval between P and P' waves of 52–62 ms (hardly readable due to overwriting by the P'R interval). After atrial pacing, the blanked portion of the AV delay extends to about 100 ms (no double counting) in contrast to its 50-ms duration after atrial sensing. Paper speed 25 mm/s; A-EGM, atrial electrogram; AS, atrial sensed; AP, atrial paced; AR, atrial refractory sensed; MI, marker intervals; VS, ventricular sensed.

Figure 15.20 Missing atrial tachyarrhythmia (AT) onset (Kappa 700™ DDD pacemaker, Medtronic). In this electrogram stored upon mode switching, an AT with a cycle length of approximately 240 ms is already present at the beginning of the tracing before onset detection; every second AT potential falls into the postventricular atrial blanking period and is unsensed (arrow; no annotation). The AT accelerates then slightly, thereby shifting the AT potentials relative to the atrial blanking period. Now the device detects the AT and activates mode switching. However, should the atrial cycle lengthen again it is conceivable that spontaneous 2 : 1 AV conduction would occur again and induce device detection of AT termination. Thus, the counter may report numerous short AT episodes during a sustained AT (presumably atrial flutter). Note atrial pacing after an unsensed atrial signal (*) before mode switching: In this device, atrial refractory sensed signals (AR, 2 cycles earlier) and atrial signals not sensed in the blanking period (atrial signal before AP) do not reset the DDD timing; therefore, atrial pacing occurs at the sensor rate (approximately 75 b.p.m., equal to 800 ms calculated from the last 'AS' marker). Paper speed 25 mm/s; VP, ventricular pace; other abbreviations as in Figure 15.19.

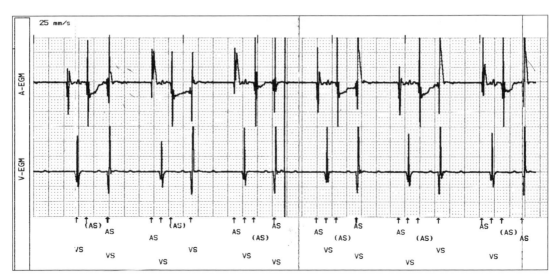

Figure 15.21 False atrial tachyarrhythmia (AT) detection due to repetitive atrial couplets (Discovery™ DDDR pacemaker, Guidant). This electrogram (EGM) was stored upon AT detection. However, the atrial EGM shows that each sinus beat is followed by two consecutive atrial premature beats (the first beat of the couplet is conducted to the ventricle but the second beat of the couplet, which is blocked in the AV node, occurs virtually simultaneously with the ventricle deflection). Rate and count AT detection algorithms including non-consecutive fast atrial cycles will add 2 to the counter for the two short atrial intervals and subtract 1 for the normal interval until rate and count criteria are met whereupon mode switching will occur [5]. Abbreviations as in Figures 15.17 and 15.18.

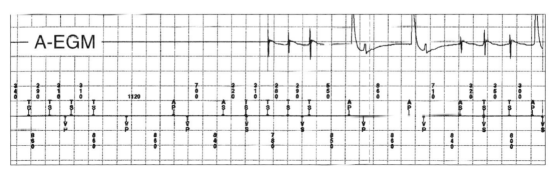

Figure 15.22 Inappropriate atrial tachyarrhythmia (AT) detection due to frequent runs of consecutive atrial premature beats (AT500™ DDDRP pacemaker, Medtronic). In this atrial electrogram (A-EGM) stored upon AT detection, short atrial runs of 4 beats alternate with 1 and 2 atrial paced cycles. 'Rate and count' and 'x out of y' AT detection algorithms would therefore interpret this sequence as AT with intermittent atrial undersensing and store it as AT. Simultaneous A-EGM with marker and cycle length annotations (TS, tachy sense; all other marker annotations as in Figures 15.19 & 15.20). Paper speed 25 mm/s.

IRAT from intermittent atrial undersensing is impossible without a stored atrial EGM (Figure 15.24). High-quality atrial EGMs may also help demonstrate the degree of AT organization and predict the success of atrial antitachycardia pacing (Figure 15.25 [14]).

Stored EGMs have only recently been introduced into pacemaker systems, primarily because they require much more memory space than histograms or other graphic representations of marker information. The first pacemaker systems offering a rate histogram had only 0.055 K random access memory (RAM) but systems offering high-resolution EGMs require 12–16 K RAM (Table 15.1).

Table 15.1 Memory capacity in pacemaker and implantable cardioverter defibrillator systems.

Device	Year of market release	Total RAM (K)	RAM for EGM storage (K)	Duration of stored EGMs (s)	Special memory function features
Pacemaker devices					
Medtronic Symbios 7008	1984	0.015	0	–	Tachycardia counter
Medtronic Elite	1990	0.055	0.05	–	Heart rate histograms
Medtronic Thera i	1994	0.76	0.512	2	No onset; 1 episode with SC-EGM, no simultaneous marker annotations, 7 arrhythmia episodes with marker annotations, atrial/ventricular rate histrograms
Medtronic Kappa 400	1996	4.2	4	2	Onset storage: 1 episode with SC-EGM + simultaneous market/CL, annotations, 8 episodes with marker annotations (onset + termination), atrial/ventricular rate histograms
Medtronic Kappa 700	1998	16	14	16	Onset storage: 1 episode with SC-EGM + simultaneous marker/CL annotations, 8 episodes with marker annotations (onset + termination), arrhythmia statistics
Medtronic AT500 Model 7253	2000	131.5	128	340	Onset storage: 35 episodes each with 2 × 48 marker annotation cycles and 4 s of annotated AEGM (arrhythmia onset and at detection/ATP therapy), 128 episodes with text information, extensive statistics (flashback, trends, AF burden, etc.)
Guidant-CPI Vigor	1993	0.61	–	–	Atrial and ventricular rate histograms
Guidant-CPI Discovery/Pulsar*	1998	12	12	40	Up to 20 episodes with DC-EGM (no onset, no marker annotations)
Guidant-CPI Discovery II/ Pulsar II*	1998	12	12	40	Onset storage: up to 20 episodes with DC-EGM and simultaneous marker/ CL annotations
Guidant Contak TR	1999‡	12	12	40	See Discovery/Pulsar II
Guidant Insignia	2002	48	12	110	See Discovery/Pulsar II
Ela Chorus	1988	2	–	–	Atrial and ventricular rate histograms
Ela Chorum	1996	8	–	–	Onset storage: 15 episodes of marker/CL annotations, arrhythmia statistics
Ela Talent	1998	8	2	9	Onset storage: 15 episodes with marker/CL annotations, 3 of these also with AV-EGM
Ela Symphony	(2003)	128	46	368	Onset storage, 23 episodes of 16 s AV-EGM, marker/CL annotations
St. Jude-Pacesetter Synchrony	1989	8	–	–	Extensive histograms and counters
St. Jude-Pacesetter Trilogy	1995	26	–	–	Extensive histograms and counters
St. Jude-Medical Affinity	1998	36	–	–	Extensive histograms and counters; events with marker annotations (e.g. patient triggered)
St. Jude-Medical Integrity	2000	36	–	–	Extensive histograms and counters: events with marker annotations (e.g. patient triggered)
St. Jude-Medical Identity	2002	128	120	144	12 episodes with A, V or AV EGM of 12 s, onset storage, marker/CL annotations (including patient triggered)

Device	Year				Description
Biotronik Actros	1997	1	–	–	Extensive arrhythmia statistics
Biotronik Inos² CLS	1998	8	–	–	Extensive arrhythmia statistics
Biotronik Philos	2000	12	2	180†	Onset storage: up to 9 DC-EGMs + simultaneous marker annotations
Implantable cardioverter/defibrillator devices					
Medtronic Jewel 7219*	1995	4	1.5	12.5	Onset storage: near-field EGM, 5 episodes with 2.5 s SC-EGM or 1 episode with 5 s SC-EGM at onset and post-therapy; simultaneous marker/CL annotations
Medtronic Jewel+ 7220*	1995	36	32	156	Onset storage: near-field of far-field EGM, programmable 16 episodes with 10 s SC-EGM without marker/CL annotations to 5 episodes with 20 s SC-EGM and simultaneous marker/CL annotations; trend data: 3000 RR intervals before onset
Medtronic MicroJewel 7221*	1996	132	128K	600	Onset storage: near-field or far-field EGM, programmable 15 min SC-EGM without marker/CL annotations to 10 min SC-EGM with marker/CL annotations; 150 episodes with CL data, 12 000 RR intervals before onset
Medtronic Gem DR*	1998	264	256	1320	Onset storage: up to 12 min DC-EGM or 22 min SC-EGM with simultaneous marker/CL annotations, CL data on 253 episodes, 3000 cycles before onset
Guidant-CPI Ventak PRx I	1990	–	–	–	No memory data available
Guidant-CPI Ventak mini	1995	128	128	315	Onset storage: up to 69 episodes with 2 SC-EGMs each, no marker annotations; separate arrhythmia statistics (CL, etc.)
Guidant-CPI Ventak AV	1996	512	512	80–960	Onset storage: programmable e.g. 16 min SC-EGM, 3–5 min TC-EGM with marker annotations: separate arrhythmia statistics (CL, etc.)
Guidant-CPI Ventak Prizm	2000	512	512	1140	Onset storage: 150 episodes with 2 TC-EGMs each, simultaneous marker/CL annotations; arrhythmia statistics
Guidant-CPI Prizm II	2000	536	512	1140	Onset storage: 150 episodes with TC-EGMs each, simultaneous marker/CL annotations: arrhythmia statistics. Patient activated EGM
Guidant Prizm AVT	2001§	548	512	1140	Onset storage: 150 episodes with TC-EGMs each, simultaneous marker/CL annotations; arrhythmia statistics
Guidant Contak CD	1999	512	512	960	Onset storage: programmable e.g. 16 min TC-EGM. 3–5 min TC-EGM with marker annotations; separate arrhythmia statistics (CL, etc.)
Guidant Renewal	2000§	536	512	1140	Onset storage: 150 episodes with TC-EGMs each, simultaneous marker/CL annotations: arrhythmia statistics, heart rate variability statistics
Guidant Renewal II	2002§	536	512	1140	Onset storage: 150 episodes with TC-EGMs each, simultaneous marker/CL annotations; arrhythmia statistics, heart rate variability statistics
Ela Defender 9001	1995	8	2	60	Onset storage: 4 episodes each with 2 AV-EGMs (arrhythmia confirmation + termination) preceded by AV marker annotations
Ela Defender 9301	1999	32	15	300	Onset storage: 12 episodes each with 2 AV-EGMs (arrhythmia confirmation + termination) and AV marker/CL annotations

Continued p. 194

Table 15.1 (cont'd)

Device	Year of market release	Total RAM (K)	RAM for EGM storage (K)	Duration of stored EGMs (s)	Special memory function features
Ela Alto DR 614	2001	128	31	460	Onset storage: 25 episodes each with 2 AV-EGMs (arrhythmia confirmation + termination) and AV marker/CL annotations
Ela Alto II	(2003)	128	50	750	Onset storage: 25 episodes each with 2 AV-EGMs (arrhythmia confirmation + termination) and AV marker/CL annotations
St. Jude-Ventritex Angstrom*	1998	128	120	960	Onset storage: up to 59 episodes with SC-EGM and simultaneous marker annotations
St. Jude-Ventritex Profile*	1998	128	120	960	Onset storage: up to 59 episodes with SC-EGM and simultaneous marker annotations
St. Jude-Medical Photon DR*	2000	128	100	1500	Onset storage: up to 60 episodes with DC-EGM and simultaneous marker/CL annotations
Biotronik mycroPhylax*	1997	160	128	1024	Onset storage: 16 SC-EGMs of 64 s with simultaneous marker annotations, up to 9 h RR intervals before arrhythmia onset
Biotronik Belos VR*	2000	512	448	3600	Onset and stability storage: configurable for SC or DC-EGM storage with additionally up to 8 h RR intervals before arrhythmia onset, or alternatively up to 1800 s EGM with up to 29 h RR intervals time controlled
Biotronik Tachos family§	2000–2002	256	128	2040	Configurable SC or DC EGM storage (including for SVTs)
Biotronik Belos DR/Belos A+	2002	512	448	1800	Onset and stability storage: configurable DC-EGM storage (including for SVTs) with additionally up to 4 h PP, PR, RR intervals before arrhythmia onset, alternatively up to 29 h PP, PR, RR intervals
Biotronik mycroPhylax*	1997	160	128	900	Onset storage: SC-EGMs with simultaneous marker annotations, up to 9 h RR intervals before arrhythmia onset
Biotronik Belos VR*	2000	512	384	3600	Onset storage: programmable, e.g. 15 DC-EGMs up to 4 min, up to 25 h RR intervals before arrhythmia onset

Year of market release in brackets: scheduled. AEGM, atrial electrogram; AF, atrial fibrillation; AV-EGM, atrioventricular compound electrogram; CL, cycle length; DC-EGM, dual channel electrogram (atrial + ventricular or ventricular near-field + far-field); K, kilobytes; RAM, random access memory; SC-EGM, single-channel electrogram; TC-EGM, triple-channel electrogram (atrial, ventricular near-field, ventricular far-field).

* Programmable electrogram duration.

† Compression algorithm stores only duration, filtered amplitudes and number of maxima of each sensed signal.

‡ Not released in the US.

§ Includes Tupos and Deikos devices.

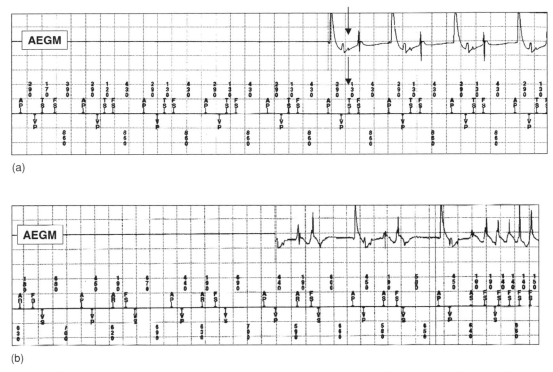

(a)

(b)

Figure 15.23 Far-field R-wave oversensing versus couplet of atrial premature beats. (a) Marker annotations stored by the device (AT500™ DDDRP pacemaker, Medtronic) immediately before atrial tachyarrhythmia (AT) onset suggest the presence of 2 consecutive atrial premature beats. However, the stored electrogram indicates ventricular far-field oversensing (arrow) to account for one of the presumed atrial deflections. (b) In this stored AT onset, marker annotations immediately before AT again suggest a couplet of atrial premature beats as in (a). The stored atrial electrogram confirms the diagnosis of a true atrial couplet. From marker and cycle length annotations alone, (a) and (b) cannot be differentiated.

AT detection algorithms

A device stores AT episodes only if they fulfill the criteria of an AT detection algorithm. AT detection algorithms are typically identical to those designed for activation of mode switching: a calculated mean atrial rate (Thera™ and Kappa 400™, Medtronic; Trilogy™, Affinity™ and Integrity™, St. Jude Medical), a certain number of atrial events above a critical rate (Discovery™ and Pulsar™, Guidant; MiniSwing™ and Living™, Sorin), 'x out of y' atrial events with a short interval (Kappa 700™ and Kappa 900™, Medtronic; Talent™, Ela Medical; Philos™, Inos™ and Logos™, Biotronik), or even single early atrial beats (Diamond™ and Selection™, Vitatron B.V. [5]). Fast-reacting mode-switching algorithms avoid sustained tracking at the upper limit during AT detection and thus seem advantageous. However, reports on AT detection in these fast algorithms may not be useful to assess the

occurrence of sustained AT episodes (see Figures 15.2, 15.4, 15.21, 15.22 & 15.23a). Some systems use a 'preliminary' AT detection response combined with a confirmation phase. Tracking of short atrial cycles (fast rate) ceases after preliminary AT detection and some form of Wenckebach behavior or rate-smoothing occurs. The device performs definitive mode switching only if criteria for AT are still met at the end of the confirmation phase. Thus, stored AT episodes are more likely to represent sustained AT. A new DDDRP device (AT500™, Medtronic, Inc.) uses a modification of the 'rate and count' principle (so-called 'evidence counter'). Whenever more than one atrial event is sensed during one ventricular cycle, the counter for rapid atrial activity is increased by 1 if far-field R-wave oversensing is excluded by an additional algorithm (PR Logic™ [15,16]). When the counter reaches 3 and the median atrial rate is above a programmed value (e.g. 180 b.p.m.), preliminary AT detection

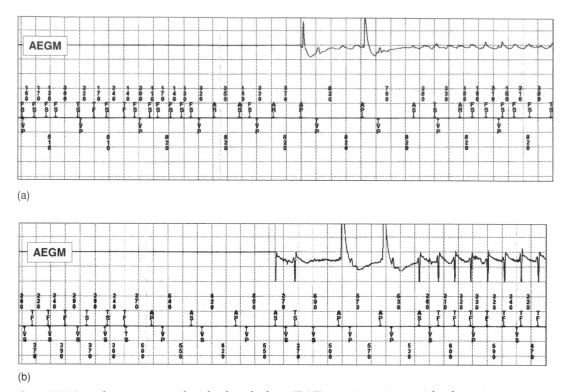

(a)

(b)

Figure 15.24 Immediate reinitiation of atrial tachyarrhythmia (IRAT) versus intermittent atrial undersensing (AT episodes stored by AT500™ DDDRP pacemakers, Medtronic). (a) After some cycles with normal intervals simulating sinus rhythm, an AT starts shortly after a prior recorded episode. However, the atrial electrogram shows intermittent atrial undersensing, so that a sustained AT episode is stored as several successive short AT episodes. (b) Another AT episode starts after some atrial cycles at normal length suggestive of sinus rhythm. However, in contrast to (a) the electrogram clearly documents the absence of intrinsic atrial signals before the start of AT, thus confirming IRAT.

and mode switching occur. However, confirmation of sustained AT detection occurs only if AT detection criteria are still met after a programmable number of ventricular cycles (e.g. 24). The episode is stored and specific interventions by the device (e.g. atrial antitachycardia pacing) may be applied only after device confirmation of sustained AT [17].

Apart from the detection algorithm, atrial sensitivity and blanking times determine the reliability of automatic AT detection. A high bipolar atrial sensitivity (≤ 0.3 mV) facilitates reliable detection of small atrial fibrillation potentials but oversensing, particularly of ventricular far-field signals, remains a potential problem. The ability of a pacemaker device to distinguish small AT potentials from noise depends on the quality of the atrial signal obtained at the time of implantation. Generally, there is a correlation between the amplitude signals from sinus

P wave and atrial fibrillation sensed by a bipolar system [18,19], implying that the better the sensing characteristics during sinus rhythm, the better the detection of atrial fibrillation. However, the amplitude of the sensed fibrillation potentials may vary by up to 300% in a given patient [20]. Thus, if a patient is in atrial fibrillation at the time of pacemaker implantation the sensing threshold should be measured after electrode fixation and the position changed if the AT cannot reliably be detected at a bipolar sensitivity of 0.25 mV. Sites with large ventricular far-field signals (filtered amplitude > 0.2 mV) limit the ability of the system to detect ATs because of longer blanking requirements.

Apart from sensing quality, atrial blanking times determine the ability of a device to detect ATs. A long postventricular atrial blanking time predisposes to 2 : 1 synchronization of atrial flutter poten-

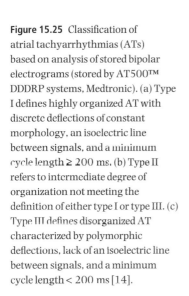

(a)

(b)

(c)

Figure 15.25 Classification of atrial tachyarrhythmias (ATs) based on analysis of stored bipolar electrograms (stored by AT500™ DDDRP systems, Medtronic). (a) Type I defines highly organized AT with discrete deflections of constant morphology, an isoelectric line between signals, and a minimum cycle length ≥ 200 ms. (b) Type II refers to intermediate degree of organization not meeting the definition of either type I or type III. (c) Type III defines disorganized AT characterized by polymorphic deflections, lack of an isoelectric line between signals, and a minimum cycle length < 200 ms [14].

tials (Figures 15.1 & 15.20). New algorithms use a dynamic atrial sensitivity maximum (e.g. 'baseline' value 0.15 mV) at the time when an atrial signal is expected and minimum (e.g. 8 times the baseline value, i. e. 1.2 mV) after a sensed or paced ventricular event [21] and use this concept to minimize atrial blanking times (Figure 15.26).

Some devices attempt to distinguish slow ATs (which may represent different types of atrial flutter) from atrial fibrillation on the basis of the AT rate: if the atrial cycle length is between an AT detection cycle or rate (e.g. 180 b.p.m.) and a second rate (e.g. 250 b.p.m.), the device assumes the presence of atrial flutter (usually referred to as 'AT') while an AT above this rate will be classified as atrial fibrillation (AF). However, different forms of atrial flutter may be faster than 250 b.p.m. while atrial fibrilla-

tion may be sensed at the site of the implanted atrial lead with a rate below 250 b.p.m.. To improve AT/AF discrimination, a rate and regularity criterion has been developed (Figure 15.27). If the AT rate is sensed within a critical zone (e.g. between 220 and 270 ms), the regularity of AT cycle length (e.g. second longest and second shortest AT cycle length are less than 25% different from the mean AT cycle length) is used for classification. However, these device classifications of AT may be wrong in the presence of atrial sensing errors (Figure 15.28). Additionally, the EGM sensed and stored by the device only reflects the type of AT at the site of the implanted atrial lead. Conceivably, a lead implanted in the lateral right atrium could sense a slow, regular AT when there is a fast irregular AT in the left atrium.

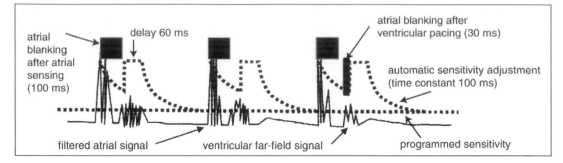

Figure 15.26 Function of an automatic atrial sensitivity adjustment algorithm. After each sensed atrial event, the device generates a short blanking period to avoid double counting while the terminal portion of the AV delay is unblanked. The sensitivity threshold increases to a predefined value (e.g. 75% of the sensed signal) and decreases again until a sensed or paced ventricular event occurs. There is a very short atrial blanking period after ventricular pacing and the atrial channel is completely unblanked after a ventricular sensed event. Following a ventricular event, a plateau phase with a higher atrial sensitivity threshold is applied and it again decreases until the next atrial event or until the programmed basic sensitivity level is reached (algorithm implemented in Medtronic AT500™ DDDRP systems).

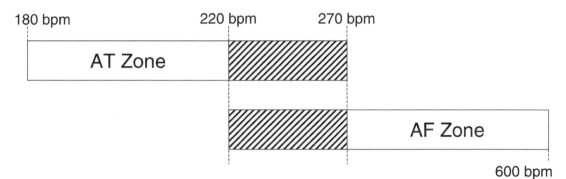

Figure 15.27 Discrimination of atrial flutter from atrial fibrillation (AF) on the basis of rate and regularity. Detected atrial tachyarrhythmias (ATs) may be sensed in the 'AT zone' (e.g. 180–270 b.p.m.) or 'AF zone' (e.g. 220–600 b.p.m.). There is a programmable 'AT/AF overlap zone' (e.g. 220–270 b.p.m., striped) in which AT classification depends on the regularity of a sensed AT (see text). This algorithm is implemented in AT500™ pacemaker systems and Jewel AF™ and GEM III AT™ cardioverter defibrillator systems (all Medtronic).

The optimal AT detection and memory function

Ideally, the AT detection algorithm should react fast and be sensitive for the identification of AT onset and preceding cycles while possessing the capability of rejecting far-field oversensing and short atrial runs. This goal is best achieved by a fast AT detection algorithm requiring confirmation of AT persistence. To avoid rapid tracking of the AT during this confirmation phase, the mode-switching algorithm may already perform a 'preliminary' switch as soon as it detects the onset of AT. Therefore, two separate counters should report the frequency of preliminary

AT detection with mode switching, and of confirmed sustained AT episodes.

Pacemaker memory function should report the number of detected AT episodes, the cumulative time in AT (AT burden), the distribution of AT duration (including data on the longest AT episode), duration of sinus rhythm between AT episodes, and the median atrial rate during AT. The maximal rate is less valuable because double counting of broad double potentials during atrial fibrillation or a single ventricular far-field signal is frequent and may induce the detection of a fast atrial rate not representative of the AT episode (cf. Figures 15.5 & 15.28). Complementary histograms of the atrial

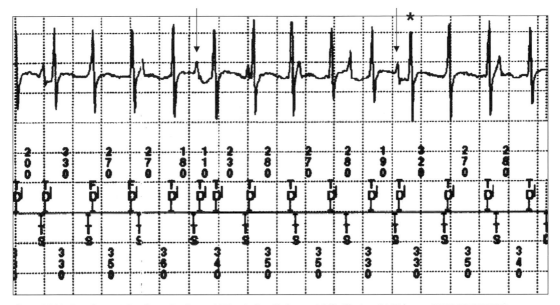

Figure 15.28 Regular atrial tachyarrhythmia (AT) misclassified as atrial fibrillation ('AF') by an AT500™ DDDRP system (Medtronic). This AT was sensed at a rate in the AT/AF overlap zone. Due to far-field R-wave oversensing (arrows), the atrial cycle length is sensed between 110 and 320 ms. Note the undersensing of the big AT potential (*) which appears after the oversensed ventricular far-field signal (second arrow) within the atrial blanking period after atrial sensing of 100 ms (cf. Figure 15.26). Due to this oversensing, this very regular AT with a cycle length of 270 ms is interpreted as irregular by the device and classified as AF.

rate (last 7 days and complete follow-up period), AT episode duration and time of day of AT detection (Figure 15.29) may be useful for clarification. However, these data are only valuable if individual AT episodes are stored for reassessment. These should provide marker/cycle length annotations, an atrial EGM and a marker for device derived AT onset detection. The detection of AT termination should be stored in the same way. The atrial EGM should have a scale to assess whether the sensed signals represent AT potentials or artifacts (e.g. giant signals in case of electrode fracture). Equipped with such memory functions, pacemaker systems become unique tools for continuous monitoring of the atrial rhythm [22,23].

Figure 15.29 Histogram illustrating the time of day when the onset of atrial tachyarrhythmia (AT) episodes were detected in a patient (AT500™ DDDRP pacemaker, Medtronic). In this example, more than 80% of 143 AT episodes detected during a 6-month period started between 9 PM and 9 AM, suggestive of vagal activity as an AT trigger ('vagally induced' AT) or an insufficient dosing interval if an antiarrhythmic drug with a short half-life is administered.

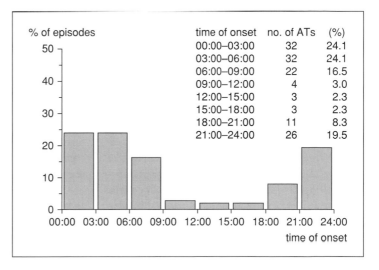

time of onset	no. of ATs	(%)
00:00–03:00	32	24.1
03:00–06:00	32	24.1
06:00–09:00	22	16.5
09:00–12:00	4	3.0
12:00–15:00	3	2.3
15:00–18:00	3	2.3
18:00–21:00	11	8.3
21:00–24:00	26	19.5

Application of AT memory functions

Pacemaker memory functions permit optimization of pacemaker programming. Advanced systems can detect intermittent atrial oversensing in the form of AT detection (Figures 15.12b, 15.16 & 15.18), and intermittent undersensing associated with numerous recorded AT episodes (Figures 15.3, 15.20 & 15.24a). If mode-switching criteria are too stringent, stored AT episodes show an already present AT episode when the AT onset is detected. Similarly, if criteria for detection of AT termination are too easy to satisfy, the stored episode may show short atrial cycles soon after detection of AT termination indicating that inappropriate detection AT termination is related to intermittent atrial undersensing (Figure 15.14).

If correct device-based AT detection is confirmed in advanced systems, the pacemaker may be used to monitor therapy directed at ATs. In patients on antiarrhythmic drugs, the system may assess the optimal drug, dosage and dosing intervals. In patients with curative ablation for AT (e.g. cavotricuspid isthmus ablation), the results of the procedure can be monitored. Evidently, the device can monitor its own efficacy if it offers pacing algorithms for prevention or termination of AT.

Memory functions may be used to assess patients' symptoms for AT. However, the majority of AT episodes in pacemaker patients seem to be asymptomatic, particularly in the setting of AV block and a stable ventricular rate with appropriate mode-switching function. In situations where ATs are not recorded by the device in symptomatic patients (e.g. underdetection of atrial fibrillation with rapid and irregular tracking), a patient-triggered storage of EGMs will often solve the problem (Figure 15.13). However, stored marker annotations without atrial EGMs in a patient-activated system are of limited diagnostic value. For example, such a system will only show markers of regular AV sequential pacing in the case of complete undersensing of atrial fibrillation, and undersensing of atrial flutter due to 2 : 1 synchronization with atrial blanking times will be depicted as regular AV synchronous ventricular pacing.

AT memory function may enhance the understanding of specific AT onset mechanisms and AT organization. AT prevention might be possible if stored AT episodes reveal an onset mechanism correctable by pacemaker reprogramming or a dedicated algorithm. For instance, if a patient develops ATs only during a sinus or paced rate of 60 b.p.m., an increase of the lower rate to 70 or 80 b.p.m. may prevent AT. If all AT episodes are preceded by short–long sequences caused by atrial premature beats with postextrasystolic pauses, an algorithm for postextrasystolic pause suppression may prevent AT. Finally, bipolar atrial EGMs may help characterize the local degree of AT organization and select those patients and AT episodes which have organized EGMs (type I [14]), for atrial antitachycardia pacing or linear ablation in the right atrium.

Clinical results of pacemaker memory functions for AT detection

Given the better ability of memory function to continuously monitor the atrial rhythm, it is not surprising that new observations have reported a much higher incidence of ATs in pacemaker patients than old data using conventional detection criteria [24–35] (Table 15.2). In fact, according to conventional diagnostic data, ATs were documented to occur in 2–16% of patients with permanent pacemakers in contrast to an incidence of approximately 50% with the advanced memory function of new pacemakers. This huge discrepancy is disconcerting because more precise knowledge is necessary to assess the effect of any antiarrhythmic interventions. It may be argued that this discrepancy was caused by the lack of specificity of AT detection by pacemaker memory functions that classified short atrial runs and ventricular far-field oversensing as AT. In a study in 46 patients with AV block and a VDD pacing system storing up to eight AT episodes with EGMs, the memory function detected 235 AT episodes during a 3-month study period [36]. Of these, only 82 (35%) were confirmed, 153 episodes (65%) demonstrating oversensing as the cause of inappropriate AT detection. Another study with 41 patients involved a DDD system storing up to eight AT episodes including one annotated EGM [37]. In 121 of 129 stored episodes, ATs fulfilled the criteria for mode switching, but 43 of these 121 AT episodes (36%) represented only atrial runs of less than 10 beats and had already terminated at the end of the stored EGM.

Pacemaker memory data were compared with 24-h Holter recordings in 17 patients with a

Table 15.2 Incidence of atrial tachyarrhythmias (ATs) in pacemaker patients according to conventional diagnostic tools versus pacemaker memory functions.

Author	Incidence of AT
Conventional diagnostic tools	
Skanes 2001 [24]	2.8% chronic AT (> 1 week) per year, 1094 patients, AAI/DDD
Connolly 2000 [25]	5.3% AT > 15 min per year, 1094 patients, AAI/DDD
Andersen 1994 [26]	14% ATs, 7% chronic AT, 102 patients, AAI
Chamberlain-Webber 1994 [27]	3% reprogramming DDD to VVI due to ATs, 771 patients, 40 months
Langenfeld 1988 [28]	2% ATs, 43 patients, DDD, 63 months
Fröhlig 1985 [29]	16% ATs, 136 patients, DDD, 14 months
Detollenaere 1992 [30]	10% sustained ATs, 252 patients, DDD, 30 months
Feuer 1989 [31]	8% ATs, 110 patients, DDD/DDI, 40 months
Pacemaker memory functions (electrograms in [32], counters/markers in [33–35])	
Israel 2002 [32]	39% ATs, 206 patients, DDD, 6 months
Sack 2001 [33]	49% ATs, 626 patients, DDD, 28 days
Defaye 1998 [34]	ATs in 51% of 354 patients under DDD during 28 days
Garrigue 1996 [35]	ATs in 49% of 213 patients with DDD during 361 days

Thera™ DR pacemaker [38]. Of 125 AT episodes occurring in 45 Holter recordings, 93 were detected by the 'atrial high rate' detection feature which was programmed in a very stringent way (40 atrial beats above 160 b.p.m.), but 32 AT episodes were too short for detection using this criterion. In contrast, 12 inappropriate AT detections occurred from far-field R-wave oversensing. Using the same 'atrial high rate' detection feature in Thera™ DR devices, a very high specificity of AT detection (99.9% in 3061 AT episodes after AV node ablation) was found if AT detection criteria were programmed to 200 beats above 180 b.p.m. [39]. However, no data about the sensitivity of this AT detection programming are available.

In a study in 56 patients, stored atrial EGMs confirmed the presence of an AT in 88% of episodes with an atrial rate greater than 250 b.p.m. and a duration greater than 10 s but the presence of an AT was only confirmed in 18% of AT episodes shorter than 10 s and in 18% of AT episodes with a rate lower than 250 b.p.m. [40].

A prospective study (*b*alanced *e*valuation of *a*trial *t*achyarrhythmias in *s*timulated patients, BEATS) evaluates the incidence of AT episodes on the basis of resting ECG at follow-up and one 24-h Holter vs. pacemaker counter data vs. stored EGMs. Preliminary results [32] in the first 206 patients (ATs known before pacemaker implant in 31 patients) show that during a mean follow-up of 6 months ATs were documented during resting ECG at follow-up visit only in 10 patients (5%); 36 patients (17%) reported symptoms suggestive of intermittent ATs. In 133 patients (65%), counter data reported that ATs had occurred in 79 patients (38%), at least one stored EGM confirmed the occurrence of an AT. In 55 of 133 patients (41%) with AT detection according to counter data, no atrial EGM confirmed this diagnosis. While atrial EGMs documented ATs in 20 of 36 patients with symptoms (56%), 59 of the 79 patients (75%) with AT documented by stored EGMs did not report any symptoms suggestive of AT. Therefore, in patients with an indication for pacing the incidence of ATs during the first 6 months after implantation seems to be as high as 38% and is severely underestimated by conventional diagnostic methods. This casts some doubt on data about AT incidence in patients under different pacing modes from megatrials which did not use stored EGMs to detect paroxysmal ATs.

Differential diagnosis of stored AT episodes

Generally, the differential diagnosis of stored AT episodes should include the following considerations (Table 15.3).

1 Does the stored AT onset show a new AT episode or an ongoing AT with intermittent undersensing? This evaluation requires an atrial EGM. Spontaneous

Table 15.3 Differential diagnosis of stored atrial tachyarrhythmia (AT) episodes.

	Counter/histogram	Markers	Annotated electrogram
Detection of AT onset			
New AT	(No characteristic information)	Long cycles before AT onset detection	Undisturbed isoelectrical line before AT onset with pacing stimuli and/or sinus P waves
Sustained AT with atrial undersensing	Numerous short ATs	No atrial markers followed by short cycles before detection of AT onset	AT potentials without annotation before recorded AT onset
Short atrial runs	Numerous short ATs	Short cycles alternating with one or two long cycles	Atrial potentials at short cycle length alternating with pacing/sinus signals
Far-field oversensing	Usually short AT	Characteristic alternation between short and long cycles, VA interval < 200 ms, 2 AA intervals sum up to normal atrial cycle length*	Narrow, large atrial sensed signal alternates with broad, usually small ventricular far-field signal
Myopotential oversensing	AT rate > 400 b.p.m.	Bursts of short atrial cycles with intervals near the minimum technical recording limit (100 ms)	Short bursts of high-frequency signals (varying amplitude), a pattern associated with baseline noise
Electromagnetic interference (EMI)	AT rate > 400 b.p.m.	Atrial cycles at intervals near the minimum technical recording limit	Bursts of high-frequency signals, noise at baseline
False detection of AT termination			
Atrial undersensing	Next AT detected within few minutes	Short cycles after AT termination detection	AT EGM signals without annotation
Atrial premature beats or runs misclassified as sustained AT	(No typical information)	Intermittent long (even paced) cycles	Intermittent sinus potentials/pacing artifacts with undisturbed isoelectric baseline
Far-field R-wave oversensing. As above	(No typical information)	Alternating short and long cycles	Narrow large atrial signals alternate with broad small ventricular far-field signals

APB, atrial premature beat; EMI, electromagnetic interference.
*For example, atrial rate 60 b.p.m. = 1000 ms; AV delay 140 ms; far-field signal 160 ms after the ventricle; atrial cycles alternate between (140 + 160 ms =) 300 ms and (1000 − 300 ms =) 700 ms.

restoration of sinus rhythm may occur for only two or three cycles and cannot usually be distinguished from intermittent atrial undersensing by marker annotations alone (Figure 15.24).

2 Far-field R-wave oversensing typically exhibiting VA intervals < 200 ms must be excluded. In systems with an unblanked terminal portion of the AV delay, ventricular far-field oversensing may also appear immediately before the spontaneous R wave is sensed in the ventricular channel [3]. Again, marker annotations alone may be suggestive of far-field R-wave oversensing in many instances, but intermittent far-field oversensing in combination with single atrial premature beats, couplets or supraventricular bigeminy will not be decipherable from marker annotations (Figure 15.23).

3 A sustained AT has to be distinguished from frequent short atrial runs at AT onset. The latter (e.g. atrial triplets alternating with one or two sinus cycles) will typically fulfill criteria for AT detection in most AT detection algorithms and cannot be distinguished from a sustained AT with intermittent atrial undersensing by marker annotations alone (Figures 15.21 & 15.22).

4 Other causes of inappropriate AT detection (myopotential oversensing, atrial exit block, atrial electrode fracture, loose atrial connector screw, insulation failure, electrocautery at a cardiac operation, external interference) are rare with atrial bipolar leads. Sensed atrial rates > 400 b.p.m. and marker annotations with intervals ranging from 100 ms to normal values may occur in lead fracture in association with typical giant signals.

5 At the end of an AT episode, another stored atrial EGM is necessary to verify correct detection of AT termination. However, this function is not yet available in market-released pacemaker systems. Therefore, there is suspicion (but not proof) of inappropriate device detection of AT termination if short atrial cycles reappear immediately after episode termination (Figures 15.14 & 15.24a). Detection of AT termination may be delayed by atrial premature beats or far-field R-wave oversensing because most algorithms require a certain number of normal atrial cycles to detect restoration of sinus rhythm.

Pacemaker memory in clinical studies on AT and pacing

An increasing number of studies on pacing interventions for prevention of ATs use pacemaker memory functions to evaluate the result of therapy. While the PA[3] studies used the device-derived time to first AT recurrence as a surrogate of the success of conventional DDDR pacing to suppress AT [41,42], the SYNBIAPACE (*synchronous biatrial pacing*) study additionally used the AT burden reported by device memory to evaluate therapy success [43]. The DAPPAF trial (dual-site atrial pacing for prevention of atrial fibrillation) used device-stored mode-switching episodes to identify AT recurrence during support pacing, single-site and dual-site overdrive pacing [44].

Also, the atrial fibrillation therapy (AFT) trial used pacemaker memory functions for evaluation of the success of preventive pacing algorithms. Using device-derived data, a significantly lower median and mean AT burden was found during preventive pacing compared to DDDR pacing [45]. Additionally, this study used dedicated memory functions for ATs to investigate AT onset patterns [46]. Using stored episodes, the study showed that 30% of AT episodes were preceded by an increase in atrial premature beat density, 26% represented AT reinitiations within 1 min of a previous AT, and 20% of episodes started during bradycardia or rate decay. Only 16% of AT episodes started during a completely regular, stable atrial rhythm. In 46%, the onset was classified as 'sudden', 7% were preceded by a single and 19% by multiple atrial premature beats, and 24% by short atrial runs. However, atrial premature beats caused short–long sequences immediately before AT onset only in 4% of AT episodes. Atrial EGM for confirmation of sensed atrial events was not available. Consequently the storage of AT episodes only with marker annotations limits the value of the conclusions.

Stored bipolar atrial EGMs have been used to assess the organization of ATs [14]. Even though they show the degree of AT organization only in a small area of the right atrium, the type of AT in the bipolar EGM can predict the success of atrial antitachycardia pacing. While regular ATs (type I, Figure 15.25a) were terminated in 62% of cases, ATs with bipolar EGMs of intermediate organization (type II, Figure 15.25b) or complete disorganization with loss of isoelectric baseline (type III, Figure 15.25c) had a much lower success rate of antitachycardia pacing (35% and 0%, respectively). EGM recordings during ATs have documented that some patients with atrial fibrillation as the only recorded AT before pacemaker implantation exhibit device-recorded highly organized ATs capable of pace termination.

Limitations of pacemaker memory functions for ATs

Pacemaker memory functions are dependent on optimal pacemaker function. If severe atrial undersensing is present, ATs cannot be detected and stored. In intermittent atrial undersensing, single AT episodes will be stored as multiple short episodes rendering useless the stored data about number of AT episodes and eventually the device-derived AT burden. This may be misleading and even lead to

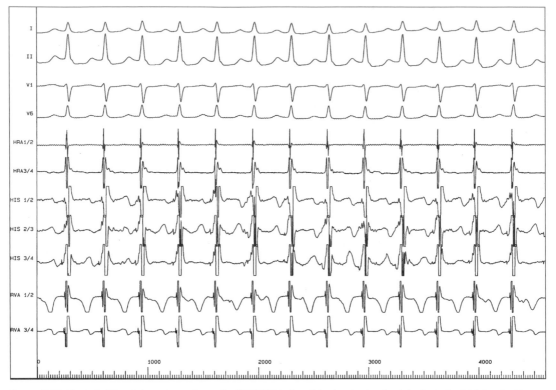

Figure 15.30 Typical AV nodal reentry tachycardia (AVNRT) induced during electrophysiologic study. Atrial activation (shown in channels HRA 1/2 and HRA 3/4) occurs at the same time as ventricular activation (channels RVA 1/2 and RVA 3/4). At this time, the atrial channel of a pacemaker is blanked (postventricular atrial blanking period) and this tachycardia will therefore be stored as VT (intrinsic ventricular rhythm sensed at 180 b.p.m. without atrial sensed events). Paper speed 50 mm/s; surface ECG leads I, II, V1 and V6; bipolar intracardiac recordings from high right atrium (HRA 1/2, HRA 3/4); His bundle (HIS 1/2, HIS 2/3, HIS 3/4); and right ventricular apex (RVA 1/2, RVA 3/4). HRA, high right atrium; RVA, right ventricular apex; HIS, His bundle recording.

inappropriate therapeutic decisions, e.g. if anticoagulant therapy is withdrawn because stored data suggest that only short AT episodes < 1 h occurred during follow-up.

A particular problem results from the use of relatively long atrial blanking times. A long blanking time may lead to 2 : 1 undersensing of atrial flutter, with resultant underdetection and misleading pacemaker memory data. Some 1 : 1 AV conducted supraventricular tachycardias such as typical AV nodal reentry tachycardia generate an atrial event within 50 ms of the ventricular event and will not be detected even with very short blanking times (< 80 ms) (Figure 15.30). On the other hand, short atrial blanking times provoke far-field R-wave oversensing that may severely limit the use of memory function. To overcome these problems, stored EGMs are necessary to reassess atrial sensing quality.

Dedicated algorithms are needed to detect far-field R-wave oversensing which typically exhibits constant and short VA intervals when the underlying rhythm decelerates or accelerates. Algorithms to dynamically reduce atrial sensitivity after ventricular events rather than completely blank these periods (Figure 15.26) may decrease the incidence of far-field R-wave oversensing and provide a higher sensitivity to atrial events during the postventricular atrial period.

Conclusions

Pacemaker memory functions offer a new dimension for monitoring patients with paroxysmal ATs. Counter data reporting AT burden or number of ATs during follow-up are useful but require corroboration by stored EGMs of AT episodes. To allow reassessment, stored AT episodes should display an atrial EGM > 3 s with marker and cycle length annotations and information about automatic algorithm function (e.g. time of AT detection and mode switching, intervention of automatic atrial sensitivity or AV delay-adjusting algorithms). This should be available at the moment of detection of AT onset as well as AT termination.

References

1 Patel AM, Westveer DC, Man KC, Stewart JR, Frumin HI. Treatment of underlying atrial fibrillation. Paced rhythm obscures recognition. *J Am Coll Cardiol* 2000; **36**: 784–7.

2 Israel CW. Automatic mode switching based on a '4 out of 7' algorithm in Medtronic Kappa 700 dual chamber pacemaker devices. *Herzschr Elektrophys* 1999; **10** (Suppl. 1): I/32 I/45.

3 Israel CW, Neubauer H, Ossowski A, Hohnloser SH. Why did mode switching occur? *Pacing Clin Electrophysiol* 2000; **23**: 1422–4.

4 Huikuri HV, Koistinen J, Petersen B, Benzer W, Appl U. A new approach to symptomatic pacemaker patients: results from the magnet stored E-gram study [abstract]. *Europace* 2000; **1** (Suppl.): D33.

5 Israel CW. Analysis of mode switching algorithms in dual chamber pacemakers. *Pacing Clin Electrophysiol* 2002; **25**: 380–93.

6 Israel CW, Ehrlich JR, Grönefeld G, Plock K, Hohnloser SH. Increased ectopic activity and short–long sequences as common mechanisms triggering paroxysmal atrial tachyarrhythmias in pacemaker patients [abstract]. *Eur Heart J* 2001; **22** (Suppl): 333.

7 Daoud EG, Hummel JD, Augostini R, Williams S, Kalbfleisch SJ. Effect of verapamil on immediate recurrence of atrial fibrillation. *J Cardiovasc Electrophysiol* 2000; **11**: 1231–7.

8 Lau CP, Lok NS. A comparison of transvenous atrial defibrillation of acute and chronic atrial fibrillation and the effect of intravenous sotalol on human atrial defibrillation thresholds. *Pacing Clin Electrophysiol* 1997; **20**: 2442–52.

9 Sra J, Biehl M, Blanck Z *et al.* Spontaneous reinitiation of atrial fibrillation following transvenous atrial defibrillation. *Pacing Clin Electrophysiol* 1998; **21**: 1105–10.

10 Timmermans C, Rodriguez LM, Smeets JLRM, Wellens HJJ. Immediate reinitiation of atrial fibrillation following internal atrial defibrillation. *J Cardiovasc Electrophysiol* 1998; **9**: 122–8.

11 Tse HF, Lau CP, Ayers GM. Incidence and modes of onset of early reinitiation of atrial fibrillation after

successful internal cardioversion, and its prevention by intravenous sotalol. *Heart* 1999; **82**: 319–24.

12 Yu WC, Lin YK, Tai CT *et al.* Early recurrence of atrial fibrillation after external cardioversion. *Pacing Clin Electrophysiol* 1999; **22**: 1614–19.

13 Israel CW, Grönefeld G, Ehrlich JR, Li YG, Hohnloser SH. Immediate reinitiation of atrial tachyarrhythmias after spontaneous restoration of sinus rhythm in patients with an implanted monitoring device. *Pacing Clin Electrophysiol* 2003; **26**: 1317–25.

14 Israel CW, Ehrlich JR, Grönefeld G *et al.* Prevalence, characteristics, and clinical implications of regular atrial tachy-arrhythmias in patients with atrial fibrillation: insights from a study using a new implantable device. *J Am Coll Cardiol* 2001; **38**: 355–63.

15 Ritz B, Justen M. Discrimination of ventricular and supraventricular tachycardia via discrimination algorithm PR Logic™ used in implantable dual-chamber cardioverter/defibrillator Gem™ DR systems. *Herzschrittmacher* 2000; **20**: 263–80.

16 Olson WH. Dual chamber sensing and detection for implantable cardioverter-defibrillators. In: Singer I, Barold SS, Camm AJ, eds. *Nonpharmacological Therapy for Arrhythmias for the 21st Century: State of the Art.* Armonk, NY: Futura Publishing Co., Inc., 1998: 385–421.

17 Israel CW, Hügl B, Unterberg C *et al.* Pace-termination and pacing for prevention of atrial tachyarrhythmias: results from a multicenter study with an implantable device for atrial therapy. *J Cardiovasc Electrophysiol* 2001; **12**: 1121–8.

18 Neuzner J, Sperzel J, Pitschner HF *et al.* Bipolar atrial sensing thresholds in sinus rhythm and atrial tachyarrhythmias. A comparative analysis in patients with DDDR pacemakers. *Europace* 1999; **1**: 135–9.

19 Wood MA, Moskovljevic P, Stambler BS, Ellenbogen KA. Comparison of bipolar atrial electrogram amplitude in sinus rhythm, atrial fibrillation, and atrial flutter. *Pacing Clin Electrophysiol* 1996; **19**: 150–6.

20 Waldfridsson H, Aunes M, Capocci M, Edvardsson N. Sensing of atrial fibrillation by a dual chamber pacemaker: how should atrial sensing be programmed to ensure adequate mode shifting? *Pacing Clin Electrophysiol* 2000; **23**: 1089–93.

21 Israel CW, Barold SS. Automatic mode switching: basic concepts. In: Israel CW, Barold SS, eds. *Advances in the Treatment of Atrial Tachyarrhythmia. Pacing, Cardioversion and Defibrillation.* Armonk, NY: Futura Publishing Co., Inc., 2002: 193–218.

22 Barold SS, Levine PA, Israel CW. Diagnostic Holter algorithms for the detection of ventricular tachycardia by implanted pacemakers. In: Santini M, ed. *Proceedings of the International Symposium on Progress in Clinical Pacing 2000.* Rome, Italy: CEPI, 2000: 483–97.

23 Israel CW, Barold SS. Advances in device memory capabilities: towards pacemaker systems as a permanent implantable cardiac rhythm monitor. *Am J Cardiol* 2001; **88**: 442–5.

24 Skanes AC, Yee R, Lee JK *et al.* Progression to chronic atrial fibrillation after pacing: The Canadian Trial of Physiologic Pacing. *J Am Coll Cardiol* 2001; **38**: 167–72.

25 Connolly SJ, Kerr CR, Gent M *et al.* Effects of physiologic pacing versus ventricular pacing on the risk of stroke and death due to cardiovascular causes. Canadian Trial of Physiologic Pacing Investigators. *N Engl J Med* 2000; **342**: 1385–91.

26 Andersen HR, Thuesen L, Bagger JP, Vesterlund T, Thomsen PE. Prospective randomized trial of atrial versus ventricular pacing in sick-sinus syndrome. *Lancet* 1994; **334**: 1523–28.

27 Chamberlain-Webber R, Petersen ME, Ingram A, Briers L, Sutton R. Reasons for reprogramming dual chamber pacemakers to VVI mode: a retrospective review using a computer database. *Pacing Clin Electrophysiol* 1994; **17**: 1730–6.

28 Langenfeld H, Grimm W, Maisch B, Kochsiek K. Atrial fibrillation and embolic complications in paced patients. *Pacing Clin Electrophysiol* 1988; **11**: 1667–72.

29 Fröhlig G, Sen S, Rettig G, Schieffer H, Bette L. Atrial flutter and atrial fibrillation by DDD stimulation. *Z Kardiol* 1985; **74**: 537–47.

30 Detollenaere M, van Wassenhove E, Jordaens L. Atrial arrhythmias in dual chamber pacing and their influence on long-term mortality. *Pacing Clin Electrophysiol* 1992; **15**: 1846–50.

31 Feuer JM, Shandling AH, Messenger JC. Influence of cardiac pacing mode on the long-term development of atrial fibrillation. *Am J Cardiol* 1989; **64**: 1376–9.

32 Israel CW, Olbrich HG, Hartung W, Wille B, Treusch S. Incidence of atrial tachyarrhythmias in paced patients: first results of the BEATS study [abstract]. *Europace* 2002; **3**: A152.

33 Sack S, Mouton E, Defaye P *et al.* Improved detection and analysis of sensed and paced events in dual chamber pacemakers with extended memory function. A prospective multicenter trial in 626 patients. *Herz* 2001; **26**: 30–9.

34 Defaye P, Dournaux F, Mouton E. Prevalence of supraventricular arrhythmias from the automated analysis of data stored in the DDD pacemakers of 617 patients: the AIDA study. *Pacing Clin Electrophysiol* 1998; **21**: 250–5.

35 Garrigue S, Cazeau S, Ritter P, Lazarus A, Gras D, Mugica J. Incidence of atrial arrhythmia in patients with long-term dual-chamber pacemakers. Contribution of the Holter function of pacemakers. *Arch Mal Coeur Vaiss* 1996; **89**: 873–81.

36 Israel CW, Gascon D, Nowak B *et al.* Diagnostic value of stored electrograms in single-lead VDD systems. *Pacing Clin Electrophysiol* 2000; **23**: 1801–3.

37 Israel CW, Böckenförde JB, Mügge A. Clinical results of a new automatic mode switch: The 'x out of y' concept [abstract]. *Pacing Clin Electrophysiol* 1999; **22**: 807.

38 Seidl K, Meisel E, van Agt E *et al.* Is the atrial high rate episodes diagnostic feature reliable in detecting paroxysmal episodes of atrial tachyarrhythmias? *Pacing Clin Electrophysiol* 1998; **21**: 694–700.

39 Fitts SM, Hill MRS, Mehra R, Gillis AM. High rate atrial tachyarrhythmia detections in implantable pulse generators: low incidence of false-positive detections. *Pacing Clin Electrophysiol* 2000; **23**: 1080–6.

40 Pollak WM, Simmons JD, Interian A *et al.* Clinical utility of intra-atrial pacemaker stored electrograms to diagnose atrial fibrillation and flutter. *Pacing Clin Electrophysiol* 2001; **24**: 424–9.

41 Gillis AM, Connolly SJ, Lacombe P *et al.* Randomized crossover comparison of DDDR versus VDD pacing after atrioventricular junction ablation for prevention of atrial fibrillation. The atrial pacing peri-ablation for paroxysmal atrial fibrillation (PA^3) study investigators. *Circulation* 2000; **15**: 736–41.

42 Gillis AM, Wyse DG, Connolly SJ *et al.* Atrial pacing periablation for prevention of paroxysmal atrial fibrillation. *Circulation* 1999; **99**: 2553–8.

43 Mabo P, Paul V, Jung W, Clémenty J, Bouhour A, Daubert JC. Biatrial synchronous pacing for atrial arrhythmia prevention: the SYNBIAPACE study [abstract]. *Eur Heart J* 1999; **20**: 4.

44 Saksena S, Prakash A, Ziegler P *et al.* Improved suppression of atrial fibrillation with dual-site right atrial pacing and antiarrhythmic drug therapy. *J Am Coll Cardiol* 2002; **40**: 1140–50.

45 Camm AJ. Results from the AFT trial. Presented at the Hotline Session, XXIII. Annual Congress of the European Society of Cardiology, Stockholm, September 3, 2001.

46 Hoffmann E, Janko S, Steinbeck G, Edvardsson N, Camm J. Onset scenarios of paroxysmal atrial fibrillation using new diagnostic pacemaker functions [abstract]. *Pacing Clin Electrophysiol* 2000; **23**: 656.

CHAPTER 16

Diagnostic Algorithms for the Detection of Ventricular Tachycardia by Implanted Pacemakers

S. Serge Barold and Michael Eldar

Antibradycardia pacemakers with memory capability can now store electrograms (EGMs) for the diagnosis of arrhythmias [1–5]. This function complements recordings of surrogates of cardiac events such as annotated markers. Stored markers in the form of marker chains are generally available in conventional pacemakers and consume little memory compared to the much larger requirements for storing EGMs of corresponding events. Marker annotations without simultaneous EGM recordings are of limited diagnostic value (Figure 16.1). The current gold standard for pacemaker diagnosis of arrhythmia is the storage of EGMs with annotations at the start of the arrhythmia or from a predetermined time before the trigger (pretrigger storage), starting for a programmable time before the trigger criteria are met.

Pacemaker EGM memory is not yet as extensive as the random access memory (RAM) in implantable cardioverter defibrillators (ICDs) and the diagnostics are not as advanced. However, it is likely that future pacemakers will eventually offer the same diagnostic memory and algorithms for arrhythmia discrimination as those available in the current generation of ICDs.

Clinical experience with the EGM storage capability of pacemakers for the diagnosis of ventricular tachycardia (VT) is still limited. There are important constraints in a pacemaker's ability to detect arrhythmias including ventricular tachycardia that would allow for EGM storage and a definitive arrhythmia diagnosis. Pacemakers have a narrower width of bandpass filter (whereas ICDs are designed to pick up low-frequency signals common in ventricular fibrillation) and may not detect some ventricular complexes with predominantly low-frequency components. Pacemakers usually have a longer refractory period and a lower ventricular sensitivity. Nominal ventricular sensitivity is generally in the range of 2–2.8 mV for pacemakers but < 1 mV for ICDs. The ventricular sensitivity of pacemakers may even be programmed at 4–5 mV in pacemaker-dependent patients to prevent oversensing, making VT recognition more difficult. Finally, the bandpass filters of contemporary devices are not programmable.

Diagnosis of ventricular tachycardia

With ICDs, algorithms must maintain a high level of sensitivity for detecting VT and ventricular fibrillation (VF) while simultaneously providing a high specificity for discriminating between supraventricular tachycardia (SVT) and VT. The first approach to discriminate SVTs and sinus tachycardia from VT was based on rate zones. ICD therapy would be delivered if the ventricular rates of the supraventricular rhythm, even sinus tachycardia, exceeded the rate zone boundary. Methods other than rate alone have evolved to differentiate SVT from VT in ICDs ('enhanced detection criteria'). These discriminators include: (i) sudden onset; (ii) interval stability; (iii) morphology discrimination; and (iv) atrioventricular (AV) relationships based on atrial sensing in

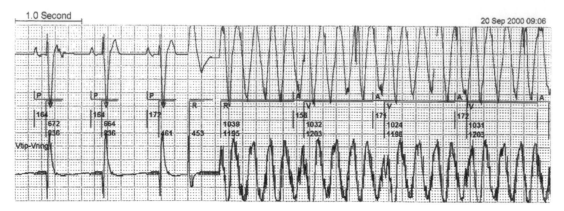

Figure 16.1 A rapid ventricular tachycardia (VT) was created using a simulator connected to a St. Jude Medical Affinity™ pulse generator while simultaneously monitoring the surface electrocardiogram, telemetered event markers and ventricular electrogram. The first isolated premature ventricular complex (PVC) is properly detected, as is the first ventricular complex of the tachycardia, both identified by 'R' markers. After that, the system reverts to asynchronous behavior at the programmed base rate consistent with its noise mode function. This is indicated by the extended horizontal line representing the atrial and ventricular refractory periods. In these devices, an event detected in the last 100 ms of the ventricular refractory period (VRP) is labeled noise and extends the VRP. If another event is detected in the extended VRP, the VRP is again extended. This continues until the atrial and ventricular escape intervals time out or the noise stops. It appears that the very wide QRS for each VT beat was being sensed on both the downslope and upslope for the VT to be labeled noise, as the rate itself would be otherwise too slow to trigger noise mode function. (Reproduced with permission from Barold SS, Levine PA, Israel CW. Diagnostic Holter algorithms for the detection of ventricular tachycardia by implanted pacemakers. In: Santini M, ed. *Progress in Clinical Pacing 2000*. Rome, Italy: CPPI-AIM Group, 2000: 483–496).

dual-chamber ICDs [6–16]. So far, the AV relationship is the only discriminator available to a limited extent in some pacemakers. The data provided by the atrial channel have not eliminated misdiagnosis of tachycardia because of atrial lead instability, atrial undersensing (failure to recognize SVT) or far-field R-wave oversensing.

Rate continues to play a major determining role in dual-chamber algorithms and in ICDs. Any rate above a given level is often interpreted as VT. Ventricular rates greater than atrial rates are used to indicate VT in both ICDs and some pacemakers. Problems arise in the design of algorithms if the rates of VT and SVT are comparable or there is 1 : 1 retrograde ventriculoatrial (VA) conduction from true VT. Analysis of atrial EGMs is important in situations involving retrograde VA conduction, unstable VT, slow VT (by virtue of detecting sinus tachycardia) and double tachycardias (VT with atrial fibrillation). In one study evaluating patients with ICDs, about 1 out of 4 exhibited retrograde 1 : 1 VA conduction at a ventricular pacing cycle length of 400 ms, creating the potential of retrograde 1 : 1 VA conduction during VT. Thus a device may interpret VT with retrograde VA conduction as SVT [17]. Visual inspection of the stored ventricular EGM

during the arrhythmia may suggest VT rather than SVT if the morphology has changed.

True atrial undersensing due to insufficient signal amplitude seems to be the major reason for VT/SVT misclassification related to atrial sensing errors and will trigger storage and diagnosis of VT because the ventricular rate exceeds the sensed atrial rate. For this reason, atrial sensitivity should be high to ensure detection of small-amplitude atrial fibrillation signals. Far-field R-wave oversensing during VT (which must be differentiated from retrograde P waves) may cause a device to label VT as SVT. Additionally, the duration of the blanking periods in both chambers should be minimized to permit sensing of as many intrinsic events as possible. By doing so, it may be necessary to accept the problem of far-field R-wave signals in the unblanked portion of the atrial channel and address it with a special far-field rejection algorithm (either by changing the atrial sensitivity after a ventricular event or by a dedicated algorithm comparing the number and coupling interval of atrial sensed events after a ventricular event) [18]. A relatively long atrial blanking period after an intrinsic ventricular event can cause sensing of only every alternate f wave in rapid atrial flutter and a resultant diagnosis of VT [19].

Technological considerations

The development of pacemakers with extensive memory capability lagged behind ICDs mostly for two reasons [20,21].

1 Low-voltage 128 K RAM chips were not available until recently. Previous 128 K chips could not retain memory at a voltage < 2.7 V, making lithium–iodine batteries unsuitable because a drop to 2.7 V occurs well before the elective replacement point. The use of a voltage doubler to accommodate the previous high-memory chips was inefficient. This has not been an issue with ICDs where the lithium silver vanadium pentoxide (LiSVO) power cell has a nominal potential of 3.5 V.

2 The large physical size, voltage requirements and large current consumption of high-memory chips have decreased. Pacemaker with 128 K of memory are now available with the power source of ICDs adapted to drive dedicated pacemakers. This memory is used for a number of functions, one of which is EGM storage.

Algorithms from several manufacturers

For VT diagnosis, one must know whether diagnostic counting includes events that occur during the pacemaker ventricular refractory period beyond the blanking period and whether atrial sensing includes detection within the postventricular atrial refractory period (PVARP) [19]. The rate and duration of EGM storage of VT should be programmable. The simple report of VT episodes becomes disconcerting, just like large number of premature ventricular complexes (PVCs). The pacemaker criteria for a PVC and VT are different from the clinician's. A pacemaker classifies every ventricular sensed event without a preceding atrial sensed or paced event as a PVC. This does not mean that a native P wave did not precede the R wave. Rather, it means that the pacemaker did not recognize the atrial event because of functional (coinciding with a blanking period or the unblanked portion of the PVARP according to algorithm design) or true atrial undersensing (Figure 16.2). Thus, atrial undersensing

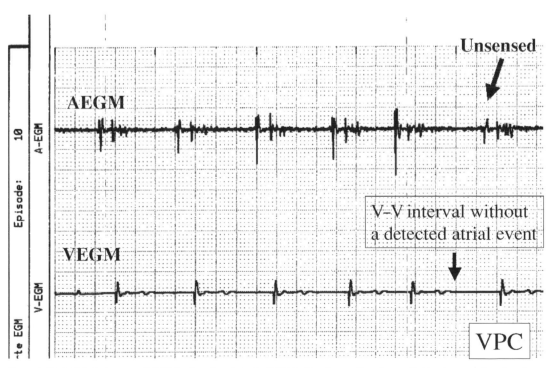

Figure 16.2 Atrial electrogram (EGM) (top) and ventricular EGM (bottom) recordings from a Guidant pacemaker showing how atrial undersensing (arrow) is interpreted as a VPC (ventricular premature complex) by the device because of a V–V cycle without a detected atrial event. No annotated markers were available in this generation of pacemaker.

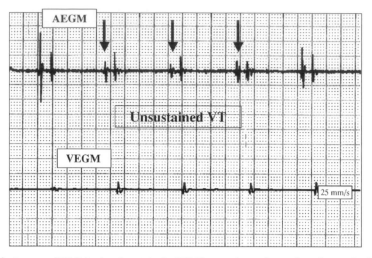

Figure 16.3 Atrial electrogram (EGM) (top) and ventricular EGM (bottom) stored recordings from a Guidant pacemaker. There is marked variability of the P-wave amplitude in sinus rhythm in the atrial EGM. Intermittent atrial undersensing of three consecutive P waves caused the false diagnosis of non-sustained VT at a rate of 68 b.p.m. In addition, there is a very discrete signal on the atrial channel coincident with the QRS that is likely to be a far-field R wave. No annotated markers were available in this generation of pacemaker. (Reproduced with permission from Barold SS, Levine PA, Israel CW. Diagnostic Holter algorithms for the detection of ventricular tachycardia by implanted pacemakers. In: Santini M, ed. *Progress in Clinical Pacing 2000*. Rome, Italy: CPPI-AIM Group, 2000: 483–496). Courtesy of Guidant Corporation.

is a common cause of inappropriate VT detection (Figure 16.3). The definition of non-sustained VT is presently arbitrary and one manufacturer has defined it as three ventricular events without an intervening sensed atrial event (Figure 16.4). Standardization is obviously required in the diagnosis of non-sustained VT. The VT diagnostic requirement that the ventricular rate be faster than the atrial rate may be useful, with the proviso that it would prevent the detection of VT with 1 : 1 VA conduction.

Several generations of pacemakers have incorporated episode-specific ventricular data such as ventricular high rate (VHR) episodes which are not specific for VT.

1 *Medtronic*. The Medtronic Kappa 700 and Kappa 900 pacemakers use a programmed trigger rate and number of consecutive beats to satisfy the VHR episode criteria. When the ventricular rate exceeds the programmed rate for the appropriate number of beats, an episode diagnostic is stored which includes date/time information and, depending on device programming, can also include marker channel information and EGM. The Kappa 700 is capable of storing an EGM for a recent high-rate episode, the Kappa 900 includes more memory and can be

configured to store somewhat shorter strips for up to eight episodes. This collection criteria is non-specific for VT and can be used for a variety of purposes including detecting rapidly conducted atrial fibrillation or capturing sensor-driven rate increases (the trigger rate can be programmed below the upper tracking rate or upper sensor rate).

The Medtronic AT 500 pacemaker was designed with the same diagnostic functions as those of dual-chamber defibrillators [22,23]. The system uses interval and stability criteria, PR logic and rate analysis. Such a sophisticated system should enhance VT detection with greater specificity.

2 *Guidant*. The device counts a ventricular sensed event and records the intervals of subsequent sensed ventricular events. The detection criteria (rate and duration) are programmable. If the VT detection criteria are set at 200 b.p.m. for a total of 8 beats, once they are met, the pacemaker will store the episode and VT is declared (Figures 16.5 & 16.6). The VT counter is an up-and-down counter so that each interval less than the programmed detection interval (rate) increments the counter and each interval greater than the programmed detection interval decrements the counter. Any ventricular paced event (Vp), PVC or sensed ventricular event

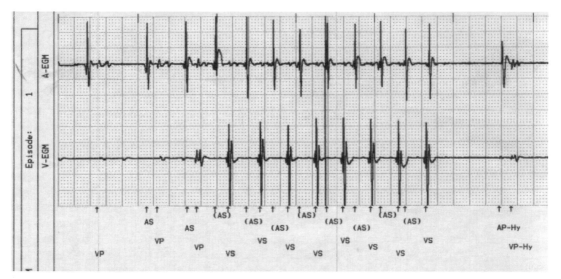

Figure 16.4 Brief salvo of supraventricular tachycardia (SVT) stored and interpreted by a Guidant pacemaker as VT because all the P waves coincided with the postventricular atrial refractory period (shown as AS in parentheses) and were not used for the identification of SVT according to the algorithm in this pacemaker. The device labeled the tachycardia as VT. The vertical line shows the trigger point. The atrial electrogram (EGM) is on top and the ventricular EGM at the bottom. AS, atrial sensed event; AP, atrial paced event; VS, ventricular sensed event; VP, ventricular paced event. (Reproduced with the permission of St. Jude Medical CRMD.)

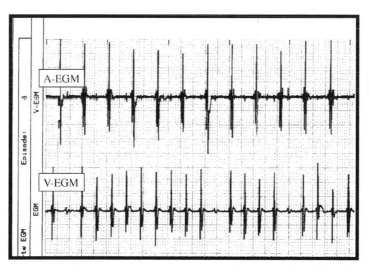

Figure 16.5 Atrial and ventricular electrogram (EGM) storage of an episode of ventricular tachycardia (VT) in a patient with a Guidant pacemaker. Since the stored EGMs are processed signals, one cannot use the relative amplitude as a guide to the size of the signal and sensing. If the small far-field signals that can be seen on this recording had been also sensed on the atrial channel, this rhythm might have been labeled supraventricular tachycardia rather than VT. Intermittent small ventricular signals represent ventricular pacing which occurred most likely after atrial events sensed outside the postventricular atrial refractory period. No annotated markers were available in this generation of pacemakers. (Reproduced with permission from Barold SS, Levine PA, Israel CW. Diagnostic Holter algorithms for the detection of ventricular tachycardia by implanted pacemakers. In: Santini M, ed. *Progress in Clinical Pacing 2000*. Rome, Italy: CPPI-AIM Group, 2000: 483–496).

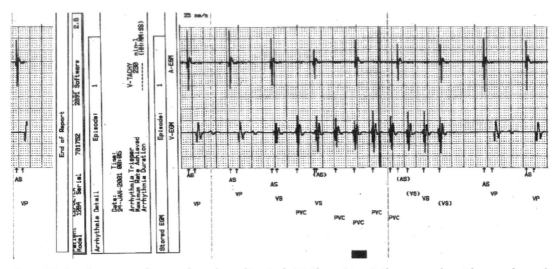

Figure 16.6 Stored unsustained ventricular tachycardia episode (230 b.p.m.) in a Guidant pacemaker with more advanced diagnostics than the function shown in Figure 16.5. The atrial electrogram (EGM) is on top and the ventricular EGM at the bottom. PVC, premature ventricular complex identified by the device after a V–V interval without intervening atrial activity; (VS), ventricular sensed event in the refractory period; PVC, premature ventricular complex. Other abbreviations are as in Figure 16.4. The vertical line shows the trigger point. (Reproduced courtesy of Guidant Corporation.)

(Vs) can start or end a ventricular cycle. A refractory sensed ventricular event cannot start a ventricular cycle, but it is used to determine the shortest V–V interval within the ventricular cycle. Thus, Vp with loss of ventricular capture can initiate a ventricular cycle for VT diagnosis and create a false diagnosis of VT by the device. In the PD2 (Pulsar Max 2, Discovery 2 family) and Insignia (Entra, Plus) designs, the pacemaker looks only at the V–V intervals and not the atrial rate (V > A rate criterion) for VT detection. PDM devices (Pulsar Max, Discovery and Meridian family) are the only ones that look at the atrial rate. In the PDM designs, the system would look at atrial events in PVARP and if the 'A to A' interval were less than the V–V interval, a VT episode would not be declared. Again, this criterion was dropped in the PD2 and Insignia.

3 *St. Jude.* The Identity pacemaker with EGM storage does not identify VT *per se.* Rather, two of the programmable triggers address this issue.

(a) The pacemaker defines a PVC as a sensed R wave without detected preceding atrial activity. With the PVC trigger, the clinician specifies the number of consecutive 'PVCs' from a minimum of 2 to a maximum of 5. P waves will still be identified, even if they coincide with the PVARP, but as long as the P is in the refractory period, the sensed R wave will be labeled a PVC. This allows

the potential detection of even slow VT or accelerated idioventricular rhythms.

(b) High ventricular rate trigger. If the ventricular rate exceeds a programmable rate for a programmable number of cycles, the system will store an EGM. It is then up to the clinician to determine whether the episode constitutes VT or SVT. On the Identity EGMs, 50% of the total EGM records pretrigger events so that initiation of the VT episode can be discerned.

Results

There is little information on the true prevalence of VT in pacemaker patients. Many non-sustained ventricular tachyarrhythmias are asymptomatic. So far, the automatic diagnosis of VT by pacemakers has been disappointing. The high incidence of incorrect pacemaker EGM diagnosis of atrial events indicates the importance of optimal device programming and the need for refining the appropriate algorithms (Table 16.1 & Figures 16.7–16.9). All detected VT episodes must be confirmed by scrutiny of the EGMs to determine the appropriateness of algorithm activation.

Defaye *et al.* [24] studied the triggered EGMs in 75 patients with a Guidant Discovery™ device, and found false-positive EGMs in 36% of non-sustained

Table 16.1 Misdiagnosis of VT by stored electrograms.

---

1 *Overdiagnosis of VT*

(a) Ventricular oversensing

Myopotential interference (including special sources from the diaphragm and intercostal muscles), T wave, etc. (Figure 16.7)

P-wave oversensing by ventricular channel

Double counting of a wide QRS signal during sinus rhythm

External interference such as electrocautery, etc.

Electrode disruption with coarse noise (Figure 16.8)

(b) Atrial undersensing

True atrial undersensing with AV conduction may be classified as VT, especially in the setting of sinus tachycardia

Functional undersensing as with P waves falling in the atrial refractory/blanking period (first-degree AV block, atrial flutter, etc.) (Figure 16.9)

'Mechanical' (atrial lead instability)

2 *Underdiagnosis of VT*

VT may not fulfil detection criteria, particularly in the presence of other pacemaker abnormalities

1 : 1 VA conduction during VT may be interpreted as SVT by some pacemakers

During double tachycardia VT may be falsely diagnosed as SVT

Absence of 'onset recording' may cause NSVT to be missed

3 *Rate regularity*

In chronic atrial fibrillation at relatively rapid ventricular responses, the ventricular rate may be regular or near-regular for the brief period that may be sufficient for an algorithm to diagnose VT

AV, atrioventricular; NSVT, nonsustained ventricular tachycardia; SVT, supraventricular tachyarrhythmia; VA, ventriculoatrial; VT, ventricular tachycardia.

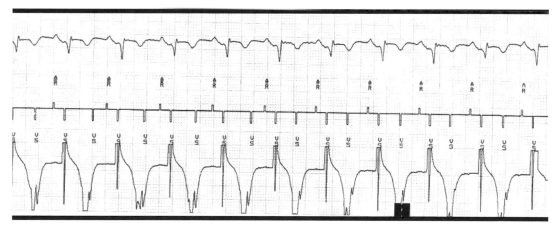

Figure 16.7 T-wave oversensing by dual-chamber pacemaker. This disturbance can be stored by a pacemaker as ventricular tachycardia because of double counting of sensed ventricular events. VS, ventricular sensed event; AR, sensed atrial event in the refractory period.

VT and 44% in sustained VT. In another study of 10 patients comparing 24-h Holter recordings with stored EGMs, 13 out of 15 episodes of registered non-sustained VT were correctly identified and two were falsely positive when P waves coincided with the postventricular refractory period and the QRS complex was labeled as being ventricular ectopic [25]. In another study involving the Guidant Pulsar™ VDD pacemaker, virtually all the cases of EGM storage upon pacemaker-defined VT detection

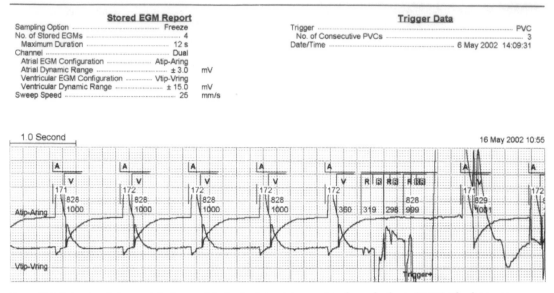

Figure 16.8 False signals from a defective ventricular lead simulate a ventricular arrhythmia (VPCs). The data were stored by an Identity (St. Jude) pacemaker. This patient had high-grade atrioventricular block and sinus node dysfunction. With the ventricular oversensing, atrial output was also inhibited. VPCs, ventricular premature complexes. (Reproduced with the permission of St. Jude Medical CRMD.)

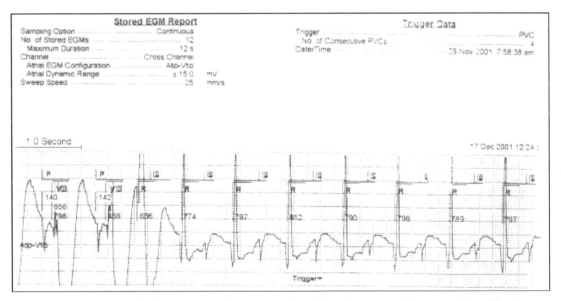

Figure 16.9 Functional atrial undersensing simulating ventricular tachycardia in a stored electrogram by an Identity (St. Jude) pacemaker. The patient had sinus rhythm with first-degree atrioventricular block. A true ventricular premature complex (VPC) occurred, with the sinus P wave coinciding with the postventricular atrial refractory period (PVARP). However, this sinus P wave was conducted. The conducted R wave was labeled a VPC, extending the PVARP in accord with the + PVARP on premature ventricular complex algorithm. Each subsequent P wave was not detected for purposes of labeling the rhythm, but each conducted R wave was again labeled a VPC. P, sensed atrial event; R, sensed ventricular event; V, ventricular paced event. The P wave in the PVARP is depicted differently. (Reproduced with the permission of St. Jude Medical CRMD.)

(≥ 3 beats at > 200 b.p.m.) were due to oversensing T waves, myopotentials and electrocautery for coronary bypass surgery [26]. In the same study, in 8% of stored EGMs no arrhythmia or sensing error could be detected either because the arrhythmia had already stopped at the time of EGM storage (no pretrigger data) or because it was undetectable from the EGM recording (e.g. oversensing of small signals).

The sensitivity of arrhythmia detection by EGM storage is unknown, simply because an EGM cannot be recorded if it is not detected. False-positive EGM atrial events reflect how a pacemaker interprets data according to its design (atrial event detection algorithms) and timing cycles, and as such do not represent pacemaker malfunction. Data from false positive EGM should not be ignored. They can be used to optimize pacemaker parameters (such as sensitivity and refractory periods). The effect of reprogramming can then be evaluated by recording a reduction of false-positive EGM atrial events during the subsequent follow-up session. It is recommended that the morphology of EGMs should be periodically recorded and incorporated in the medical record for comparative purposes to facilitate future interpretation of recorded data.

Conclusion

The increasing random access memory capability of pacemakers has added a new dimension to device diagnosis of arrhythmias and pacemaker malfunction by allowing for EGM storage in a manner similar to that of ICDs. This modality is still in its infancy and lagging behind that of ICDs for a variety of technical limitations that are being actively addressed by industry. The recent development of pacemaker pretrigger EGM storage and the addition of annotated markers with EGM storage represent two major advances in this field. This new pacemaker technology will also provide important data about the incidence and natural history of asymptomatic ventricular arrhythmias that are detected by the devices based on criteria established and programmed by the monitoring physician. Proper clinical applicability and limitations need to be further defined based on practical experience with this technology. State-of-the-art pacemaker technology will continue to be incorporated into ICDs, and advanced ICD memory systems will be incorporated into pacemakers. With the availability of patient-triggered event recordings [27–29], and transtelephonic data transmission of recorded events, a pacemaker would function much like an external event recorder or implantable loop recorder. Industry continues to require the active input of the clinical community to define the optimal duration of EGM recording in pacemakers required for useful information and how best to use it by means of programmability in various clinical situations.

References

1 Plummer CJ, Henderson S, Gardener L et al. The use of permanent pacemakers in the detection of cardiac arrhythmias. Europace 2001; 3: 229–32.

2 Nowak B. Pacemaker stored electrograms: teaching us what is really going on in our patients. Pacing Clin Electrophysiol 2002; 25: 838–49.

3 Huikuri H. Effect of stored electrograms on management in the paced patient. Am J Cardiol 2000; 86 (9 Suppl. I): K101–K103.

4 Guilleman D, Scanu P, Citerne O et al. Clinical value of stored intracardiac electrograms [abstract]. Europace 2000; 1 (Suppl. D): D28.

5 Petersen B, Huikiri H, Benzer W et al. Specificity of pacemaker diagnostics verified by stored E-grams [abstract]. Europace 2000; 1 (Suppl. D): D214.

6 Wilkoff BL, Kuhlkamp V, Volosin K et al. Critical analysis of dual-chamber implantable cardioverter-defibrillator arrhythmia detection: results and technical considerations. Circulation 2002; 103: 381–6.

7 Unterberg C, Stevens J, Vollmann D et al. Long-term clinical experience with the EGM width detection criterion for differentiation of supraventricular and ventricular tachycardia in patients with implantable cardioverter defibrillators. Pacing Clin Electrophysiol 2000; 23: 1611–17.

8 Swerdlow CD, Schols W, Dijkman B et al. Detection of atrial fibrillation and flutter by a dual chamber cardioverter defibrillator. Circulation 2000; 101: 878–85.

9 Dijkman B, Wellens HJ. Importance of the atrial channel for ventricular arrhythmia therapy in the dual chamber implantable cardioverter defibrillator. J Cardiovasc Electrophysiol 2000; 11: 1309–19.

10 Swerdlow CD. Supraventricular tachycardia–ventricular tachycardia discrimination algorithms in implantable cardioverter defibrillators: state-of-the-art review. J Cardiovasc Electrophysiol 2001; 12: 606–12.

11 Gronefeld GC, Schulte B, Hohnloser SH et al. Morphology discrimination: a beat-to-beat algorithm

for the discrimination of ventricular from supra-ventricular tachycardia by implantable cardioverter defibrillators. *Pacing Clin Electrophysiol* 2001; **24**: 1519–24.

12 Hintringer F, Schwarzacher S, Eibl G *et al.* Inappropriate detection of supraventricular arrhythmias by implantable dual chamber defibrillators: a comparison of four different algorithms. *Pacing Clin Electrophysiol* 2001; **24**: 835–41.

13 Deisenhofer I, Kolb C, Ndrepepa G *et al.* Do current dual chamber cardioverter defibrillators have advantages over conventional single chamber cardioverter defibrillators in reducing inappropriate therapies? A randomized, prospective study. *J Cardiovasc Electrophysiol* 2001; **12**: 134–42.

14 Schimpf R, Wolpert C, Luderitz B. Algorithms for better arrhythmia discrimination in implantable cardioverter defibrillators. *Curr Cardiol Rep* 2001; **3**: 467–72.

15 Boriani G, Biffi M, Frabetti L *et al.* Clinical evaluation of morphology discrimination: an algorithm for rhythm discrimination in cardioverter defibrillators. *Pacing Clin Electrophysiol* 2001; **24**: 994–1001.

16 Dijkman B, Wellens HJ. Dual chamber arrhythmia detection in the implantable cardioverter defibrillator. *J Cardiovasc Electrophysiol* 2000; **11**: 1105–15.

17 Militianu A, Salacata A, Meissner MD *et al.* Ventriculoatrial conduction capability and prevalence of 1 : 1 retrograde conduction during inducible sustained monomorphic ventricular tachycardia in 305 implantable cardioverter defibrillator recipients. *Pacing Clin Electrophysiol* 1997; **20**: 2378–84.

18 Wood MA, Swerdlow C, Olson WH. Sensing and arrhythmia detection in implantable devices. In: Ellenbogen K, Kay N, Wilkoff B, eds. *Clinical Cardiac Pacing and Defibrillation*, 2nd edn. Philadelphia PA: W. B. Saunders, 2000: 68–126.

19 Barold SS. Timing cycles and operational characteristics of pacemakers. In: Ellenbogen K, Kay N, Wilkoff B, eds. *Clinical Cardiac Pacing and Defibrillation*, 2nd edn. Philadelphia PA: W. B. Saunders, 2000: 727–825.

20 Barold SS, Bornzin G, Levine P. Development of a true pacemaker Holter. In: Vardas PE, ed. *Cardiac Arrhythmias, Pacing and Electrophysiology. The Expert View.* Boston, MA: Kluwer, 1998: 421–6.

21 Israel CW, Barold SS. Pacemakers systems as implantable cardiac rhythm monitors. *Am J Cardiol* 2001; **15**: 442–5.

22 Vollmann D, Stevens J, Buchwald AB *et al.* Automatic atrial antitachy pacing for the termination of spontaneous atrial tachyarrhythmias: clinical experience with a novel dual-chamber pacemaker. *J Interv Card Electrophysiol* 2001; **5**: 477–85.

23 Israel CW, Hügl B, Unterberg C *et al.* Pace-termination and pacing for prevention of atrial tachyarrhythmias: results from a multicenter study with an implantable device for atrial therapy. *J Cardiovasc Electrophysiol* 2001; **12**: 1121–8.

24 Defaye P, Hazard JR, Besson B *et al.* Contribution of pacemaker stored electrograms to patient management [abstract]. *Pacing Clin Electrophysiol* 2000; **23**: 681.

25 Hamel E, Hudelo C, Maillard L *et al.* Appropriate detection of Guidant pacemaker stored electrograms assessed by 24-hour surface ECG [abstract]. *Europace* 2000; **1** (Suppl. D): D214.

26 Israel CW, Gascon D, Nowak B *et al.* Diagnostic value of stored electrograms in single-lead VDD systems. *Pacing Clin Electrophysiol* 2000; **23**: 1801–3.

27 Machado C, Johnson D, Thacker JR *et al.* Pacemaker patient-triggered event recording: accuracy, utility, and cost for the pacemaker follow-up clinic. *Pacing Clin Electrophysiol* 1996; **19**: 1813–18.

28 Huikuri HV, Koistinen J, Petersen B *et al.* A new approach to symptomatic pacemaker patients results from the magnet stored E-gram study [abstract]. *Europace* 2000; **1** (Suppl. D): D32.

29 Rebollo JMG, Madrid AH, Megias MA *et al.* Externally patient-activated devices in pacemaker patients. Clinical utility [abstract]. *Europace* 2000; **1** (Suppl. D): D31.

CHAPTER 17

Evaluation of the Pacing Function of Dual- and Triple-Chamber ICDs

Sergio L. Pinski

Introduction

Several factors explain the increased use of dual- and triple-chamber implantable cardioverter defibrillators (ICDs). Up to 30% of ICD patients have concomitant bradyarrhythmic indications for dual-chamber pacing [1–4]. Dual-chamber, rate-responsive ICDs have eliminated the need for a separate pacemaker in these populations. This has resulted in fewer intravascular leads, elimination of device–device interactions, better cosmetic results, and simplified follow-up [5]. Dual-chamber ICDs have the potential to improve tachyarrhythmia discrimination [6,7], and so they could also be beneficial in patients without pacing indications. Two-thirds of ICDs implanted in the US are dual chamber, and an ongoing randomized trial is investigating the relative merits of single- versus dual-chamber ICDs in patients without bradyarrhythmias [8]. Additionally, many ICD candidates with heart failure can benefit from resynchronization pacing therapy [9,10]. Finally, atrioventricular ICDs may be valuable in selected patients with drug-refractory atrial fibrillation [11].

As clinical experience with these devices grew, some shortcomings and idiosyncrasies became apparent. Addition of full-featured pacing is technically complex, and the resultant product is not simply the sum of a DDDR (or DDDRV [12]) pacemaker and a tiered-therapy ICD. Manufacturers have endeavored to avoid intradevice interactions between pacing and arrhythmia detection algorithms that could cause underdetection or spurious detection of ventricular tachyarrhythmia. Thus, especially in early devices, compromises were made

between pacing versatility and safe defibrillator function [5]. Many of the initial shortcomings have been corrected in successive device generations, but defibrillation safety considerations will always restrict the range of pacing rates and blanking and refractory periods that can be programmed in ICDs. These restrictions at times still result in suboptimal pacemaker function. Furthermore, as the ICD becomes more of a 'stand-by' device [13], attempts at tachyarrhythmia prevention by multi-site pacing and sophisticated pacing algorithms make analysis of its pacing function more complex than in the conventional antibradycardia pacemaker.

All manufacturers incorporate in their latest ICDs most (but not all) diagnostic and therapeutic functions available in their top-of-the-line pacemakers (Table 17.1). Up to now, all rate-adaptive sensors have been of the activity or accelerometer type. Minute ventilation, intracardiac impedance or multisensor units have not been developed. All devices incorporate differential AV/PV intervals, automatic mode switching for atrial tachyarrhythmias, and algorithms to prevent and terminate endless-loop tachycardia. ICDs do not yet incorporate automatic capture management algorithms [14]. Among current devices, the Prizm 2 DR provides the most comprehensive set of specific algorithms (e.g. AV interval search hysteresis, rate search hysteresis), that may be useful in individual patients.

In this chapter, we evaluate the pacing function of current dual- and triple-chamber ICDs, describe potential problems and provide guidelines for their prevention, both at time of implant (and initial programming) and during follow-up.

Table 17.1 Programmability of pacing functions in some current dual- and triple-chamber implantable cardioverter defibrillators.

Function	Tachos DR[a]	Defender IV DR	Contak CD 1823	Prizm 2 DR 1861	GEM III DR, InSync 7272	GEM III AT 7276	Marquis DR 7274	Photon/Atlas
Pacing mode								
Oil, ODO			✓	✓		✓	✓	✓
AAI(R)	✓ (no R)		✓	✓		✓	✓	✓
VVI(R)	✓	✓	✓	✓	✓	✓	✓	✓
VDD(R)	✓		✓	✓	✓			
DDD(R)	✓	✓	✓	✓	✓	✓	✓	✓
DDI(R)	✓	✓	✓	✓	✓	✓	✓	✓
Lower/upper rate								
Rate hysteresis	✓[b]	✓	✓	✓	✓[j]		✓[j]	✓
Night rate	✓							
Rest rate								
Search hysteresis	✓[c]			✓[g]				✓[m]
MTR	160 b.p.m.	NP[d]	175 b.p.m.	175 b.p.m.	150 b.p.m.	150 b.p.m.	150 b.p.m.	150 b.p.m.
MSR	180 p.p.m.	142 b.p.m.[e]	175 p.p.m.	175 p.p.m.	150 p.p.m.	150 p.p.m.	150 p.p.m.	150 p.p.m.
Rate response								
Sensor	Accel	Accel	Accel	Accel	Piezoelectric	Piezoelectric	Accel	Accel
Threshold	✓		✓	✓	✓	✓	✓	✓
Gain (slope)		✓	✓	✓	✓	✓	✓	✓
Reaction time		✓	✓	✓	✓	✓	✓	✓
Recovery time			✓	✓	✓	✓	✓	✓
AV delay								
Dynamic	✓	✓	✓	✓	✓	✓	✓	✓
Separate AV/PV	✓	✓	✓	✓	✓	✓	✓	✓
Search hysteresis				✓				
Automatic mode								
Detection rate	NP (MTR + 20 b.p.m.)	= MTR	P: 100–200 b.p.m.	P: 100–200 b.p.m.	P: 120–176 b.p.m.	= AT (or AF) detection rate (or MTR)	P: 120–175 b.p.m.	P: 110–220 b.p.m.

Duration	P: 4–8 cycles	P: 8, 16, 32, 2016 cycles	P: 0–2000 intervals	P: 0–2000 intervals[h]	NP	NP	NP	NP
Fallback mode	P: DDI or DDIR	VDIR	VDIR	P: VDIR or DDIR	DDIR	DDIR	DDIR	P: DDIR, VVIR
Fallback rate	P: 31–110 b.p.m. (or SIR)	LRL (or SIR)	P: 40–175 b.p.m. (or SIR)[f]	P: 30–175 b.p.m. (or SIR)[i]	SIR	SIR[k]	SIR	LRL (SIR)

Accel, accelerometer; b.p.m., beats per minute; LRL, lower rate limit; MSR, maximum sensor rate; MTR, maximum tracking rate; NP, not programmable; P, programmable; p.p.m., pulses per minute; SIR, sensor-indicated rate.

Tachos DR

[a] Some features (e.g. repetitive hysteresis, scan hysteresis) are locked out in the version commercialized in the US.

[b] A programmable repetitive hysteresis function allows pacing at the hysteresis rate for a programmable number of cycles before switching back to the basic rate.

[c] When scan hysteresis is enabled, the pacemaker will pace at the basic rate for 180 cycles, and will then scan for intrinsic rhythm by pacing again at the hysteresis rate for a programmable number of cycles.

Defender IV

[d] The MTR is not programmable independently. It is always ≥ 12 b.p.m. lower than the VT detection zone.

[e] The MSR can be programmed in the slow VT zone.

Contak CD

[f] A programmable (0 s–5 min) ATR fallback time determines how quickly the rate will decrease from the MTR to the programmed fallback rate.

Prizm 2 DR

[g] When rate search hysteresis is enabled the pulse generator will lower the escape rate to the programmed hysteresis rate after a programmable number of cycles (256–4096) for up to 8 cardiac cycles.

[h] P entry and exit count intervals also influence how fast atrial tachyarrhythmia is detected and how quickly the pacemaker returns to an atrial tracking mode.

[i] A programmable (0 s–5 min) ATR fallback time determines how quickly the rate will decrease from the MTR to the programmed fallback rate.

GEM III DR, InSync

[j] Hysteresis is only available in AAI or VVI modes.

GEM III AT 7276

[k] During the mode switch, ventricular rate is continuously smoothed.

Marquis DR 7274

[l] Hysteresis is only available in AAI or VVI modes.

Photon/Atlas

[m] When rate hysteresis with search is enabled, the pulse generator extends the pacing interval to the hysteresis rate every 5 min for 1 pacing cycle to search for intrinsic activity.

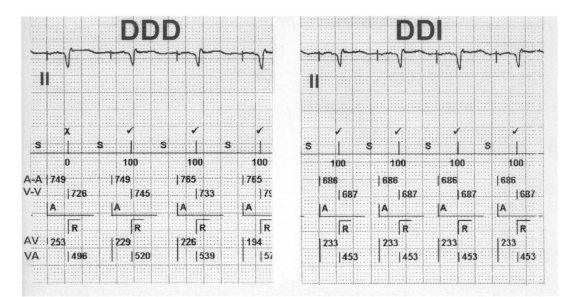

Figure 17.1 Different lower rate timing according to programmed mode in a St. Jude ICD. Real-time lead II and event markers displaying A–A, V–V, AV and VA intervals. The left panel depicts DDD pacing and the right panel DDI pacing. The lower rate is programmed to 80 b.p.m. (750 ms) and the paced AV delay to 300 ms during both modes. There is intrinsic conduction with an AV interval of ~ 230 ms. Due to ventricular-based timing in DDI mode, the pacing rate accelerates by the difference between the conducted and programmed AV intervals.

Timing cycles of dual- and triple-chamber ICDs

Basic bradycardia pacing operation

In general, DDDR lower-rate timing is atrial based or modified ventricular based (i.e. the pacing rate does not increase after Ap–Vs cycles). However, in many devices timing is ventricular based in DDIR mode (Figure 17.1). Different from other devices, the Biotronik Tachos DR has atrial-based timing also after a ventricular premature depolarization (VPD). Therefore, the postextrasystolic pause can violate the lower rate limit.

In dual-chamber ICDs, the timing cycles during AAIR pacing may be modified in comparison to dual-chamber pacemakers. Ventricular sensing and tachyarrhythmia detection still occur during single-chamber atrial pacing, and so sensed ventricular events can interfere with atrial pacing. In Guidant devices, for example, atrial events falling during the cross-chamber blanking after ventricular sensed events initiated by a VPD are not seen and competitive atrial pacing can ensue [15]. Because during AAIR pacing a ventricular sensed event does not inhibit delivery of the next atrial pulse, the pulse may be delivered within the tachycardia detection

interval. This may cause inappropriate tachyarrhythmia detection if crosstalk from atrial pacing occurs, or tachyarrhythmia underdetection if arrhythmic ventricular events are missed due to cross-chamber blanking [16].

Blanking and refractory periods

Timing intervals are more complicated in dual-chamber ICDs than in conventional dual-chamber pacemakers (Figure 17.2; Tables 17.2 & 17.3). Understanding the function and programmability of the different blanking and refractory periods available in a device is often the key to successful troubleshooting of oversensing or functional undersensing.

Blanking periods, during which the ICD does not sense electrical signals, are necessary to avoid sensing ICD outputs, postpacing polarization, T waves and multiple sensing of the same event. However, the need to detect rapid rhythms in both chambers precludes the relatively long blanking periods used in standard pacemakers. Most devices implement longer blanking periods following paced events (to avoid sensing the depolarizations signal on the electrodes), while the blanking periods after sensed events are short or even absent. Some devices also

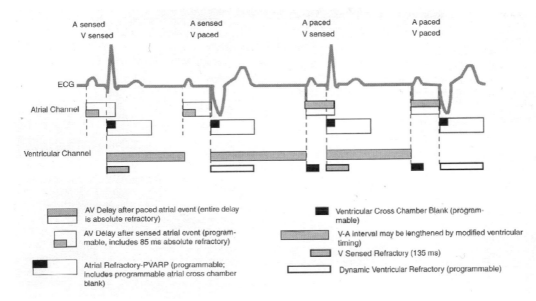

A sensed   A sensed   A paced   A paced
V sensed   V paced   V sensed   V paced

ECG

Atrial Channel

Ventricular Channel

■ AV Delay after paced atrial event (entire delay is absolute retractory)

□ AV Delay after sensed atrial event (programmable, includes 85 ms absolute refractory)

■ Atrial Refractory-PVARP (programmable; includes programmable atrial cross chamber blank)

■ Ventricular Cross Chamber Blank (programmable)

■ V-A interval may be lengthened by modified ventricular timing)

■ V Sensed Refractory (135 ms)

□ Dynamic Ventricular Refractory (programmable)

Figure 17.2 Refractory periods for dual-chamber pacing modes in the Guidant Prizm 2 DR. (Reproduced with permission.)

present different blanking periods for antibradycardia pacing and antitachycardia function. In theory, up to 16 different blanking periods (8 atrial, 8 ventricular) could occur [17].

During a refractory period a signal can be sensed but cannot start certain pacing timing intervals. The way the terminology is used differs among manufacturers. For practical purposes, however, if a signal sensed during a refractory period is ignored by *all* timing cycles in the device, the refractory period operates as a blanking period. Although the traditional definition of the postventricular atrial refractory period (PVARP) as the time period after a paced or sensed ventricular event during which an atrial sensed event does not inhibit an atrial pace nor trigger a ventricular pace still applies, devices differ regarding the behavior of other functions in response to events sensed during this window.

Nomenclature can be confusing. For example, in Medtronic devices, the so-called postventricular atrial blanking period (PVAB) refers only to the bradycardia function. It is important for functions such as the non-competitive atrial pacing algorithm and the mode-switching algorithm, and as the shortest value that the PVARP can adopt when programmed to the 'varied' mode. Telemetered annotations may also be confusing. For example, far-field atrial sensing of an R wave is depicted as an A_R, although there is no tachycardia refractory period

(i.e. the events are used for tachycardia discrimination) and they fall inside the bradycardia blanking and would otherwise be ignored by a dual-chamber pacemaker of similar design [17].

Rate-smoothing or rate stabilization algorithms

Rate-smoothing or rate stabilization algorithms have been incorporated into ICDs with the goal of preventing the onset of atrial or ventricular tachyarrhythmias. The evidence regarding their efficacy with routine use is still sparse [18–20]. However, there is no doubt that in individual cases (e.g. in patients with QT prolongation and torsades de pointes) [21], ventricular rate stabilization algorithms are useful. Two algorithms (the one in Guidant devices and the one in GEM DR and Marquis DR devices) aim primarily at regularizing the ventricular rate. The atrial rate stabilization algorithm available in the GEM III AT ICD aims at regularizing the atrial rate.

The ventricular rate stabilization (VRS) algorithm in Medtronic devices has the simplest operation. It functions as a continuous rate-smoothing algorithm to suppress postextrasystolic pauses. Two parameters are programmable: (a) the VRS minimum pacing interval (programmable between 500 and 900 ms in 50-ms steps, but subject to programmer interlocks); and (b) the interval increment (programmable between 50 and 400 ms in 10-ms

Table 17.2 Atrial blanking and refractory periods in some current dual- and triple-chamber implantable cardioverter defibrillators.

Model	Postatrial paced blanking	Postatrial sense blanking	Postventricular paced blanking	Postventricular sense blanking	PVARP	PVARP on PVC
Biotronik Tachos DR	P: 150–400 ms (*300 ms)	Fixed at 102 ms	P: 23–200 ms (*23 ms)	P: 0–120 ms (*0 ms)	P: 200–500 ms (*250 ms)	P extension: 125–300 ms (*150 ms)
Ela Medical Defender IV DR	Fixed at the entire AV delay	Fixed at 47 ms	P: 78*, 94, 109, 125, 141, 156	P: 47*, 63, 78, 94, 109, 125, 141, 156	P: 281–563 (*391)	NP at 469 ms
Guidant Contak CD 1823	Fixed at the entire AV delay	Fixed at 86 ms	Fixed at 66 ms	Fixed at 66 ms	P: 150–500 ms (*250 ms)	P: OFF*, 150–500 ms
Guidant Prizm 2 DR 1861	Fixed at the entire AV delay	Fixed at 85 ms	P: 45, 65, 85*	P: 45, 65, 85*	P: fixed (150–500 ms) or dynamic (P max: 160–500 ms; P min: 150–490 ms)	P: OFF*, 150–500 ms
Medtronic GEM III DR 7275, InSync 7272	P: 200–250 ms (*240 ms)	Fixed at 100 ms	Fixed at 30 ms (tachy) P PVAB: 100–350 ms (*150 ms) (brady)	None (tachy) P PVAB: 100–350 ms (*150 ms) (brady)	P: varied or fixed 150–500 ms (*310 ms)	P: OFF or ON (at 400 ms)
Medtronic GEM III AT 7276	P: 200–250 ms (*240 ms)	Fixed at 100 ms	Fixed at 30 ms	None	P: 150–500 ms (*310 ms) P PVARP for ARS: 100–500 ms (*200 ms)	NP at 400 ms
Medtronic Marquis DR 7274	P: 150–250 ms (*200 ms)	Fixed at 100 ms	Fixed at 30 ms (tachy) P PVAB: 100–310 ms (*150 ms) (brady)	None (tachy) P PVAB: 100–310 ms (*150 ms) (brady)	P: varied or fixed 150–500 ms (*310 ms)	P: OFF or ON (at 400 ms)
St. Jude Photon DR V-230, Photon μ DR V-232, Atlas DR V-240	Fixed at 190 or 220 ms depending on atrial output	P: 93*, 125 or 157 ms	NP PVAB: at 30 or 60 ms depending on programmed V output, and max paced rate (brady) P: 'far R suppression': OFF*, 20–200 ms	P 'far R suppression': OFF*, 20–200 ms	P: 125–470 ms	P: OFF*, or 'pace on PVC' at 330 ms

* Nominal setting.

ARS, atrial rate regularization; AV, atrioventricular; brady, bradycardia; max, maximum; min, minimum; NP, not programmable; P, programmable; PVARP, postventricular atrial refractory period; PVAB, postventricular atrial blanking; PVC, premature ventricular complex; tachy, tachycardia.

Table 17.3 Ventricular blanking and refractory periods in some current dual- and triple-chamber implantable cardioverter defibrillators.

Model	Postatrial paced blanking	Postventricular paced blanking	Postventricular sense blanking
Biotronik Tachos DR	Fixed at 23 ms No VSP	P: 250–400 ms (*250 ms)	Fixed at 121 ms
Ela Medical Defender IV DR 612	Fixed at 47 ms NP VSP[1]	Fixed at 219 ms	Fixed at 94 ms
Guidant Contak CD 1823	Fixed at 66 ms No VSP	P: fixed (150–500 ms; *250 ms) or dynamic (max: 160–500 ms; min: 150–490 ms)	Fixed at 135 ms (40-ms noise detection window)
Guidant Prizm 2 DR 1861	P: 45, 65*, 85 ms No VSP	P: fixed (150–500 ms; *250 ms) or dynamic (P max: 160–500 ms; P min: 150–490 ms)	Fixed at 135 ms (40-ms noise detection window)
Medtronic GEM III DR 7275, GEM III AT 7276, InSync 7272, Marquis DR 7274	Fixed at 30 ms P VSP[2]; ON*, OFF	P: 150–440 ms (*200 ms)	Fixed at 120 ms
St. Jude Photon DR V-230, Photon μ DR V-232, Atlas DR V-240	NP: 32–44 ms Set by programmer based on atrial pulse amplitude, width and maximum pacing rate P VSP[3]: ON, OFF*	P: 125–470 ms (*250 ms) P: Rate responsive: OFF*, Low, Medium, High Min: 125–470 ms P: 'arrhythmia unhiding': OFF, 2–15 intervals (*3 intervals)	P: *125 or 157 ms

* Nominal.

max, maximum; min, minimum; NP, not programmable; P, programmable; VSP, ventricular safety pacing.

[1] Crosstalk detection window fixed for 47 ms after end of blanking. VSP occurs 94 ms after the atrial pulse.

[2] Crosstalk detection window equals the current VSP interval. VSP occurs at 110 ms if ventricular rate is lower than VSP switch rate or at 70 ms if ventricular rate is at or above the VSP. With nominal settings, the VSP switch rate is 96 b.p.m.

[3] Crosstalk detection window 64 ms – postatrial pace ventricular blanking. VSP occurs at 120 ms (or at the programmed AV delay if shorter). A signal in the AV delay after the crosstalk window inhibits VSP.

steps). Each ventricular event begins a VRS escape interval equal to the previous ventricular interval plus the programmed interval incremental value (but not shorter than the VRS minimum interval). If this escape interval expires before a ventricular sensed or escape event occurs, the ICD delivers a pacing pulse. In dual-chamber pacing modes, VRS automatically shortens the atrial pacing interval according to the programmed AV delay, so the ventricular pacing pulse is delivered at the required VRS escape interval. Competitive atrial pacing can result, especially if the non-competitive atrial pacing function is not enabled [22]. The VRS escape interval is then recalculated based on the last ventricular interval. The VRS escape interval lengthens, from beat to beat, by a value equal to the programmed VRS interval increment. Once the rate

generated by VRS operation slows to the intrinsic sensor-indicated, or lower rate, the device returns to normal pacing operation.

The rate-smoothing algorithm in Guidant devices is more complex. It will not only suppress postextrasystolic pauses (i.e. 'rate-smoothing down'), but it will also limit the ventricular tracking rate in response to APDs or the onset of atrial tachyarrhythmias (i.e. 'rate-smoothing up'). The rate-smoothing down and up parameters are independently programmable in percentage of the previous R–R interval (3–25%). The rate-smoothing up parameter defaults to 12% when rate-smooth down in enabled but rate-smoothing up is OFF. The rate-smoothing algorithm operates between the LRL (or the hysteresis rate if programmed) and the MTR (or MSR if programmed faster). In the DDI or DVI mode, a

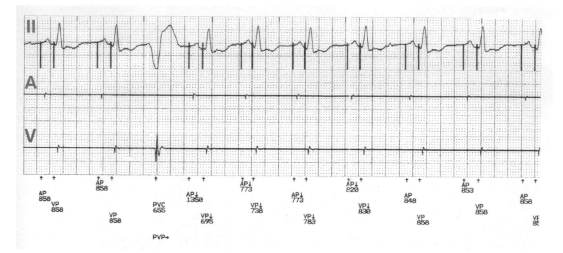

Figure 17.3 Rate-smoothing algorithm in the Prizm DR device. Real-time lead II, atrial (A) and ventricular (V) electrograms. Pacing is programmed DDD 70–125, atrioventricular delay 200 ms, rate-smoothing down 6% and up 25%. After a PVC with coupling interval of 655 ms, the following AP↓–VP↓ cycle results in a pause of only 695 ms (i.e. 655 ms + 6%).

maximum pacing rate for the rate-smoothing down algorithm needs to be programmed. After each cycle, two synchronization windows are set up. The atrial synchronization window equals [(previous R–R) ± (rate-smoothing)] – (AV delay). The ventricular window equals (previous R–R) ± (rate-smoothing). Pacing activity, if is to occur, must occur within the appropriate synchronization window. Competitive atrial pacing often results from this algorithm. Intrinsic beats faster than the maximal tracking rate (e.g. VPDs) will not reset the rate-smoothing down escape any faster than by the rate-smoothing up percentage (or 12% if OFF). Thus, maximum obliteration of a postextrasystolic pause is obtained when rate-smoothing down is programmed at 3% and rate-smoothing up to 25% (Figure 17.3). When rate-smoothing is enabled in AAI mode, it acts as an atrial rate stabilization algorithm.

The atrial rate stabilization (ARS) programmable feature in the Medtronic GEM III AT is designed to inhibit the onset of atrial tachyarrhythmias by eliminating the long sinus pause that commonly follows an atrial premature depolarization (APD) (Figure 17.4). ARS is available in DDDR and AAIR modes. Three parameters are programmable: (a) the minimum pacing interval for ARS (programmable between 400 and 700 ms in 10-ms steps, but subject to programmer interlocks); (b) the interval increment (programmable at 12.5, 25 or 50%); and

(c) the PVARP for ARS (programmable between 100 ms and the standard PVARP). When ARS is enabled, each atrial event outside the PVARP for ARS begins an ARS escape interval equal to the last A–A interval plus the percentage increment (but up to the minimum pacing interval for ARS). If the escape interval expires, the ICD delivers an atrial pace and recalculates its ARS interval using the current A–A interval. If dual-chamber pacing is programmed, the device delivers a ventricular pulse after the programmed AV delay.

In addition, the GEM III AT also allows programming of an atrial preference pacing algorithm, designed to reduce the incidence of atrial tachyarrhythmias by providing rate-variable continuous pacing closely matching the intrinsic sinus rate whenever it exceeds the sensor-indicated rate. Three parameters are programmable: (a) the minimum pacing interval (which is shared with the ARS algorithm); (b) the interval decrement (programmable between 30 and 150 ms in 10-ms steps); and (c) the number of search beats (programmable between 5 and 50 in 5-beat steps). When the feature is enabled, on every non-refractory atrial sensed event the ICD shortens its pacing escape by the programmed decrement value (but up to the minimum pacing interval), accelerating the pacing rate. If the next atrial event is another non-refractory sensed event, the pacing interval is again decremented.

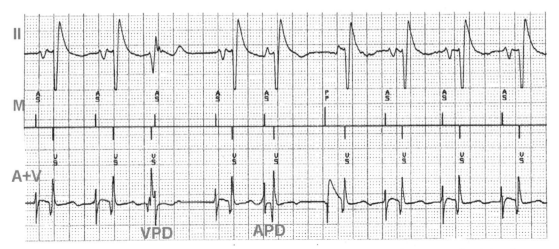

Figure 17.4 Atrial rate stabilization algorithm in the Medtronic GEM III AT. Real-time lead II, event marker (M), and composite atrial and ventricular electrogram (A + V). The device is programmed in the AAI mode at a lower rate of 60 b.p.m. Following the atrial premature depolarization, atrial pacing occurs early (PP). There is no attempt at ventricular rate stabilization after the ventricular premature depolarization.

This progression continues until the pacing rate exceeds the intrinsic rate, resulting in an atrial paced rhythm. When the number of consecutive paced atrial events reaches the programmed search beats value, the ICD adds 20 ms to the pacing escape interval, slowing the pacing rate. After the same number of consecutive paced atrial events at the new rate, the escape interval is again decremented. This process continues until pacing reaches the lower rate limit or the sensor-indicated rate, or is interrupted by intrinsic atrial activity. At the next, non-refractory atrial sensed event, atrial preference pacing rate acceleration resumes. If ARS and atrial preference pacing are both enabled, the more aggressive of the two algorithms (shorter escape interval) is applied on each atrial cycle.

Automatic mode switching during ventricular arrhythmia detection and therapy

High-rate DDDR pacing during a ventricular arrhythmia could interfere with appropriate detection and reconfirmation of ventricular arrhythmia. Most devices provide for some type of automatic mode switching during ongoing ventricular tachyarrhythmias. The earliest mode switch is achieved in St. Jude ICDs. As soon as three tachycardia intervals are binned, the device forces a mode switch to a non-tracking pacing mode (called 'episodal pacing mode' and programmable to DDI (nominal) or VVI),

disables rate-adaptive pacing, rate-adaptive AV delay and ventricular safety standby, and changes the bradycardia sensing threshold to the tachycardia sensing threshold if programmed differently. This pacing mode persists until sinus rhythm is redetected (Figure 17.5).

In Guidant devices, an automatic mode switch to VVI pacing occurs only after a ventricular tachyarrhythmia is detected (i.e. during capacitor charging). Pacing occurs at the programmed ATR/VTR fallback LRL (same as the fallback rate during automatic mode switch for atrial tachyarrhythmias) and uses the programmed antitachycardia pacing pulse width and amplitude values. In the latest model (Prizm DR 2), VVI pacing continues until the shock is aborted or the postshock pacing parameters take effect.

In Medtronic devices, switching to VVI pacing occurs only after the end of capacitor charging and the 300-ms postcharging blanking period (i.e. during the reconfirmation window). Pacing occurs at the interval used before capacitor charging started. (No pacing occurs during committed defibrillation shocks, as the escape interval of 1200 ms is longer than the synchronization window of 900 ms after which the committed shock is delivered if there are no sensed ventricular events.) If the device aborts a defibrillation therapy, it reverts immediately to the programmed bradycardia pacing settings.

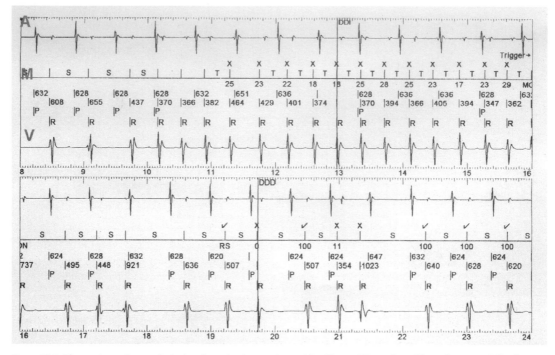

Figure 17.5 Change in pacing mode during detection in a patient with a Photon DR implantable cardioverter defibrillator. Stored event markers (M), atrial (A) and ventricular (V) electrograms of an episode of ventricular tachyarrhythmia. The device switches from DDD to DDI after 3 consecutive tachycardia beats are detected. The tachycardia self-terminates. The device switches back to DDD pacing the first cycle after redetection of sinus rhythm (RS).

Postshock bradycardia pacing

Most devices transiently change their pacing function after delivery of a high-energy shock (Table 17.4). In devices from Biotronik, Guidant and St. Jude, initiation of postshock pacing is delayed by a programmable postshock pacing delay or pause. Transient undersensing can occur after a high-energy shock [23]. The delay before pacing initiation maximizes the chances of early arrhythmia redetection after a failed shock. Additionally, if arrhythmia termination was not 'clean', transient after-shock undersensing could result in asynchronous pacing and proarrhythmia. However, in pacemaker-dependent patients programmed with nominal settings, the additional 2 or 3 s of asystole following tachyarrhythmia termination could contribute to syncope. In these patients, the programmable postshock pacing delay should be minimized. Medtronic devices present a fixed single escape cycle in VVI mode at 50 b.p.m. before postshock pacing parameters take effect.

High-energy shocks often induce a transient increase in pacing threshold that can lead to non-capture. This phenomenon was first described after epicardial shocks in patients with separate ICD and pacemaker systems [24], but it is also common with current systems in which a multipurpose lead is used for pacing, sensing and biphasic defibrillation. It is not clear whether its severity varies with the type of lead used. Kudenchuk *et al.* [25] studied 57 patients with Medtronic Transvene 'true bipolar' leads and found that pacing at a pulse width 3 times the preshock threshold always achieved ventricular capture within 1 s of defibrillation. Small changes in threshold were not related to defibrillation energy, number of shocks, lead chronicity, shock orientation or clinical factors. In contrast, Welch *et al.* [26] observed failure to capture at twice preshock voltage threshold 2.5 s following a shock in 8 of 20 patients with 'true bipolar', steroid-eluting Medtronic Sprint leads, which persisted in 3 when the output was increased threefold over threshold. Kessler *et al.* [27] found an increase in pacing threshold (1.5- to fourfold) in 6 of 10 patients (60%) 2.5 s after biphasic endocardial shocks via Endotak 'integrated bipolar' leads.

Table 17.4 Programmability of postshock pacing function in some current dual- and triple-chamber implantable cardioverter defibrillators.

Model	Mode	Rate	Postshock pacing delay	Postshock pacing duration	Postshock atrial pacing amplitude	Postshock ventricular pacing amplitude	Postshock atrial pacing pulse width	Postshock ventricular pacing pulse width
Biotronik Tachos DR	*DDDR, DDIR, VDDR, VVIR, AOO, AAI	31–110 p.p.m. (*60 p.p.m.)	1–10 s (*1 s)	30 s–30 min (*30 s)	0.1–7.2 V (*7.2 V)	0.1–7.2 V (*7.2 V)	0.2–1.5 ms (*1.0 ms)	0.2–1.5 ms (*1.0 ms)
Ela Medical Defender IV	Same as normal bradycardia	Same as normal bradycardia	1–10 s (*1 s)	N/A	Same as normal bradycardia	Same as normal bradycardia	Same as normal bradycardia	Same as normal bradycardia
Guidant Prizm series/Contak CD	Off, AAIR, VVIR, VDDR, DVIR, DDIR, DDDR, OOOR	30–175 p.p.m. (*60 p.p.m.)	1.5–10 s (*3 s) Must be > 275 ms longer bradycardia escape interval	15 s–60 min	0.2–5.0 V (*3.5 V)	0.2–7.5 V (*7.5 V)	0.06–2.0 ms (*0.4 ms)	0.06–2.0 ms (*1.0 ms)
Medtronic GEM, InSync and Marquis series	Same as normal bradycardia	Same as normal bradycardia	Single VVI cycle at 1200 ms (with 520 ms blanking)	Fixed	1–6 V	1–*6 V	0.03–*1.6 ms	0.03–*1.6 ms
St. Jude Photon DR/Atlas DR	Off, AAI, VVI, DDI, or DDD (*programmed mode with sensor passive)	35–100 p.p.m. (*programmed rate)	1–7 s (*2 s)	30 s, 1, 2.5, 5, 7.5 or 10 min (*30 s)	From permanent atrial pacing amplitude to 10 V (*7.5 V)	From permanent atrial pacing amplitude to 10 V (*7.5 V)	0.05–*1.9 ms	0.05–*1.9 ms

* Nominal setting.

p.p.m., pulses per minute.

To counteract this phenomenon, all current ICDs (with the exception of the Defender IV) allow independent programming of higher pacing outputs immediately after shock delivery. However, they differ in the extent of programmability (Table 17.4). For example, Medtronic ICDs do not allow independent programming of the postshock pacing mode or rate. At the other extreme, Guidant devices allow independent programming of the entire set of pacing parameters (including blanking periods and rate-smoothing). Unexpected postshock pacing behavior could occur if one omits to individualize these parameters. In most devices, the postshock pacing parameters take effect immediately after the postshock delay (or an initial VVI cycle at 50 b.p.m. in Medtronic). In St. Jude ICDs, postshock pacing mode and rate begins only after sinus rhythm is redetected (nominally, 5 intervals). However, postshock pacing outputs are immediately operative after the postshock pacing delay.

The longest reported instances of non-capture after internal shocks have been > 50 s [28,29], but there was no significant increase in pacing thresholds measured 1 min after defibrillation in seven patients with a prototype Endotak lead [30]. Therefore, programming higher pacing outputs for ~ 1 min after shocks is recommended to ensure consistent capture. In Medtronic generators, the duration of postshock higher-output pacing is fixed. Higher-output pulses are delivered until the episode is terminated (8 consecutive V–V intervals below the lowest tachycardia detection interval) or a total of 25 events have occurred. Transient loss of capture could in theory occur because of the short duration of postshock bradycardia pacing parameters.

Biventricular pacing

Although a large number of scenarios could exist, current ICDs capable of biventricular pacing sense and trigger timing cycles from the composite biventricular electrogram (Contak CD) or from the right ventricular electrogram alone (InSync, Tupos LV) (Figure 17.6). Currently, pacing is delivered simultaneously to both ventricles. Recent studies suggest that earlier activation of the left ventricle could be hemodynamically beneficial, and devices undergoing clinical research allow limited programming of an interventricular (LV–RV) delay [31]. Wang *et al.* [32] have published a comprehensive discussion of advantages and limitations of many possible biventricular pacing timing cycles scenarios.

Unresolved issues and limitations of the pacing function of ICDs

Increased incidence of hardware and software design problems

It appears that the increased complexity of ICDs makes them more prone than pacemakers to flaws in hardware or software design that can result in (at times unheralded) pacing failure [33]. Recent examples include an idiosyncratic form of crosstalk inhibition with the original Ventak AV device due to an inadvertent < 2-ms hiatus during the non-programmable 66-ms ventricular blanking period after atrial pacing [34]. In Ventak AV II and III ICDs sudden failure to pace for up to 24 h could occur due to an interaction of the device's internal timing sequences [35]. The observed frequency of the problem was 0.035% per month [36]. A manufacturing flaw (a solder connection that may weaken over time) in some Medtronic GEM II DR defibrillators could result in loss of telemetry and device output [37]. Although most of these malfunctions were rapidly corrected (with software upgrades or appropriate reprogramming), they highlight the possibility of unexpected interactions between different components in complex ICDs.

Long-term lead reliability

The incidence, causes and prevention of pacing lead failure (conductor fracture, insulation breakdown) have been the subject of intense investigation. Leads differ in their long-term reliability [38]. The best are associated with > 95% 10-year survival, while several models with a failure rate ≥ 10% at 5 years have been identified [39]. There is less information on long-term performance of transvenous defibrillator leads [40]. Design features, including larger size and complex multielectrode configurations, make defibrillator leads more susceptible to structural failure. Failure of the pacing/sensing components of a defibrillator lead can be associated with severe symptoms (or death) in pacemaker-dependent patients [41]. Non-dependent patients usually present with inappropriate aborted or delivered shocks [42].

Rapid evolution in transvenous ICD lead design makes assessment of long-term performance difficult [43]. Current leads have been available for

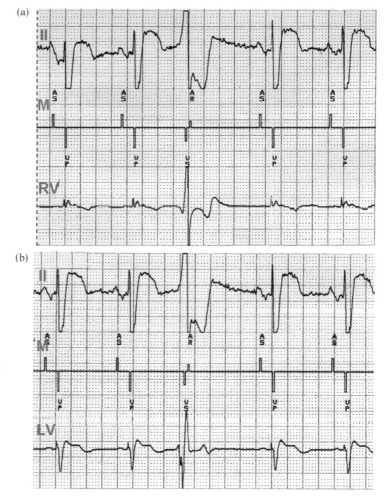

Figure 17.6 Sensing of ventricular premature depolarizations in a patient with a biventricular ICD with right ventricular (RV) timing (Medtronic InSync 7276). Depicted are surface lead II, event marker channel (M), and RV electrogram (a) or left ventricular (LV) electrogram (b). The strips were obtained a few seconds apart. There are frequent VPDs originating from the LV. Sensing occurs simultaneously with the RV signal. Notice that the LV electrogram is earlier but is not used for sensing.

< 3 years. Ongoing surveillance is crucial because excellent performance during the first few years postimplant does not guarantee long-term reliability [39]. Table 17.5 summarizes available information on medium-term performance of early lead designs [44–49]. Current pectoral leads with multi-lumen body design may reduce failure rates [50]. As with pacemaker leads, it appears that lead breakdown at the level of the thoracic inlet is less common with insertion through cephalic vein cutdown compared to subclavian puncture [49]. Using a modified Seldinger technique [51], defibrillation leads can be implanted via a small cephalic vein most of the time. Extrathoracic (axillary) vein puncture is a safe alternative [52]. Medial subclavian punctures should be avoided. Abrasion of lead insulation inside the pocket has also been a common mechanism of ICD

lead failure, particularly with abdominal devices [53]. Abrasions seem less frequent with shorter leads and smaller generators implanted pectorally [54].

Uncertainties about the long-term performance of defibrillation leads should be taken into account in pacemaker-dependent patients. Although automatic capacitor reformation permits widely spaced clinic visits, these patients should be seen more often (probably every 3–4 months). Abnormalities in electrical parameters, including lead impedance, can be an early sign of lead failure [55]. Routine radiologic surveillance is low yield [56,57]. Current systems perform daily automatic measurements of lead impedance that are retrievable in a trend format upon interrogation. Medtronic devices can be programmed to warn the patients with an alarm

Table 17.5 Failure rate of defibrillator leads.

Study	Lead(s)	Number	Failure rate (%)*	Follow-up (months)
Lawton *et al.* [42]	Endotak (60 and 70 series)	348	2.8	15 ± 11
Jones *et al.* [44]	Transvene 6996	159	1.3	21 ± 10
Tyers *et al.* [45]	Intermedics Intervene	269	1.2	> 36 (up to 72)
Degeratu *et al.* [46]	Endotak (60 and 70 series)	140	4.3	26 ± 14
Peralta [47]	Endotak (60 and 70 series) —Abdominal	146	16	47 (18–78)
Medtronic Chronic Lead Study [48]	Transvene 6936, 6966	1322	21	90
	Sprint 6932	378	1.5	42
	Sprint 6943	643	3	30
Kron *et al.* (AVID Trial) [49]	Various	539	6	36
Luria *et al.* (Mayo Clinic) [50]	Various			48
	Abdominal ICD	29	38	
	Pectoral ICD	362	12	

* Indicates proportion of leads that failed during follow-up except for [47], [49] and [50] which reported actuarial rate of failure.

tone if the measurement is out of range [58]. Enabling the alarm should be considered in pacemaker-dependent patients. However, there are no long-term data on effectiveness of this measure. The short-interval (120–130-ms) counter available in Medtronic ICDs may provide an early warning of impending lead failure [59]. Algorithms for automatic identification of lead problems from analysis of the intracardiac electrograms are also being developed [60]. More complex leads capable of shocking, pacing and sensing both atrium and ventricle are under clinical investigation [61,62]. It may be prudent to avoid using those leads in pacemaker-dependent patients until their long-term reliability is established.

Increased current drain causing reduced device longevity

ICDs are inefficient pacemakers. Constant pacing will reduce longevity twofold compared to bradycardia pacemakers of similar battery size. This results in part from differences in battery chemistry. The deliverable energy density of the lithium–iodine (Li/I) battery used in pacemakers is about 10% greater than that of a lithium–silver vanadium oxide battery of similar size used in most ICDs. Pacemaker batteries are optimized to generate 1–10 μJ pulses needed for cardiac stimulation, whereas ICD batteries are optimized to deliver up to 40 J, a current drain 100 000 times greater. Fundamentally different internal designs result in more ICD battery waste space, and hence a much lower deliverable energy density, a prime determinant of device longevity. The use of separate batteries with different chemistries for shocking and pacing could help extend ICD longevity in patients with frequent pacing. The Tachos DR has two batteries: a 6.3-V lithium–manganese oxide (Li/MnO_2) used only by the high-voltage circuit and a 2.8-V Li/I used for pacing and monitoring.

Current drain increases with lower pacing impedance. In 'integrated' bipolar defibrillation leads, pacing occurs between the distal tip and the large-surface right ventricular coil. The pacing impedance of these leads is in the 400–700 Ω range (lower than average for standard bipolar pacing leads). For example, during clinical trials the mean pacing impedance for the Medtronic 6945 lead ('integrated' bipolar) was 692 Ω, versus 1169 Ω for the otherwise similar 6943 ('dedicated' bipolar) [63]. This problem can be minimized by using a higher-impedance 'integrated' bipolar defibrillation lead with a smaller active tip electrode surface area (e.g. Endotak Reliance) or a 'true bipolar' lead in which pacing pulses are delivered between a tip and ring electrode.

In first-generation ICDs capable of biventricular pacing, the two ventricular leads are connected to the circuit in parallel configuration, creating a dual-cathodal system [64]. The coil (Medtronic, Guidant) or ring (Biotronik) in the right ventricular (RV) lead constitute the common anode. The total impedance (typically $250–400\,\Omega$) is thus lower than that of each lead alone. This lower pacing impedance and the impossibility to adjust pacing outputs independently may cause accelerated battery depletion. This is especially likely to happen when the pacing threshold in one lead is high and the impedance in the other lead is lower. When the output is increased to ensure capture on the higher-threshold lead, the majority of the current will be diverted to the lower-impedance lead. Because in general the chronic capture threshold is higher when pacing the left ventricle (LV) via a coronary vein than the RV endocardially, the use of a high-impedance RV lead would promote greater efficiency of current biventricular ICD systems [65]. On the other hand, the pacing threshold of a coronary vein lead is lower when the anode is the RV coil versus the smaller ring in a 'true bipolar' lead [66]. Future versions of these devices with independent ventricular channels will circumvent these problems, but they may require a short separation (e.g. 1 ms) between the pacing pulses to maintain low individual site capture thresholds [67].

Estimation of pulse generator longevity is more complex in ICDs than in pacemakers because it depends upon capacity and efficiency of power source(s), frequency and energy of shocks, static current drain, frequency and efficiency of pacing, and ancillary functions (e.g. electrogram storage) [68]. There are no standard criteria to predict device longevity, and different manufacturers' estimates are not comparable. Their scenarios may be constructed to amplify strengths and minimize weaknesses [68]. Manufacturers' estimates suggest that 100% pacing decreases battery longevity by 20–40%. For example, in a Medtronic Marquis DR with quarterly maximum energy charging, 100% AV sequential pacing at 60 b.p.m. (2.5 V at 0.4-ms pulse width, pacing load $500\,\Omega$) will decrease expected longevity by 20% (from 7.5 years with

100% sensing to 6 years). With similar programming, a pacing impedance of $900\,\Omega$ would extend longevity by 10% (to 6.6 years). Pacing at 3 V on the 500-Ω leads further reduces longevity to 5.5 years [69].

Thoughtful programming of pacing parameters (mode, rates, AV delays and outputs) is more critical to optimize battery longevity for ICDs than for standard pacemakers [70]. In patients with sinus node dysfunction and intact AV conduction, pacing in the AAIR mode [71] or, better yet, in the DDDR with AV interval search hysteresis should be considered [72]. Postshock ventricular pacing should always be enabled for a short period because of the risk of arrhythmia- or shock-induced AV block. It should be noted that Medtronic devices do not allow programming of different baseline and postshock pacing modes.

Loss of tracking during biventricular pacing

In standard-demand bradycardia pacing, stimulation is performed only when the rate is not fast enough or the AV interval is too long. In contrast, effective cardiac resynchronization therapy requires continuous pacing of both ventricles. The restrictions imposed on the timing cycles of biventricular ICDs by the need to maintain arrhythmia detection windows may make this goal a little more difficult than with biventricular pacemakers.

It appears important to maintain 1 : 1 atrial-synchronous biventricular pacing during the sinus tachycardia of exercise. However, in ICDs the tachycardia detection rate and the ventricular blanking periods restrict the MTR. With usual programming, upper rate behavior is more likely to be initiated by an atrial rate above the MTR than above the total atrial refractory period (TARP) (AV delay + PVARP). If there is intact AV conduction, atrial rates exceeding the MTR will result in continuous inhibition of biventricular pacing. However, tracking will not be restored until the atrial rate is below the intrinsic TARP (intrinsic PR + PVARP), creating therapy hysteresis [32,73]. Furthermore, in devices with biventricular sensing, if the timing between RV and LV sensing exceeds the postventricular sense blanking (a frequent occurrence in patients with severe intraventricular conduction delay when leads are optimally placed), double counting could result in spurious tachyarrhythmia detection and therapy [74,75]. Pharmacologic blunting of the maximum sinus rate with beta-blocker or amiodarone is important to avoid this complication. Double counting of intrinsic events is unlikely in biventricular pacemakers, as the postsense refractory period is much longer (e.g. nominal 230 ms in the Medtronic InSync 8040 pacemaker).

In the setting of a very long PR interval, even a single VPD could lead to prolonged inhibition of tracking and loss of biventricular pacing [76]. Especially if the PVC option is enabled, the next P wave can fall in the PVARP and not be tracked. A long PR interval in the conducted beat will place the next sinus beat shortly after the sensed QRS and the cycle will autoperpetuate. In Guidant devices, timing cycles are automatically reset after a VPD is detected; thus, the PVARP will be extended no more frequently than every other cycle, preventing autoperpetuation. Double counting of the VPD and conducted QRS in a device with biventricular sensing will make the sequence more likely to occur (even without PVARP extension), as the second ventricular deflection retriggers the PVARP and moves it further out. A similar scenario could be triggered by double counting of a conducted APD, as the second deflection will be interpreted as a 'PVC' by most algorithms (i.e. two sensed ventricular events without an intervening atrial event). In general, to maximize tracking after VPDs or other sensed intrinsic events, the PVARP should be programmed short and the PVC option disabled in patients with biventricular ICDs.

A biventricular trigger function that would trigger pacing on the opposite ventricular chamber upon sensing of a spontaneous ventricular event (conducted beat or VPD) would alleviate many of these considerations and could even be antiarrhythmic by initiating a collision wavefront that might prevent reentrant excitation. Such an operating mode is available in the Biotronik Triplos LV pacemaker. It has been tentatively named DDT/V by the manufacturer, and corresponds to the $\frac{A}{V-V}D\frac{D}{T}$ mode in the split format proposed by Barold [77]. It should be noted that this mode is not operative in the Tupos LV ICD, which only senses via the right ventricular lead. When implemented in ICDs, triggered pacing will require programming a maximum pacing rate limit and also a limit on the number of consecutive cycles in which the function may be triggered to avoid interfering with tachyarrhythmia detection.

Ventricular oversensing

A basic requirement of ICDs is reliable sensing of low-amplitude ventricular depolarization signals during ventricular fibrillation (VF), while simultaneously avoiding T-wave sensing and extracardiac noise. In contrast to antibradycardia pacemakers with fixed sensitivity, this technically challenging process is accomplished by an automatic adjustment of either the gain or sensing threshold [78,79]. Generally, these autoadjusting algorithms function adequately. Life-threatening tachyarrhythmias are correctly detected, while spurious device activations due to oversensing are infrequent.

However, in the absence of sensed complexes, the ICD faces a dilemma. Two potentially life-threatening diagnoses must be considered: asystole (requiring pacing); and fine VF (requiring amplifier gain adjustments for proper detection). To ensure VF detection, pacing onset triggers a rapid increase in ventricular channel sensitivity in most devices (Table 17.6; Figure 17.7). These very high sensitivity levels can promote oversensing of intra- or extracardiac signals. Oversensing can lead to spurious ICD discharges (with associated psychologic morbidity [80], battery consumption and occasional proarrhythmia [28]) and to potentially catastrophic inhibition of pacing. If the patient is pacemaker dependent, oversensing perpetuates because the absence of spontaneous large-amplitude escape beats maintains the high operating sensitivity.

Oversensing of diaphragmatic myopotentials

Oversensing of intermittent, high-frequency signals representing diaphragmatic myopotentials during ventricular pacing was first identified as a clinical problem in patients with Ventritex Cadence defibrillators [81,82]. Similar instances of oversensing were reported soon after the clinical introduction of dual-chamber ICDs (Figure 17.8) [83,84]. Sweeney *et al.* [85] evaluated oversensing of diaphragmatic myopotentials with provocative maneuvers during both intrinsic rhythm and ventricular pacing in 329 patients with Guidant or Medtronic ICDs with right ventricular apical leads (including some patients with dual-chamber units). Spontaneous oversensing compatible with respirophasic transients had occurred in 12 patients (4%)—in 11 during pacing—during a follow-up of 7 ± 10 months. Syncope due to pacing inhibition had occurred in 2 patients. The incidence of provoked oversensing

Table 17.6 Ventricular sensing algorithms of some current dual- and triple-chamber implantable cardioverter defibrillators.

Device	Ventricular sensitivity during pacing at nominal settings	Programmability
Biotronik Tachos DR	Threshold automatically set to 50% of signal (but not > 2 mV) at the end of 250-ms refractory period. The threshold is cut in half every 125 ms thereafter. The minimum threshold is fixed at 0.5 mV	Maximum sensitivity: 0.25 mV–3.0 mV in 0.125-mV steps (*0.5 mV) 'T-wave suppression': *Normal, Large T, Long QT, Large T + Long QT
Ela Defender IV	Set at 1.2 mV [i.e. programmed value (0.4 mV) + postpacing margin (0.8 mV)] for 500 ms after ventricular pacing before returning to the programmed value	Maximum sensitivity: 0.4 mV–4.0 mV in 0.2-mV steps (*0.4 mV) Ventricular postpacing sensitivity margin from 0 to 2.0 mV in 0.2-mV steps (*0.8 mV)
Guidant Contak CD	Set at 2.5 mV at the end of the ventricular pace blanking. Threshold starts to automatically decrease to ensure that sensitivity reaches 0.18 mV 150 ms before the end of the ventricular escape interval	Maximum sensitivity: 'nominal' = 0.18 mV; 'less sensitive' = 0.27 mV; 'least sensitive' = 0.44 mV
Guidant Prizm 2 DR	Set at 3.5 mV at the end of the ventricular pace blanking. Threshold starts to automatically decrease to ensure that sensitivity reaches 0.27 mV 150 ms before the end of the ventricular escape interval	Maximum sensitivity: 'most sensitive' = 0.18 mV; 'nominal' = 0.27 mV; 'least sensitive' = 0.44 mV
Medtronic GEM III DR 7275, GEM III AT 7276, InSync 7272, Marquis DR 7274	Set at 1.35 mV at the end of the postventricular pace blanking. Decays toward 0.3 mV with a 450-ms constant. Additionally, the threshold is increased by 0.45 mV after atrial pacing it then decays with a 60-ms constant until the preceding 450-ms decay, or the programmed threshold is restored	Maximum sensitivity 0.15 mV–1.2 mV in 0.15-mV steps (*0.3 mV) Sensitivity is set at 4.5 times maximum at the end of the postpace blanking (but only up to 1.8 mV) Threshold is not adjusted after atrial pacing if maximum sensitivity programmed value exceeds 0.3 mV
St. Jude Photon DR, Atlas DR	Threshold start and decay delay automatically adjusted after the end of the postpace refractory period according to a 'look-up table' to provide increased sensitivity at faster rates (e.g. at a rate of 70 b.p.m., the threshold start is set at 1.6 mV and the decay delay at 187 ms; at a rate of 103 b.p.m., the threshold start is set at 1.5 mV and the decay delay at 62 ms). Threshold decays at a rate of 3 mV/s towards 0.6 mV	*Maximum sensitivity* Defibrillator: 0.2–0.6 mV (*0.3 mV) Pacemaker: 0.2–2.0 mV (*same as defibrillator) *Decay delay:* Postsense: 0–220 ms (*0 ms) Postpace: auto, 0–220 ms (*auto) *Threshold start:* Postsense: 50, 62.5, 75, 100% of maximum peak amplitude, but between 1 and 3 mV (*50%) Postpace: auto, 0.2 to 3.0 mV (*auto)

* Nominal settings.

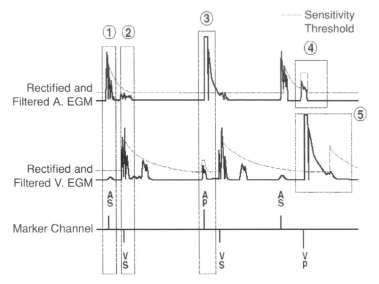

Figure 17.7 Auto-adjusting sensitivity thresholds in the Medtronic Marquis DR implantable cardioverter defibrillator.
1. After an atrial sensed event, the atrial sensitivity threshold increases to 75% of the electrogram (EGM) peak (maximum: 8 times the programmed value; decay constant: 200 ms). 2. After a ventricular sensed event, the ventricular sensitivity increases to 75% of the EGM peak (maximum: 8 times the programmed value, decay constant: 450 ms). 3. After an atrial paced event, the device does not adjust the atrial sensitivity threshold. The ventricular sensitivity threshold increases by 0.45 mV (decay constant: 60 ms). (If the programmed sensitivity value exceeds 0.3 mV, the threshold is not adjusted.) 4. After a ventricular paced event, the atrial sensitivity threshold increases to 4 times the programmed value (maximum: 1.8 mV, immediate return after 60 ms). (If the programmed sensitivity value exceeds 1.2 mV, the threshold is not adjusted.) 5. After the ventricular pace blinking period is finished, the ventricular threshold increases to 4.5 times the programmed value (maximum: 1.8 mV, decay constant: 450 ms).

was 1% during intrinsic rhythm and 10% during pacing. Provoked manifest or concealed oversensing was more common in patients with spontaneous oversensing, in men, with devices with automatic gain control sensing algorithm (i.e. Guidant), and with 'integrated' bipolar leads. Among 140 patients with dual-chamber ICDs programmed at nominal sensitivity reported by Kopp *et al.* [86], oversensing of myopotentials occurred in 10 of 102 (10%) with Guidant devices and in none of 38 with Medtronic devices. All cases of oversensing occurred during ventricular pacing, and at 21 ± 25 weeks after implant. Pacing inhibition produced symptoms in four pacemaker-dependent patients.

It may be difficult to differentiate myopotential oversensing from structural lead failure requiring operative lead replacement [87]. Oversensing exclusively during deep breathing favors the former, while reproduction of oversensing by pocket manipulation and measurement of abnormal or changing lead parameters (impedance, pacing threshold, electrogram amplitude) suggest lead failure. In unclear

cases, frequent follow-up may elucidate the cause [88]. With some leads, incomplete deployment of an active fixation screw can also produce oversensing of non-physiologic signals ('chatter'). In some cases, this can subside as the lead matures [89,90].

Oversensing of intracardiac signals
Despite a short postsense refractory period, oversensing of T waves after spontaneous beats is rare, as long as the R wave has an adequate voltage. The sensing threshold is adjusted according to the R-wave voltage, and then decreases exponentially (with variable time constants) in most devices. The Biotronik Tachos DR instead implements a two-level sensing threshold to 'hop' over the T wave. St. Jude devices and the Tachos DR allow additional fine programming of the decay in sensitivity after a sensed QRS (Figure 17.9). These features can be useful in patients with long QT syndrome.

A high operating sensitivity makes T-wave oversensing much more common after ventricular paced beats, despite the longer blanking (or refractory)

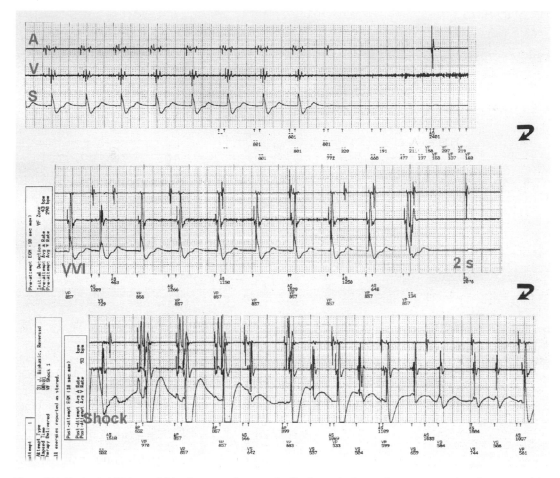

Figure 17.8 Pacing inhibition and false detection of ventricular fibrillation (VF) secondary to oversensing of myopotentials during defecation. Stored electrograms (A, atrium; V, rate-sensing; S, shocking electrodes) of a delivered shock in a patient with a Ventak AV III implantable cardioverter defibrillator (ICD) implanted for VT and complete heart block. Myopotentials are detected during AV sequential, resulting first in pacing inhibition and then in fulfilment of VF detection criteria (first strip). Myopotentials cease during device charging (second strip). During charge, the device switches to VVI pacing at 70 b.p.m. (857 ms). Pacing stops for 2 s at the end of charging. Ventricular asystole is present, and a 'committed' shock is delivered after this confirmation period. Postshock pacing at 70 b.p.m. starts after a 1.5-s delay. (The confirmation algorithm in the Prizm 2-DR would have aborted this shock.) Myopotential oversensing at the programmed settings could be provoked in the clinic during Valsalva, and was remedied by decreasing the maximum sensitivity. A sensing safety margin had been confirmed during implantation.

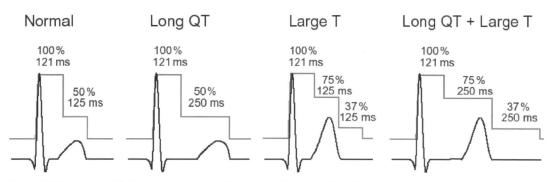

Figure 17.9 Programmable T-wave suppression algorithms in the Biotronik Tachos DR.

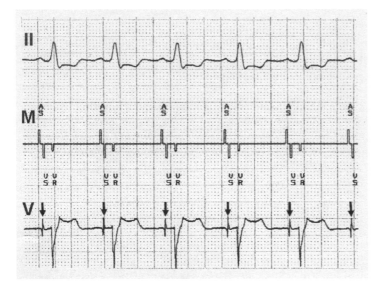

Figure 17.10 Inhibition of ventricular pacing secondary to oversensing of the atrial depolarization in a patient with a resynchronization pacemaker that senses from the composite biventricular electrogram (Medtronic InSync). The real-time recording shows lead II, telemetered event markers (M) and ventricular electrogram (V). The left ventricular lead had migrated to the main coronary sinus. Sensing by the ventricular channel of the large (~ 5 mV) left atrial deflection (arrows) inhibits ventricular output. The conducted beat is then sensed in the refractory period (V_R). Asystole would have resulted if complete heart block were present.

period present after pace than after sensed ventricular events [91]. In patients with AV sequential pacing, T-wave oversensing can result in inhibition of the next pacing stimulus, consequently lengthening the effective pacing escape interval. Most instances are of little clinical consequence, but the resulting bradycardia may become symptomatic. In patients with long QT syndrome, the slower paced rate further prolongs the QT interval, and may perpetuate oversensing [92,93] and lead to development of torsades de pointes. Loss of tracking of sinus rhythm can also occur, as T-wave oversensing can trigger an extended PVARP and result in functional undersensing of the following P wave [94]. If there is no spontaneous conduction, ventricular pacing could then maintain non-re-entrant AV synchrony [95]. Oversensing of paced T waves can also invoke 'rate stabilization' algorithms and perpetuate pacing in patients without bradycardia [96].

Oversensing of the far-field atrial activation is uncommon, but can be life-threatening when it results in prolonged inhibition of pacing. Several investigators [97–99] have reported cases of inappropriate sensing of atrial depolarizations during atrial flutter with continuous or intermittent ventricular pacing. Oversensing resulted in spurious shocks and (in one case) prolonged asystole. Ensuring that the distal coil of 'integrated' bipolar leads lies entirely within the right ventricular chamber can minimize oversensing of atrial signals. In biventricular ICDs that sense and time from both ventricular channels (i.e. composite electrogram), proximal migration of the LV lead toward the main coronary sinus (where a sizable atrial electrogram is recorded) will lead to continuous ventricular inhibition (Figure 17.10). A drastic decrease in ventricular sensitivity (useful when the problem occurs in patients with biventricular pacemakers [100]) is not a viable solution in patients with biventricular ICDs.

Oversensing of electromagnetic interference

Because of their higher operating sensitivity, ICDs may be more vulnerable to electromagnetic interference (EMI) than permanent pacemakers [101]. To be clinically relevant, studies of the interactions between sources of EMI and ICDs should create a 'worst-case scenario' by ensuring maximum sensitivity during pacing. The report by Santucci *et al.* [102] highlighted the potential risk of EMI in patients who depend on their ICD for bradycardia pacing. A patient with complete heart block and a Ventak AV ICD developed multiple shocks and near-fatal inhibition of pacing upon exposure to EMI from an antitheft device. Provocative testing with similar equipment in a controlled environment reproduced the interaction. The maximum distance at which ventricular oversensing occurred was 30 cm. When sensitivity was reprogrammed from 'nominal' to 'least sensitive', the interaction only occurred at closer proximity. Groh *et al.* [103] studied the interaction between ICDs and three models of antitheft devices (two electromagnetic and one acoustomagnetic) in 169 patients who were not pacemaker dependent. No spurious detections occurred during a 10–15-s walk through the gates. False VF detection occurred in three patients during a 2-min exposure to the acoustomagnetic system. The incidence of oversensing was much higher (15%), when the 2-min exposure was repeated during continuous pacing. Oversensing was severe (complete or prolonged pacing inhibition) in 6%. In 12 patients (9%), intermittent delayed pacing (compatible with noise-augmented T-wave oversensing) was seen. All the patients with serious interactions had an abdominal implant, but by multivariate analysis, diminished R-wave amplitude and a Ventritex ICD were the only predictors of interactions. It seems prudent to recommend that ICD recipients do not linger in close proximity to antitheft devices. Cellular phones appear safe for patients with ICDs. During *in vitro* testing, interference only occurred with some devices very close to the source [104,105]. *In vivo* 'worst-case scenario' testing has not disclosed instances of significant oversensing [104,106].

Prevention of ventricular oversensing
Several measures can minimize the likelihood of oversensing. The larger length and surface area of the right ventricular coil electrode compared to a ring could increase the opportunity for oversensing with 'integrated bipolar' leads. In at least one clinical study, ventricular oversensing was indeed more common with 'integrated bipolar' than with 'true bipolar' defibrillator leads [107]. However, many implanters prefer 'integrated' bipolar leads because they incorporate two defibrillation coils in the same lead and increase defibrillation efficiency [108]. 'True bipolar' dual-coil leads (i.e. quadripolar) now available from Biotronik (Kainos SL), Medtronic (Sprint Quattro) and St. Jude (Riata) make the trade-off between optimal sensing and defibrillation efficiency no longer necessary. It should be noted that the long-term performance of these more complex leads will remain unknown for several years.

Placement of the defibrillation lead in the right ventricular outflow tract minimizes myopotential oversensing. Limited evidence suggests that this lead location does not compromise defibrillation efficiency [109,110]. Therefore, the high septum or outflow tract should be considered in patients with

'integrated bipolar' defibrillation leads who will rely intensively on the ICD for pacing. Careful testing of the defibrillation threshold appears prudent in this instance.

A decrease in the programmed maximum sensitivity (i.e. to a higher value) is the first maneuver to attempt in patients who present with oversensing of diaphragmatic myopotentials. Because their amplitude is generally low, decreasing the maximum sensitivity by just a level is often sufficient to eliminate this oversensing. After disabling tachyarrhythmia therapy, oversensing is first elicited with provocative maneuvers (deep inspiration, forced exhalation, cough and the Valsalva maneuver), while ventricular pacing is forced by shortening the AV delay, and real-time electrograms and event markers are monitored. Once oversensing is documented, the maximum sensitivity is then gradually decreased until oversensing is eliminated.

In the study by Sweeney *et al.* [85], reducing the sensitivity eliminated provoked oversensing during intrinsic rhythm in all cases and eliminated provoked oversensing during ventricular pacing in 69% of cases. Niehaus *et al.* [111] studied 14 patients with Guidant devices who had spurious ventricular fibrillation detection due to oversensing of myopotentials. In 9 of them oversensing could be reproduced with provocative maneuvers. After reprogramming the sensitivity to 'less' (5 patients) or 'least' (9 patients), clinical oversensing was almost completely eliminated during a follow-up of 4 months. Among the 10 patients with oversensing reported by Kopp *et al.* [86], reprogramming was able to eliminate oversensing in 7 (5 at 0.27 mV and 2 at 0.43 mV). It should be noted that the Guidant devices included in the above studies have a higher nominal sensitivity (roughly similar to the 'most' level of current models). The incidence of oversensing is now reduced. However, it is possible that in patients with Prizm ICDs who present myopotential oversensing at the already reduced nominal sensitivity, reprogramming of the sensitivity may be less effective in eliminating it.

When sensitivity is decreased, it is crucial to ensure detection of VF. A randomized crossover study with Guidant devices showed no difference in the time required to detect VF with sensitivity programmed at maximum (0.18 mV) or minimum (0.43 mV) settings [112]. However, clinical experience indicates that some patients can have delayed or failed VF detection when the maximum sensitivity is reprogrammed to values above nominal, especially with devices that allow programming the maximum sensitivity over a wide range. For example, in Medtronic ICDs the nominal maximum sensitivity is 0.3 mV and the next programmable steps are 0.45 and 0.6 mV. Thus, when reprogramming is done to avoid oversensing, reproducible prompt detection of induced VF must be verified. It is highly recommended to program a 'worst-case' sensing scenario (e.g. 1.2 mV in Medtronic, sensitivity 'least' with Guidant devices) during intraimplant device-based defibrillation testing. Such testing provides information about the 'safety margin' for VF detection and allows safe reprogramming during follow-up without the need for arrhythmia reinduction. It should be noted that the relation between induced and spontaneous VF has not been investigated extensively. In general, the cycle length of spontaneous VF is slower than the cycle length of induced VF in the same patient. Thus, at least in terms of cycle length, VF induced during testing may represent a worst-case scenario [113,114].

In recalcitrant cases of myopotential oversensing, safe reprogramming of the sensitivity may not be sufficient. Surgical revision, including change of the generator to a model with a different autoadjusting algorithm (most appealing when the battery is close to depletion), repositioning of the defibrillation lead away from the diaphragm, or addition of a separate bipolar sensing lead then becomes necessary [85,86].

Programming a longer postpace blanking period usually circumvents T-wave oversensing [115]. However, a fixed long postpace blanking period during the fast rates achievable with dual-chamber or rate-adaptive pacing may delay tachyarrhythmia detection (see p. 243). Oversensing of paced T waves may be difficult to eliminate in patients with QT prolongation, as the T wave may fall outside the maximum programmable ventricular blanking period. Alternatively, decreasing the ventricular pulse voltage, pulse width or maximum sensitivity —or modifying the parameters of the autoadjusting algorithm when possible—can also help eliminate T-wave oversensing (Figure 17.11).

Far-field R-wave oversensing

The phenomenon of far-field R-wave oversensing (FFRWOS) was recognized shortly after the introduction of atrial and dual-chamber pacemakers [116]. However, it had little clinical consequence and could be abolished by decreasing the atrial sensitivity, extending the blanking periods, or both. With the incorporation of automatic mode-switching algorithms in pacemakers, however, FFRWOS became clinically important.

The diagnostic performance of dual-chamber ICDs critically depends on appropriate atrial sensing [117]. Unlike pacemakers, dual-chamber ICDs require accurate atrial sensing during high ventricular rates. FFRWOS is a frequent phenomenon that can have adverse consequences depending on the type of device and programmed parameters. FFRWOS does not trigger ventricular pacing, as the signals invariably fall in PVARP, but can lead to spurious detection of atrial tachyarrhythmia [118]. Unwarranted mode switching, spurious atrial tachyarrhythmia detection and therapies [119,120], and even underdetection of ventricular tachyarrhythmia could result. The PR Logic® algorithm in Medtronic ICDs can make a positive diagnosis of sinus tachycardia or atrial tachyarrhythmia with FFRWOS when a certain number of ventricular intervals contain two atrial events with a short–long pattern *and* a short A–V interval (< 60 ms) or a short V–A interval (< 160 ms). More intermittent FFRWOS during sinus tachycardia, however, can result in spurious detection of VT [121].

The programmed sensitivity, the atrial sensing algorithm (fixed vs. autoadjusting [122]), the interelectrode spacing in the atrial lead, and the atrial lead position all influence the likelihood of FFRWOS. The incidence of FFRWOS increases greatly when the sensitivity is fixed and programmed at < 0.3 mV [123]. With RV apical leads, the window of FFRWOS occurs later after paced events than after sensed events. In some patients with wide intrinsic QRS, FFRWOS can occur even before ventricular sensing [123]. The incidence of FFRWOS may be higher with bipolar leads with longer interelectrode spacing (i.e. > 30 mm) [124,125]. Reducing the interelectrode spacing from 15 mm to 5 mm may further improve the signal-to-noise ratio [126]. However, permanent leads with such a close bipole are not commercially available, and there is concern that a stiffer distal portion would make them more prone to dislodgment, perforation or high capture thresholds. The far-field R-wave signal recorded by a bipolar right atrial lead is larger in

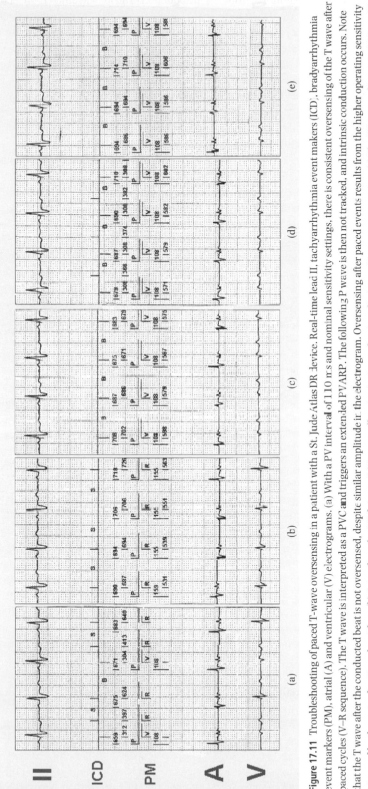

Figure 17.11 Troubleshooting of paced T-wave oversensing in a patient with a St. Jude Atlas DR device. Real-time lead II, tachyarrhythmia event makers (ICD), bradyarrhythmia event markers (PM), atrial (A) and ventricular (V) electrograms. (a) With a PV interval of 110 ms and nominal sensitivity settings, there is consistent oversensing of the T wave after paced cycles (V–R sequence). The T wave is interpreted as a PVC and triggers an extended PVARP. The following P wave is then not tracked, and intrinsic conduction occurs. Note that the T wave after the conducted beat is not oversensed, despite similar amplitude in the electrogram. Oversensing after paced events results from the higher operating sensitivity triggered by the autoadjusting algorithm. (b) Extending the PV delay to 180 ms to allow intrinsic conduction eliminates T-wave oversensing. (c) The PV interval is again 110 ms. T-wave oversensing was also eliminated when extending the postventricular pace blanking period to 340 ms. (d) Programming of different maximal sensitivity (0.3 mV for ICD, 2 mV for pacemaker) results in selective suppression of oversensing in the bradycardia channel. Note that the T wave is still detected at ~ 380 ms in the ICD channel. but this does not interfere with timing cycles. (e) Maximum sensitivity is again 0.3 mV in both channels. T-wave oversensing is eliminated by programming a postventricular pace decay delay of 60 ms and a postventricular pace threshold start of 2 mV (instead of the nominal auto settings).

the appendage than in the lateral wall [127]. The signal-to-noise ratio is even worse in the septal region [126]. This creates a trade-off, as a septal lead position can protect against the development of atrial fibrillation [19,128] and may optimize AV timing during resynchronization therapy [129]. Israel [130] discusses advantages and limitations of different right atrial lead positions.

Weretka *et al.* [131] studied the incidence, determinants and consequences of FFRWOS in 48 patients with a Medtronic Jewel 7250 device followed for a total of 797 months, using follow-up strip charts, 12-channel Holter recordings and, in some cases, Holter recordings with intracardiac markers. FFRWOS was documented in 21% of patients. Compared to other lead locations, the right atrial appendage lead position was most frequently associated with FFRWOS. Patients with FFRWOS had significantly more treated and non-treated atrial episodes, many of which appeared to have been detected inappropriately. In one case, inappropriate atrial antitachycardia pacing due to R-wave oversensing triggered sustained VT, which was terminated eventually with a high-energy shock.

In most cases, FFRWOS can be eliminated by optimization of atrial sensing parameters without inducing atrial undersensing. A cross-chamber blanking period or a reduction in atrial sensitivity are the main tools used to prevent FFRWOS, but devices differ greatly in the way these features are implemented and in the extent of their programmability (Tables 17.3 & 17.7). In general, a longer cross-chamber atrial blanking period prevents FFRWOS, but can cause underdetection of atrial tachyarrhythmia during high ventricular rates [132]. When the ventricular rate is below 100 b.p.m., extending the postventricular atrial blanking may not compromise detection of atrial fibrillation [133]. However, a long cross-chamber blanking is more likely to interfere with the detection of atrial tachycardia or atrial flutter. In those cases, decreasing the atrial sensitivity may be preferred to extending the cross-chamber blanking.

In devices with autoadjusting atrial sensitivity, FFRWOS is more common after an atrial paced event than after an atrial sensed event [134]. Therefore, a postatrial pace blanking that supersedes the AV delay (or PR interval) can help avoid FFRWOS without the need for a long cross-chamber blanking interval. Blanking periods or changes in sensitivity triggered by ventricular sensing are not protective when FFRWOS occurs before the sensed ventricular event. The Tachos DR has an 'early far-field tolerance function' aimed at this situation. A second atrial sensing occurring before the ventricular sensing by the programmed tolerance (programmable from 0 to 16 ms; nominal 8 ms) is ignored (i.e. not used for tachyarrhythmia detection).

Undersensing resulting in asynchronous pacing and tachyarrhythmia induction

Competition between asynchronous pacing and the spontaneous rhythm may induce ventricular tachyarrhythmias if the pacemaker stimulus captures the ventricle during its vulnerable period [135]. This is extremely uncommon with antibradycardia pacemakers (attested to by the routine magnet used to check pacemaker function). ICD patients may have a more vulnerable substrate. Saeed *et al.* [136] studied stored electrograms from 268 episodes of monomorphic VT, and found that 12 (4.5%) were induced by asynchronous ventricular pacing after undersensing the previous beat.

Interactions between spontaneous variation in signal amplitude and the autoadjusting amplifier mechanism make transient undersensing relatively common in patients with ICDs. The electrogram amplitude of a sinus beat following a premature beat is often significantly lower than the preceding beat [137]. Depending on the coupling interval and the time constant of the autoadjusting mechanism (200–400 ms in different devices), the sensitivity may not be sufficiently high to sense the postpause beat. A 'dual sensing level' using a large time constant for the period immediately after detection (to 'hop' over T waves) and a shorter time constant afterwards could reduce this problem [138]. The two sensing steps present in the Tachos DR result in an immediate increase in sensitivity after the end of the first step and could also make undersensing less likely.

To prevent crosstalk inhibition in the absence of 'safety pacing' options, Guidant devices have a relatively long postatrial paced ventricular blanking (e.g. 65 ms nominal in Prizm II). If the AV delay is programmed long (i.e. $\geq$ 200 ms), undersensing of a late-coupled VPD falling during ventricular blanking followed by ventricular capture in the vulnerable period can result in arrhythmia induction

Table 17.7 Atrial sensing algorithms of some current dual- and triple-chamber implantable cardioverter defibrillators.

Device	Atrial sensitivity at nominal settings	Programmability
Biotronik Tachos DR	Set at 50% of the EGM peak (but not > 2 mV) at the end of the 102-ms postsense blanking (or 300-ms postpace blanking). After 82 ms, threshold further decreased to 25% of the EGM peak (but no less than 0.375 mV)	Maximum sensitivity: 0.25 mV–3.0 mV in 0.125-mV steps (*0.375 mV) 'Raise atrial threshold' (*OFF, 2 times, Max)[1]
Ela Defender IV	Fixed atrial sensitivity at 0.4 mV	Sensitivity: 0.2 mV–4.0 mV in 0.2-mV steps (*0.4 mV)
Guidant Contak CD	Sensing threshold automatically adjusted after each sensed event. Additionally, a floating gain control mechanism changes the amplifier gain one step (i.e. by a factor of 1.2) when 3 out of the last 4 sensed events over- or underscale the A-D converter. The threshold is set at 2.5 mV at the end of the atrial pace blanking. Threshold starts to automatically decrease to ensure that sensitivity reaches 0.18 mV 150 ms before the end of the atrial escape interval	Maximum sensitivity: 'nominal' = 0.18 mV; 'less sensitive' = 0.24 mV; 'least sensitive' = 0.29 mV
Guidant Prizm 2 DR	Sensing threshold automatically adjusted after each sensed event. Additionally, a floating gain control mechanism changes the amplifier gain in one step (i.e. by a factor of 1.2) when 3 out of the last 4 sensed events over- or underscale the A-D converter. The threshold is set at 3.5 mV at the end of the atrial pace blanking. Threshold starts to automatically decrease to ensure that sensitivity reaches 0.24 mV 150 ms before the end of the atrial escape interval	Maximum sensitivity: 'most sensitive' = 0.18 mV; 'nominal' = 0.24 mV; 'least sensitive' = 0.29 mV
Medtronic GEM III DR 7275, GEM III AT 7276, InSync 7272, Marquis DR 7274	Set at 75% of the EGM peak but not more than 8 times the programmed maximum sensitivity (i.e. 2.4 mV). It decays towards 0.3 mV with a time constant of 200 ms. The atrial sensing threshold is not adjusted after an atrial paced event (i.e. most of the time will be at maximum sensitivity at the end of the postpace atrial blanking). Additionally, the threshold is increased by 4 times the programmed maximum sensitivity, but no more than 1.8 mV (i.e. 1.2 mV) after ventricular pacing with immediate return to the preceding decay after 60 ms	Maximum sensitivity: 0.15 mV–2.1 mV (*0.3 mV). Threshold is not adjusted after ventricular pacing if maximum sensitivity programmed value exceeds 1.2 mV
St. Jude Photon DR/Atlas DR	Sensing threshold is automatically set at 50% of the measured peak P wave (but not < 0.3 mV or > 1.5 mV) at the end of the postsense refractory. It then decays towards 0.2 mV at a rate of 1.5 mV/s. The threshold is set at 0.8 mV at the end of atrial refractory period after an atrial-paced event	Atrial sensing mode: fixed or automatic (*) Atrial sensitivity/maximum sensitivity: 0.2–1.0 mV (*0.2 mV) *Decay delay* Postsense: 0–220 ms (*0 ms) Postpace: 0–220 ms *Threshold start* Postsense: 50, 62.5, 75, 100% of maximum peak amplitude (*50%) Postpace: 0.2–3.0 mV (*0.8 mV)

* Nominal setting.

[1] When this function is enabled the atrial sensing threshold is doubled or raised to 2 mV after the postventricular sensed or paced atrial blanking period.

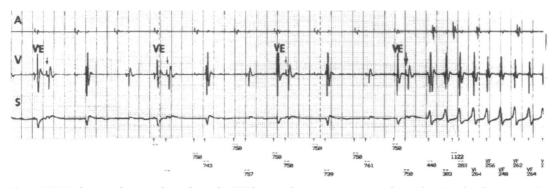

Figure 17.12 Induction of ventricular tachycardia (VT) by asynchronous pacing secondary to functional undersensing of ventricular premature depolarization. Stored atrial (A), ventricular (V) and shocking (S) electrograms show ventricular trigeminy with late ventricular extrasystoles (VE) falling 40 ms after the atrial artifact (ventricular blanking period). There is consistent ventricular capture by the 'committed' pulses (small arrows). The AV delay was programmed at 200 ms and rate-smoothing was enabled at 9%. The last asynchronous pulse (large arrow) triggers a run of rapid monomorphic VT (cycle length 260 ms), that the ICD appropriately detects and terminates (not shown). (Reproduced from [5] with permission.)

(Figure 17.12). Shortening of the blanking period or of the paced AV delay to ensure delivery of committed ventricular pacing during the myocardial effective refractory period would solve this type of proarrhythmia. In other dual-chamber ICDs the postatrial pacing ventricular blanking is shorter (Table 17.3). Ventricular sensing during the AV delay (but after the blanking) invokes ventricular safety pacing.

A long PVARP during conducted sinus tachycardia can also promote ventricular asynchronous pacing as competitive atrial pacing initiates a cross-chamber blanking period. Depending on the device and the timing of the conducted QRS, 'safety pacing' or pacing at the end of the AV delay will occur. If the ventricular rate stabilization algorithm is enabled, the sequence tends to autoperpetuate, as the ventricular pacing pulse recycles the stabilization escape interval, even if it is ineffectual in achieving capture [15]. Programming maneuvers that extend the atrial and ventricular alert periods, like shortening of the PVARP and AV delays or increasing the minimum rate stabilization interval, reduce the risks of asynchronous pacing. Enabling of noncompetitive atrial pacing (when available) also helps, by delaying the scheduled atrial pulse and allowing the intrinsic QRS to reset the timers.

Biventricular ICDs that allow pacing with an interventricular delay are now being developed. In these devices, competitive pacing after a sensed event will be more likely at fast pacing rates, when

the intrinsic interventricular delay is long and the paced interventricular delay is also long but of opposite sign, and if the second component of the sensed event does not retrigger the timing cycles (i.e. falls in blanking or the device times from the other ventricle only). It is expected that programming of most potentially dangerous timing combinations will be prevented by parameter interlocks [32].

Failure to abort shocks after non-sustained arrhythmias

Adding reconfirmation capabilities to ICDs dramatically decreased shock delivery for non-sustained ventricular arrhythmias [139]. However, in some devices pacing interferes with the reconfirmation algorithm because of conservative reconfirmation algorithms designed to avoid withholding therapy for low-amplitude VF. In pacemaker-dependent patients, the algorithms cause shock delivery after self-terminating ventricular arrhythmias [140].

The Tachos DR suppresses pacing after capacitor charge and delivers a shock at the end of the 'shock confirmation period' if asystole is present. The confirmation period during which the device looks for spontaneous beats can be short (4 times the slowest programmed tachycardia zone as default; 8 times if the 'extended confirmation period' feature is selected). Thus, the algorithm can result in delivery of committed shocks in patients with even mild or transient bradycardia. When programming only one VF zone (or a very fast VT zone), the extended confirmation period is recommended because it improves the chances to abort a shock in the event of sudden bradycardia after spontaneous arrhythmia termination. However, the extended confirmation period will not prevent 'committed' shocks in pacemaker-dependent patients with complete heart block and the longer period of asystole can cause syncope. In these cases, one could disable the default 'fine VF' function. When 'fine VF' is disabled, the device assumes that asystole (and not fine VF) is the cause for the lack of sensing. The shock is aborted and bradycardia pacing starts at the end of the confirmation period. It should be noted that programming of the 'fine VF' function is locked out in Tachos DR devices commercialized in the US.

Guidant defibrillators prior to Prizm II (including the Contak CD) also functioned *de facto* as committed in pacemaker-dependent patients [141]. Upon detection of tachyarrhythmias, the devices switch their pacing mode to VVI at the programmed fallback lower rate (nominal 70 b.p.m.). During capacitor charge, shock diversion for non-sustained arrhythmias requires the presence of four ventricular *sensed* events at a rate below the tachycardia cut-off rate, but ventricular paced events count as tachycardia beats. The shock can also be aborted after completion of capacitor charge if two spontaneous ventricular events below the rate cut-off are sensed during the 2 s in which the pacing function is suspended. However, if two spontaneous ventricular beats do not occur (a likely scenario in pacemaker-dependent patients), the shock is delivered upon expiration of the 2-s timer (Figure 17.13).

Programming strategies aimed at eliminating this problem are limited. The duration parameter can be extended to decrease the likelihood of capacitor charging for non-sustained VT. However, this could result in syncope before shock delivery if the tachyarrhythmia sustains. It may be necessary to pharmacologically suppress the non-sustained VT or change the device for one with non-committed behavior.

Delayed tachyarrhythmia detection secondary to a short detection window

As stated previously, it is often necessary to program a relatively long (> 250-ms) postpace ventricular blanking period to avoid oversensing the pacing-evoked repolarization response. Ventricular tachyarrhythmias that emerge during relatively rapid

pacing due to tracking or sensor activation may be temporarily masked by a lengthy blanking period thereby delaying detection. During AV sequential pacing, the postatrial paced ventricular blanking further shortens the detection window. A similar phenomenon can occur when the initial tachycardia beats trigger rate-smoothing pacing at or close to the upper rate limit [142]. In Medtronic devices, parameter interlocks prevent pacing in the detection zone. However, atrial pacing in the detection zone can occur in Guidant devices when the rate-smoothing option is programmed aggressively. Underdetection of VT can occur if its rate is not very fast and the programmed AV delay is long, as this demands delivery of the atrial pulses shortly after the tachycardia sensed beats (Figure 17.14). Glikson *et al.* [143] routinely programmed rate-smoothing down during arrhythmia induction in 16 patients with Guidant Prizm devices. The algorithm did not interfere with the detection of VF. However, detection of induced VTs with cycle length between 300 and 350 ms was often delayed or prevented by the algorithm. In these cases, the AV delay had been programmed long (250–300 ms) and rate-smoothing down at 9–12%. In extensive simulation testing, the same authors addressed the impact of different parameters on VT non-detection. Non-detection was more likely with longer programmed AV delays, higher maximal pacing rates, or more aggressive rate-smoothing down. In these simulation studies the cross-chamber and ventricular postpace blanking were left at nominal settings (see below). Enabling the dynamic AV delay feature prevented the interaction in most cases. However, the clinical impact of such maneuver is difficult to predict, because the dynamic AV delay is not adjusted by a PVC cycle or when the previous cycle was affected by rate-smoothing or by maximal tracking rate. Importantly, in every case of non-detection, the programmer issued a parameter warning. However, the absence of interlocks still allowed programming of the parameters. The authors recommended adjusting parameters to avoid programming warning messages when using rate-smoothing. If a warning is intentionally ignored, safe functioning should be demonstrated via repeated induction of VT. In future iterations of the algorithm, automatic shortening of the AV delay during rate-smoothing could minimize the risk of non-detection of VT [144].

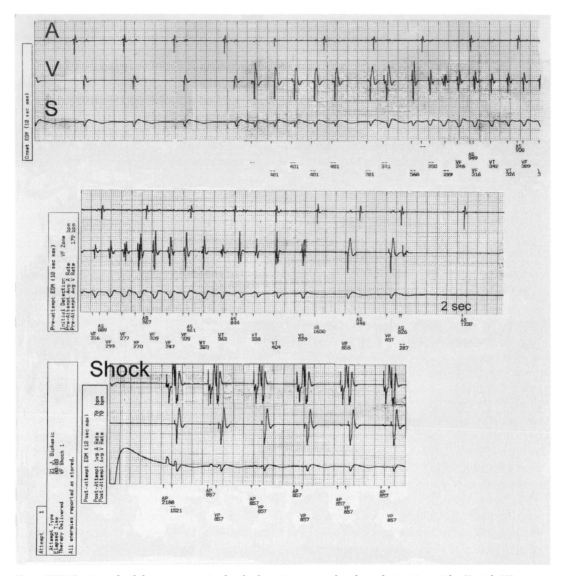

Figure 17.13 Spurious shock for a non-sustained arrhythmia in a pacemaker-dependent patient with a Ventak AV implantable cardioverter defibrillator. Stored atrial (A), ventricular (V) and shocking (S) electrograms show onset of rapid ventricular tachyarrhythmia that terminates during capacitor charging. There is VVI pacing at 70 b.p.m. for 2 beats after VT termination. Upon completion of charging, pacing is suspended for 2 s with consequent asystole. A shock is delivered. After the shortest programmable delay of 1.5 s, AV sequential pacing is restored.

When the postpaced blanking is fixed, the upper rate limit(s) may need to be lowered to ensure maintenance of a tachycardia detection window during ventricular pacing [145]. Although current ICDs allow MTR and MSR > 140 b.p.m. (Table 17.1), the maximum achievable pacing rate is limited by a series of parameter interlocks. In GEM devices, for example, parameter interlocks ensure that: (i) the minimum paced V–V interval is 60 ms longer than the tachycardia detection interval; (ii) in dual-chamber pacing modes, the shortest V–A interval must be equal to or longer than the tachycardia detection interval; and (iii) no more than 50% of the ventricular pacing interval is blanked. If ventricular safety pacing is enabled, the minimum ventricular pacing interval must be $\geq 2 \times$ (ventricular pace blanking + 50 ms). Although disabling ventricular safety pacing is a possible way to resolve a

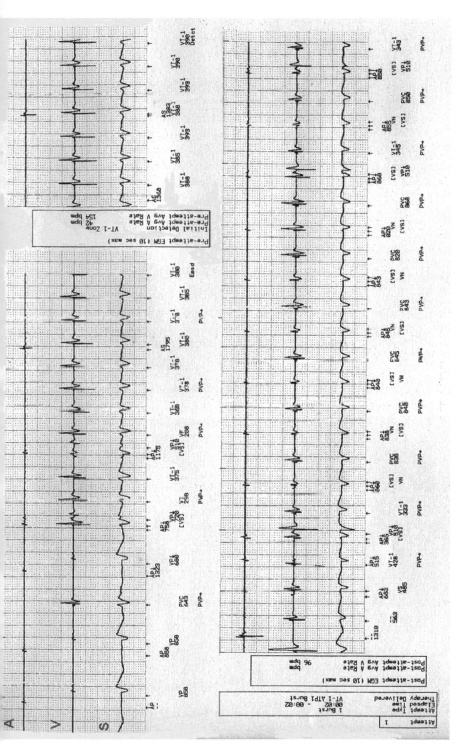

Figure 17.14 Underdetection of ventricular tachyarrhythmia (VT) secondary to rate-smoothing down algorithm in an inpatient with a Prizm DR implantable cardioverter defibrillator. Stored atrial (A), ventricular (V) and shocking (S) electrograms. The VT-1 detection zone had been programmed at 140 b.p.m., the VT zone at 190 b.p.m. and the ventricular fibrillation zone at 230 b.p.m. Bradycardia pacing was programmed DDD 70–125 b.p.m. with rate-adaptive AV delay (200–120 ms), V-blank after A-pace 65 ms (nominal) and rate-smoothing up at 25% and down at 3%. The initial panel shows onset of VT with cycle length ~ 380 ms. The rate-smoothing down algorithm is operative (AP↓-VP↓ cycles). Some of the initial beats fall in the cross-chamber ventricular blanking after atrial pacing (VS). VT is eventually detected and an initial unsuccessful antitachycardia pacing sequence is delivered (not shown). Lower panel shows failed redetection. Every other VT beat falls in the cross-chamber blanking and is ignored (VS). During most beats a second component of the signal falls in the noise sampling period (VN) and prevents delivery of an ineffectual VP↓ (which would have reset the cycles and possibly broken the sequence). Each VT beat outside blanking is interpreted as a PVC with a coupling interval of ~ 840 ms, and triggers the rate-smoothing down algorithm. The synchronization windows and the programmed AV delay cause the delivery of the AP↓ pulse synchronous with the next VT beat. Note that the dynamic AV delay does not operate on a PVC cycle. The device eventually considers the episode terminated with a postattempt average ventricular rate of 96 b.p.m. The patient developed hypotension and external cardioversion was required.

parameter interlock [146], it is risky in patients with complete heart block in view of the short postatrial pace ventricular blanking.

Shorter ventricular blanking periods can maintain a wider alert window during rapid pacing. The cross-chamber ventricular blanking after atrial pace shows little programmability among different models. The postventricular paced blanking is more extensively programmable (Table 17.3). The QT interval shortens at faster paced rates. Guidant and St. Jude devices take advantage of this phenomenon via programmable dynamic ventricular paced blanking periods. In Guidant devices, this feature results in automatic linear shortening of the ventricular blanking period from the programmed baseline value (at the lower rate limit) down to the minimum 'dynamic' value at the upper rate limit. In St. Jude ICDs, the rate-responsive ventricular pace refractory period starts to shorten when the filtered atrial rate (in DDD mode) or sensor-indicated rate (other modes) exceeds 90 b.p.m. The slope of the decrease is programmable 'low' (shortening of 1 ms for each b.p.m.), 'medium' (2 ms for each b.p.m.) or 'high' (3 ms for each b.p.m.). Shortening continues until the MSR, the MTR or the shortest refractory period (also programmable) is reached.

The Guidant algorithm has been tested clinically. Worst-case scenario testing (maximum pacing output and ventricular sensitivity, shortest blanking period of 150 ms, maximum rate of 120 b.p.m.) suggests that this feature prevents oversensing of paced T waves while maintaining a wide tachyarrhythmia detection window [147]. Safe detection of VF occurring in the setting of rapid paced rates in devices with a dynamic postpace ventricular blanking was confirmed by Ellenbogen et al. [148]. They compared the detection time for induced VF during DDD pacing at 150 b.p.m. and DDDR pacing at 175 b.p.m. in 26 patients with Ventak AV ICDs. All VF episodes were detected with mean times of 2.35 and 2.85 s, respectively. The minimum dynamic ventricular blanking was programmed at 150 ms in all patients except the first two. In a patient with minimum ventricular blanking programmed at 240 ms, detection of a slower episode of polymorphic VT induced during pacing at 175 b.p.m. was delayed up to 10.5 s, due to a combination of intermittent undersensing plus tachycardia beats falling in the blanking period. There is little safety information on tachyarrhythmia detection during rapid pacing by ICDs with fixed postpace ventricular blanking.

St. Jude devices allow programming of an additional 'arrhythmia unhiding' function that increases the alert period (through an adaptive relative refractory period) to unmask arrhythmias hidden by pacing. An adaptive relative refractory period is enabled when the ventricular pacing cycle length is less than 2 times the longest tachycardia detection interval or 2 times the pacing refractory period, whichever is shorter. If a sensed event occurs during the adaptive relative refractory period and the next event is paced, the adaptive relative refractory period is enabled again. If no sense event occurs during the adaptive relative refractory period or the next event is not paced, the pace refractory period returns to normal. Once the number of intervals with a sensed event during the adaptive relative refractory period specified by the arrhythmia unhiding function have occurred consecutively, the pacing cycle length is extended for six cycles in an attempt to reveal the arrhythmia. If no arrhythmia is revealed during the extended pacing interval, the adaptive relative refractory period will not be re-enabled for 10 cycles in order to prevent unnecessary extension of the pacing interval.

In future biventricular ICDs with biventricular sensing and an interventricular pacing interval (e.g. pace LV first, then RV), the need to have a prolonged total blanking interval may further shorten the window for detection. Likewise, a longer cross-chamber blanking may interfere with atrial tachyarrhythmia detection.

Lack of magnet-triggered and programmable asynchronous pacing modes

ICD magnet responses generally inhibit tachyarrhythmia therapy without affecting bradycardia pacing (Table 17.8). Thus, pacemaker-mediated tachycardia (PMT) will not terminate with magnet application in dual-chamber ICDs [145]. When the automatic algorithms are not activated, termination of PMT requires reprogramming or pharmacologic blockade of VA conduction.

Some ICDs lack programmable asynchronous pacing modes (DOO, VOO) that are useful in pacemaker-dependent patients during procedures involving sources of EMI. (Ventak ICDs have temporary asynchronous pacing modes, but they require a continuous telemetry link with the programmer.)

Table 17.8 Noise reversion, asynchronous pacing and electrical reset responses of some current dual- and triple-chamber implantable cardioverter defibrillators.

Model	Noise reversion	Programmable asynchronous mode	Electrical reset
Biotronik Tachos DR	Asynchronous pacing in the chamber with noise	AOO	VVI 70 b.p.m., 7.2 V @ 1 ms Single zone at 150 b.p.m., 30 J × 6
Ela Medical Defender IV	Asynchronous ventricular pacing, ventricular sensitivity ↓ until noise (i.e. cycle < 63 ms) no longer detected	None	VVI 60 b.p.m., 4.8 V, 0.37 ms Single zone at 297 ms, 33 J × 4
Guidant Ventak AV III, Contak CD	Programmable: AOO, DOO*, VOO, Inhibit	AOO(R)†, VOO(R)†, DOO(R)†	VVI 60 b.p.m., 7.5 V @ 1 ms Single zone at 165 b.p.m., maximum energy × 5
Guidant Prizm DR, Prizm 2 DR	Programmable: AOO, DOO*, VOO, Inhibit	AOO(R)†, VOO(R)†, DOO(R)†	Non-rate responsive mode (i.e. DDDR to DDD) 60–120 b.p.m. 7.5 V @ 1 ms Single zone at 165 b.p.m. maximum energy × 5
Medtronic GEM III DR 7275, InSync 7272	None	None	VVI 65 b.p.m., 6 V, 1.6 ms Single zone at 320 ms, 30 J × 6 High-urgency alert sounds every 20 h until cleared
Medtronic GEM III AT 7276	None	Programmable¶: DOO, VOO	VVI 65 b.p.m., 6 V, 1.6 ms Single zone at 320 ms, 30 J × 6
Marquis DR 7274	None	Programmable¶: DOO, VOO	VVI 65 b.p.m., 6 V, 1.6 ms Single zone at 320 ms, 30 J × 6 High-urgency alert sounds every 9 or 20 h (depending on type of electrical reset) until cleared
St. Jude Photon/Atlas	Programmable: VVI(R); VOO or OFF*; DDD(R), DDI(R); VOO, DOO or OFF* Fixed rate of 50 b.p.m.	Programmable¶: AOC, VOO, DOO	VVI 60 b.p.m., 5 V Defib only: detection rate 146 b.p.m.; 800 V × 3

* Nominal setting.

¶ Available only when tachyarrhythmia detection is disabled.

† Requires continuous telemetry link.

(R), pacing at the sensor-indicated rate if rate-responsive pacing enabled.

In Guidant devices a noise response mode can be programmed to the DOO, VOO (nominal) or OOO. A 40-ms retriggerable noise reversion window starts early after each sensed event. Recurrent noise activity in this window would result in asynchronous pacing at the end of the escape interval. Programming an asynchronous mode in pacemaker patients should prevent asystole in response to external interference. However, reversion may not occur reliably in response to common sources of interference such as electrocautery [5]. St. Jude's ICDs, the Biotronik Tachos DR and the Defender IV also allow programming of an asynchronous pacing noise reversion mode, but differ in the required frequency and duration of the signals. Medtronic devices do not incorporate a noise reversion mode.

Manufacturers' reluctance to provide asynchronous pacing in patients with the substrate for sustained ventricular tachyarrhythmias is understandable. However, as more of these devices are implanted in pacemaker-dependent patients, the inability to program asynchronous pacing modes (under strict monitoring) may become clinically detrimental.

Conclusions

Current ICDs capable of dual- and triple-chamber, rate-responsive pacing provide state-of-the-art therapy. Many shortcomings present in early-generation devices [5] have been corrected. If current and future trials expand the prophylactic indications for defibrillator implant, it is possible that a majority of patients in need of a pacing device for bradycardia or heart failure will receive (at least in the most developed countries) an ICD [149,150]. Cost considerations aside, this would have a profound impact on the way cardiac rhythm management devices are designed, marketed, implanted and followed up.

The limitations of these complex devices can be partially countered by heightened awareness and understanding. In patients who will pace frequently from the ICD, the type of device, sensing lead configuration and lead position are crucial to avoid adverse outcomes. Pacemaker-dependent patients are especially vulnerable. De facto committed devices should be avoided in them. A dedicated bipolar configuration is preferable. Worst-case scenario testing at implantation and during follow-up can

ensure necessary sensing 'safety margins'. Initial programming should not be standardized but based instead on patient needs. For patients without bradycardia or conduction system disease, promotion of intrinsic activation by programming in DDI or VVI mode at a low back-up rate is desirable. In these patients, the forced DDD pacing that results with nominal settings in Guidant and Medtronic units is detrimental, as it accelerates battery depletion and could impair hemodynamics [151]. (Nominal settings are VVI at 60 b.p.m. in the Defender IV St. Jude devices and VVI at 50 b.p.m. in the Tachos DR.) Thereafter, changes in pacing parameters or addition of more complex pacing algorithms (e.g. rate stabilization) can be introduced according to clinical needs. This approach to programming will promote use of only the features likely to benefit the individual patient.

In patients with bradycardia, the pacing mode, rate, AV intervals and outputs should be carefully individualized. For pacemaker-dependent patients, we recommend programming of maximum sensitivity to less than nominal after testing confirms reproducible VF detection. In resynchronization devices, ensuring of permanent biventricular pacing requires thoughtful programming of maximum tracking rate, AV delay and PVARP. The addition of alpha-blockers is very helpful in this scenario.

Periodic clinic follow-up and prompt device interrogation after shocks can identify problems and suggest appropriate reprogramming maneuvers. Logical interactions between the pacing and tachyarrhythmia detection algorithms of modern ICDs are more likely to occur when the spontaneous heart rate is fast, a circumstance during which the detection window becomes critically dependent on the duration of blanking and refractory periods. Therefore, exercise testing and Holter recordings, together with induction of ventricular and atrial arrhythmias, are valuable for studying the functioning of the different algorithms and their interactions.

References

1 Geelen P, Lorga Filho A, Chauvin M et al. The value of DDD pacing in patients with an implantable cardioverter defibrillator. Pacing Clin Electrophysiol 1997; **20**: 177–81.

2 Iskos D, Fahy GJ, Lurie KG et al. Physiologic cardiac pacing in patients with contemporary implantable

cardioverter-defibrillators. *Am J Cardiol* 1998; **82**: 66–71.

3 Higgins SL, Williams SK, Pak JP *et al.* Indications for implantation of a dual-chamber pacemaker combined with an implantable cardioverter-defibrillator. *Am J Cardiol* 1998; **81**: 1360–2.

4 Best PJM, Hayes DL, Stanton MS. The potential usage of dual chamber pacing in patients with implantable cardioverter-defibrillators. *Pacing Clin Electrophysiol* 1999; **22**: 79–85.

5 Pinski SL, Trohman RG. Permanent pacing via implantable defibrillators. *Pacing Clin Electrophysiol* 2000; **23**: 1667–82.

6 Dorian P, Newman D, Thibault B *et al.* A randomized clinical trial of a standardized protocol for the prevention of inappropriate therapy using a dual chamber implantable cardioverter-defibrillator. *Circulation* 1999; **100**: I-766 [abstract].

7 Sadoul N, Jung W, Jordaens L *et al.* Diagnostic performance of a dual-chamber cardioverter defibrillator programmed with nominal settings: a European prospective study. *J Cardiovasc Electrophysiol* 2002; **13**: 25–32.

8 Wilkoff BL. Should all patients receive dual chamber pacing ICDs? The rationale for the DAVID trial. *Curr Control Trials Cardiovasc Med* 2001; **2**: 215–7.

9 Stellbrink C, Auricchio A, Diem B *et al.* Potential benefit of biventricular pacing in patients with congestive heart failure and ventricular tachyarrhythmia. *Am J Cardiol* 1999; **83**: 143D–50D.

10 Kühlkamp V, for the InSync 7272 ICD World Wide Investigators. Initial experience with an implantable cardioverter-defibrillator incorporating cardiac resynchronization therapy. *J Am Coll Cardiol* 2002; **39**: 790–7.

11 Pinski SL. Implantable device therapy of atrial tachyarrhythmias: ready for prime time? *J Cardiovasc Electrophysiol* 2001; **12**: 1254–5.

12 Bernstein AD, Daubert JC, Fletcher RD *et al.* The revised NASPE/BPEG generic code for antibradycardia, adaptive-rate, and multisite pacing. *Pacing Clin Electrophysiol* 2002; **25**: 260–4.

13 Saksena S. Implantable defibrillators in the third millennium: increasingly relegated to a standby role? *J Am Coll Cardiol* 2000; **36**: 828–31.

14 Splett V, Trusty JM, Hayes DL *et al.* Determination of pacing capture in implantable defibrillators: benefits of evoked response detection using RV coil to can vector. *Pacing Clin Electrophysiol* 2000; **23**: 1645–50.

15 Dijkman B, Wellens HJJ. Interactions between pacing and arrhythmia detection algorithms in the dual chamber implantable cardioverter-defibrillator. *J Interv Card Electrophysiol* 2001; **6**: 299–308.

16 *GEM III DR 7275 System Reference Guide*. Minneapolis, MN: Medtronic, Inc., 2000: 6–6.

17 Barold SS, Cantens F. Characterization of the 16 blanking periods of the Medtronic GEM DR dual chamber defibrillators. *J Interv Card Electrophysiol* 2001; **5**: 319–25.

18 Gold MR, Sulke N, Schwartzman DS *et al.* Clinical experience with a dual-chamber implantable cardioverter defibrillator to treat atrial tachyarrhythmias. *J Cardiovasc Electrophysiol* 2001; **12**: 1247–53.

19 Padeletti L, Pieragnoli P, Ciapetti C *et al.* Randomized crossover comparison of right atrial appendage pacing versus interatrial septum pacing for prevention of paroxysmal atrial fibrillation in patients with sinus bradycardia. *Am Heart J* 2001; **142**: 1047–55.

20 Canby RC, Zhou X, Pulling CC *et al.* Reduction of tachyarrhythmias by ventricular rate stabilization in patients with ICD. *Pacing Clin Electrophysiol* 2001; **24**: 585 [abstract].

21 Viskin S, Glikson M, Fish R *et al.* Rate smoothing with cardiac pacing for preventing torsade de pointes. *Am J Cardiol* 2001; **86**: 111K–115K.

22 Barold SS. Complex arrhythmia in a patient with a dual chamber defibrillator. *Pacing Clin Electrophysiol* 2001; **24**: 1689–91.

23 Cooklin M, Tummala RV, Peters RW *et al.* Comparison of bipolar and integrated sensing for redetection of ventricular fibrillation. *Am Heart J* 1999; **138**: 133–6.

24 Guarnieri T, Datorre SD, Bondke H *et al.* Increased pacing threshold after an automatic defibrillator shock in dogs: effects of class I and class II antiarrhythmic drugs. *Pacing Clin Electrophysiol* 1988; **11**: 1324–30.

25 Kudenchuk PJ, Poole JE, Dolack GL *et al.* Prospective evaluation of the effect of biphasic waveform defibrillation on ventricular pacing thresholds. *J Cardiovasc Electrophysiol* 1997; **8**: 485–95.

26 Welch PJ, Joglar JA, Hamdan MH *et al.* The effect of biphasic defibrillation on the immediate pacing threshold of a dedicated bipolar, steroid-eluting lead. *Pacing Clin Electrophysiol* 1999; **22**: 1229–33.

27 Kessler DJ, Canby RC, Horton RP *et al.* Effect of biphasic endocardial countershock on pacing thresholds in humans. *Am J Cardiol* 1996; **77**: 527–8.

28 Pinski SL, Fahy GJ. The proarrhythmic potential of implantable defibrillators. *Circulation* 1995; **92**: 1651–64.

29 Calkins H, Brinker J, Veltri EP *et al.* Clinical interactions between pacemakers and automatic implantable cardioverter-defibrillators. *J Am Coll Cardiol* 1990; **16**: 666–73.

30 Winkle RA, Bach SM Jr, Mead RH *et al.* Comparison of defibrillation efficacy in humans using a new catheter and superior vena cava spring-left ventricular patch electrodes. *J Am Coll Cardiol* 1988; **11**: 365–70.

31 Mortensen P, Sogaard P, Mansour H *et al.* European study on safety and efficacy of sequential biventricular pacing. *Pacing Clin Electrophysiol* 2002; **25**: 694 [abstract].

32 Wang P, Kramer A, Estes NAM III *et al.* Timing cycles for biventricular pacing. *Pacing Clin Electrophysiol* 2002; **25**: 62–75.

33 Maisel WH, Sweeney MO, Stevenson WG *et al.* Recalls and safety alerts involving pacemakers and implantable cardioverter-defibrillators. *JAMA* 2001; **286**: 793–9.

34 Wilkoff BL, Ching EA, Chung MK *et al.* Dual chamber pacemaker defibrillators: a unique form of crosstalk inhibition. *Pacing Clin Electrophysiol* 1998; **21**: 847 [abstract].

35 Coppess MA, Miller JM, Zipes DP *et al.* Software error resulting in malfunction of an implantable cardioverter-defibrillator. *J Cardiovasc Electrophysiol* 1999; **10**: 871–3.

36 De Vries DW. Medical device safety alert. Guidant Corporation, December 4, 1998.

37 Tremmel J. Important patient management information. Medtronic, Inc., February 11, 2000.

38 Helguera ME, Maloney JD, Pinski SL *et al.* Long-term performance of endocardial pacing leads. *Pacing Clin Electrophysiol* 1994; **17**: 56–64.

39 Maloney JD, Hayes DL, Timmis GC *et al.* Report of the policy conference of NASPE on device/lead performance and the development of a postmarket surveillance database. *Pacing Clin Electrophysiol* 1991; **16**: 1945–52.

40 Bracke FALE, Meijer A, van Gelder LM. Malfunction of endocardial defibrillator leads and lead extraction: where do they meet? *Europace* 2002; **4**: 19–24.

41 Helguera ME, Maloney JD, Fahy GJ *et al.* Clinical presentation of endocardial pacing lead malfunction. *Am J Cardiol* 1996; **78**: 1297–9.

42 Lawton JS, Ellenbogen KA, Wood MA *et al.* Sensing-lead related complications in patients with transvenous implantable cardioverter-defibrillators. *Am J Cardiol* 1996; **78**: 647–51.

43 Lawton JS, Wood MA, Gilligan DM *et al.* Implantable cardioverter-defibrillator leads: the dark side. *Pacing Clin Electrophysiol* 1996; **19**: 1273–8.

44 Jones GK, Bardy GH, Kudenchuk PJ *et al.* Mechanical complications after implantation of multiple-lead nonthoracotomy defibrillator systems: implications for management and future system design. *Am Heart J* 1995; **130**: 327–33.

45 Tyers GFO, Sanders R, Jacqmein W. Reliability of coated wire defibrillation leads. *Pacing Clin Electrophysiol* 1999; **22**: 174–8.

46 Degeratu FT, Khalighi K, Peters RW *et al.* Sensing lead failure in implantable defibrillators: a comparison of two commonly used leads. *J Cardiovasc Electrophysiol* 2000; **11**: 21–4.

47 Peralta AO, John RM, Martin DT *et al.* Long-term performance of the Endotak C defibrillator lead. *Pacing Clin Electrophysiol* 2000; **23**: 753 [abstract].

48 *Tachyarrhythmia Products Performance Report*, 2nd edn, no. 10. Minneapolis, MN: Medtronic, Inc., 2001.

49 Kron J, Herre J, Renfroe EG *et al.* Lead- and device-related complications in the Antiarrhythmics Versus Implantable Defibrillator Trial. *Am Heart J* 2001; **141**: 92–8.

50 Luria D, Glikson M, Brady PA *et al.* Predictors and mode of detection of transvenous lead malfunction in implantable defibrillators. *Am J Cardiol* 2001; **87**: 901–4.

51 Ong LS, Barold SS, Lederman M *et al.* Cephalic vein guide wire technique for implantation of permanent pacemakers. *Am Heart J* 1987; **14**: 753–6.

52 Calkins H, Ramza BM, Brinker J *et al.* Prospective randomized comparison of the safety and effectiveness of placement of endocardial pacemaker and defibrillator leads using the extrathoracic subclavian vein guided by contrast venography versus the cephalic approach. *Pacing Clin Electrophysiol* 2001; **24**: 456–64.

53 De Lurgio DB, Sathavorn C, Mera F *et al.* Incidence and implication of abrasion of implantable cardioverter-defibrillator leads. *Am J Cardiol* 1997; **79**: 1409–11.

54 Mehta D, Nayak HM, Singson M *et al.* Late complications in patients with pectoral defibrillator implants with transvenous defibrillator lead systems: high incidence of insulation breakdown. *Pacing Clin Electrophysiol* 1998; **21**: 1893–900.

55 Schibgilla V, Diem B, Mahmout O *et al.* Impedance rise, only clue to severe insulation damage in a transvenous single-lead AICD-system. *Pacing Clin Electrophysiol* 1998; **21**: 1322–4.

56 Gupta A, Zegel HG, Dravid VS *et al.* Value of radiography in diagnosing complications of cardioverter-defibrillators implanted without thoracotomy in 437 patients. *Am J Roentgenol* 1997; **168**: 105–8.

57 Coyne RF, Winters SL, Curwin JH *et al.* Non-electrode related surprises at radiographic surveillance of implantable defibrillator systems. *Circulation* 2001; **104** (Suppl. II): II-656.

58 Murphy J, Haw J, McMillan H *et al.* Initial clinical experience with automatic audible alerts in ICD patients. *Pacing Clin Electrophysiol* 2001; **24**: 578 [abstract].

59 Dorwath U, Frey B, Matis T *et al.* High failure rate of transvenous defibrillator sensing leads during long-term follow-up: presentation and strategies for early identification. *Pacing Clin Electrophysiol* 2002; **25**: 691 [abstract].

60 Gunderson B, Patel A, Bounds C *et al.* Automatic identification of ICD lead problems using electrograms. *Pacing Clin Electrophysiol* 2002; **25**: 664 [abstract].

61 Butter C, Auricchio A, Schwarz T *et al.* Clinical evaluation of a prototype passive fixation dual chamber single pass lead for dual chamber ICD systems. *Pacing Clin Electrophysiol* 1999; **22**: 169–73.

62 Niehaus M, Schuchert A, Thamasett S *et al.* Multicenter experiences with a single lead electrode for dual chamber ICD systems. *Pacing Clin Electrophysiol* 2001; **24**: 1489–93.

63 Model 6945 RV-SVC lead. Clinical report. Minneapolis, MN: Medtronic, Inc., 1998.

64 Barold SS, Levine PA. Significance of stimulation impedance in biventricular pacing. *J Interv Card Electrophysiol* 2002; **6**: 67–70.

65 Ricci R, Ansalone G, Toscano S *et al.* Cardiac resynchronization: materials, technique and results. *Eur Heart J* 2000; **20** (Suppl. J): J6–15.

66 Worley SJ, Gohn DC, Mandalakas NJ *et al.* Biventricular pacing: the size of the anode is critical for successful capture of the LV. *Pacing Clin Electrophysiol* 2001; **24**: 618 [abstract].

67 Stahmann J, Belalcazar A, Spinelli JC. Staggered pacing pulses are required to maintain low individual site capture thresholds during simultaneous independent output biventricular stimulation. *Pacing Clin Electrophysiol* 2002; **25**: 623 [abstract].

68 Crossley GH, Fitzgerald DM. Estimating defibrillator longevity: a need for an objective comparison. *Pacing Clin Electrophysiol* 1997; **20**: 1897–901.

69 *Marquis DR 7274 Reference Manual.* Minneapolis, MN: Medtronic, Inc., 2002: 7.

70 Crossley GH, Gayle DD, Simmons TW *et al.* Reprogramming pacemakers enhances longevity and is cost-effective. *Circulation* 1996; **94** (Suppl. II): II245–7.

71 Andersen HR, Nielsen JC, Thomsen PE *et al.* Long-term follow-up of patients from a randomised trial of atrial versus ventricular pacing for sick-sinus syndrome. *Lancet* 1997; **350**: 1210–6.

72 Barold SS. Permanent single chamber atrial pacing is obsolete. *Pacing Clin Electrophysiol* 2001; **24**: 271–5.

73 Bode F, Wiegand U, Katus HA *et al.* Inhibition of ventricular stimulation in patients with dual chamber pacemakers and prolonged AV conduction. *Pacing Clin Electrophysiol* 1999; **22**: 1425–31.

74 Garcia-Moran E, Mont L, Brugada J. Inappropriate tachycardia detection by a biventricular implantable cardioverter-defibrillator. *Pacing Clin Electrophysiol* 2002; **25**: 123–4.

75 Pavia SV, Saliba WI, Chung MK *et al.* Matching approved hardware to obtain biventricular pacing and defibrillation: feasibility and trouble-shooting. *Pacing Clin Electrophysiol* 2001; **24**: 613 [abstract].

76 Fu EY, Wood MA, Ellenbogen KA. Loss of atrial tracking following dual chamber ICD implantation. *Pacing Clin Electrophysiol* 2000; **23**: 402–4.

77 Barold SS. Multisite cardiac pacing: a proposal for a simple code. *Acta Cardiol* 2001; **56**: 253–4.

78 Jones GK, Bardy GH. Considerations for ventricular fibrillation detection by implantable cardioverter defibrillators. *Am Heart J* 1994; **127**: 1107–10.

79 Brumwell DA, Kroll K, Lehmann MH. The amplifier: sensing the depolarization. In: Kroll MW, Lehmann MH, eds. *Implantable Cardioverter-Defibrillator Therapy: the Engineering–Clinical Interface.* Norwell, MA: Kluwer Academical Publishers, 1996: 275–302.

80 Dunbar SB, Warner CD, Purcell JA. Internal cardioverter defibrillator device discharge: experiences of patients and family members. *Heart Lung* 1993; **22**: 494–501.

81 Kelly PA, Mann DE, Damle RS *et al.* Oversensing during ventricular pacing in patients with a third-generation implantable cardioverter-defibrillator. *J Am Coll Cardiol* 1994; **23**: 1531–4.

82 Rosenthal ME, Paskman C. Noise detection during bradycardia pacing with a hybrid nonthoracotomy implantable cardioverter-defibrillator system: incidence and clinical significance. *Pacing Clin Electrophysiol* 1998; **21**: 1380–6.

83 Deshmukh P, Anderson K. Myopotential sensing by a dual chamber implantable cardioverter-defibrillator: two case reports. *J Cardiovasc Electrophysiol* 1998; **9**: 767–72.

84 Babuty D, Fauchier L, Cosnay P. Inappropriate shocks delivered by implantable cardioverter-defibrillators during oversensing of activity of diaphragmatic muscle. *Heart* 1999; **81**: 94–6.

85 Sweeney MO, Ellison KE, Shea JB *et al.* Provoked and spontaneous high-frequency, low amplitude respirophasic noise transients in patients with implantable cardioverter-defibrillators. *J Cardiovasc Electrophysiol* 2001; **12**: 402–10.

86 Kopp DE, Burke MC, Lin AC *et al.* Oversensing in dual chamber implantable cardioverter-defibrillators. *Pacing Clin Electrophysiol* 2000; **23**: 591 [abstract].

87 Mortensen PT, Hansen PS, Jensen HK *et al.* Oversensing by implantable defibrillators is most often caused by sensing lead failure as verified by surgical exploration. *Pacing Clin Electrophysiol* 2000; **23**: 630 [abstract].

88 Pinski SL, Trohman RG. Letter to the editor. *Pacing Clin Electrophysiol* 2001; **24**: 1834–5.

89 Gelder RN, Galvin JM, Albert CM *et al.* Lead noise with an active-fixation defibrillation lead. *Pacing Clin Electrophysiol* 2000; **23**: 2113–16.

90 Doshi RN, Goodman J, Naik AM *et al.* Initial experience with an active-fixation defibrillation electrode and the presence of nonphysiological sensing. *Pacing Clin Electrophysiol* 2001; **24**: 1713–20.

91 Reiter MJ, Mann DE. Sensing and tachyarrhythmia detection problems in implantable cardioverter defibrillators. *J Cardiovasc Electrophysiol* 1996; **7**: 542–58.

92 Perry GY, Kosar EM. Problems in managing patients with long QT syndrome and implantable cardioverter-defibrillators: a report of two cases. *Pacing Clin Electrophysiol* 1996; **19**: 863–7.

93 Böhm A, Pintér A, Préda I. QT dependent T wave sensing. *Pacing Clin Electrophysiol* 1998; **21**: 1290–1.

94 Pinski SL. 2 : 1 tracking of sinus rhythm in a patient with a dual-chamber ICD: what is the mechanism? *J Cardiovasc Electrophysiol* 2001; **12**: 503–4.

95 Barold SS, Levine PA. Pacemaker repetitive non-reentrant ventriculoatrial synchronous rhythm. A review. *J Interv Card Electrophysiol* 2001; **5**: 45–58.

96 Pinski SL. Inappropriate pacing due to autoperpetuation of the ventricular rate stabilization algorithm: a manifestation of T-wave oversensing by ICDs. *Pacing Clin Electrophysiol* 2000; **23**: 1446–7.

97 Curwin JH, Roelke M, Ruskin JN. Inhibition of bradycardia pacing caused by far-field atrial sensing in a third-generation cardioverter defibrillator with an automatic gain feature. *Pacing Clin Electrophysiol* 1996; **19**: 124–6.

98 Schecter SO, Greenberg SM, Hoch DH *et al.* Inappropriate discharges of an implantable cardioverter defibrillator secondary to automatic adjustable gain of atrial tachycardia. *Pacing Clin Electrophysiol* 1997; **20**: 1721–2.

99 Peters W, Kowallik P, Wittenberg G *et al.* Inappropriate discharge of an implantable cardioverter-defibrillator during atrial flutter and intermittent ventricular antibradycardia pacing. *J Cardiovasc Electrophysiol* 1997; **8**: 1167–74.

100 Lipchenca I, Garrigue S, Glikson M *et al.* Inhibition of biventricular pacemakers by oversensing of far-field atrial depolarization. *Pacing Clin Electrophysiol* 2002; **25**: 365–7.

101 Pinski SL, Trohman RG. Interference with cardiac pacing. *Cardiol Clin* 2000; **18**: 219–39.

102 Santucci PA, Haw J, Trohman RG *et al.* Interference with an implantable defibrillator by an electronic antitheft-surveillance device. *N Engl J Med* 1998; **339**: 1371–4.

103 Groh W, Boschee S, Engelstein E *et al.* Interactions between electronic article surveillance systems and implantable cardioverter-defibrillators. *Circulation* 1999; **100**: 387–92.

104 Fetter JG, Ivans V, Benditt DG *et al.* Digital cellular telephone interaction with implantable cardioverter-defibrillators. *J Am Coll Cardiol* 1998; **31**: 623–8.

105 Bassen HI, Moore HJ, Ruggera PS. Cellular phone interference testing of implantable cardiac defibrillators in vitro. *Pacing Clin Electrophysiol* 1998; **21**: 1709–15.

106 Sanmartín M, Feranández Lozano I, Márquez J *et al.* Ausencia de interferencia entre teléfonos móviles GSM y desfibriladores implantables: estudio in vivo. *Rev Esp Cardiol* 1997; **50**: 715–19.

107 Gunderson BD, Pratt T, Johnson WB *et al.* Ventricular oversensing in ICD patients: true bipolar versus integrated bipolar sensing. *Pacing Clin Electrophysiol* 2001; **24**: 560 [abstract].

108 Gold MR, Olsovsky MR, Pelini MA *et al.* Comparison of single- and dual-coil active pectoral defibrillation lead systems. *J Am Coll Cardiol* 1998; **31**: 1391–4.

109 Wolfhard UF, Jäger HP, Knocks M *et al.* Alternative lead positioning in the right ventricular outflow tract in transvenous implantation of ICDs. *Pacing Clin Electrophysiol* 1995; **18**: 179–81.

110 Giudici MC, Paul DL, VanWhy KJ. Permanent right ventricular outflow septal placement of active-fixation pacing-defibrillation leads: safety and efficacy for pacing and defibrillation. *Pacing Clin Electrophysiol* 1999; **22**: 801 [abstract].

111 Niehaus M, Neuzner J, Vogt J *et al.* Adjustment of maximum automatic sensitivity (automatic gain control) reduces inappropriate therapies in patients with implantable cardioverter-defibrillators. *Pacing Clin Electrophysiol* 2002; **25**: 151–5.

112 Schulte B, Sperzel J, Schwarz T *et al.* Detection of ventricular fibrillation in implantable defibrillators with automatic gain control amplifiers: effects of programming sensitivity. *Europace* 2000; **2**: 160–2.

113 Bollmann A, Langberg JJ. The relationship between induced and spontaneous ventricular fibrillation. *Circulation* 1997; **96**: I-529 [abstract].

114 Taneja T, Goldberger J, Passman R *et al.* Ventricular fibrillation characteristics of induced and spontaneous ventricular fibrillation. *Circulation* 2001; **104** (Suppl. II): II-381 [abstract].

115 Mann DE, Damle RS, Kelly PA *et al.* Comparison of oversensing during bradycardia pacing in two types of implantable cardioverter-defibrillator systems. *Am Heart J* 1998; **136**: 658–63.

116 Brandt J, Fahraeus T, Schuller H. Far-field QRS complex sensing via the atrial pacemaker lead. I. Mechanism, consequences, differential diagnosis and countermeasures in AAI and VDD/DDD pacing. *Pacing Clin Electrophysiol* 1988; **11**: 1432–8.

117 Israel CW, Gronefeld G, Iscolo N *et al.* Discrimination between ventricular and supraventricular tachycardia by dual chamber cardioverter defibrillators: importance of the atrial sensing function. *Pacing Clin Electrophysiol* 2001; **24**: 183–90.

118 Plummer CJ, Henderson S, Gardener L *et al.* The use of permanent pacemakers in the detection of cardiac arrhythmias. *Europace* 2001; **3**: 229–32.

119 Wolpert C, Jung W, Scholl C *et al.* Electrical proarrhythmia: induction of inappropriate atrial therapies due to far-field R wave oversensing in a new dual chamber defibrillator. *J Cardiovasc Electrophysiol* 1998; **9**: 859–63.

120 Swedlow CD, Schöls W, Dijkman B *et al.* Detection of atrial fibrillation and flutter by a dual-chamber implantable cardioverter-defibrillator. *Circulation* 2000; **29**: 878–85.

121 Dijkman B, Wellens HJ. Dual chamber arrhythmia detection in the implantable cardioverter defibrillator. *J Cardiovasc Electrophysiol* 2000; **11**: 1105–15.

122 Lam CT, Lau CP, Leung SK *et al.* Improved efficacy of mode switching during atrial fibrillation using automatic atrial sensitivity adjustment. *Pacing Clin Electrophysiol* 1999; **22**: 17–25.

123 Brandt J, Worzewski W. Far-field QRS complex sensing: prevalence and timing with bipolar atrial leads. *Pacing Clin Electrophysiol* 2000; **23**: 315–20.

124 Fröhlig G, Helwani Z, Kusch O *et al.* Bipolar ventricular far-field signals in the atrium. *Pacing Clin Electrophysiol* 1999; **22**: 1604–13.

125 Brown ML, Mehra R. Reduced interelectrode spacing improves far field ventricular electrogram rejection in chronic canine study. *J Am Coll Cardiol* 2001; **77** (Suppl. A): 90A [abstract].

126 Van Gelder B, Bracke F, Meijer A. Farfield R-wave sensing: the role of the interelectrode distance, electrode location and ventricular activation. *Pacing Clin Electrophysiol* 2002; **25**: 645 [abstract].

127 Kantharia BK, Wilbur SL, Padder FA *et al.* Effect of different location of atrial lead position on nearfield and farfield electrograms in dual chamber pacemaker-defibrillators. *J Interv Card Electrophysiol* 2001; **5**: 59–66.

128 Bailin SJ, Adler S, Giudici M. Prevention of chronic atrial fibrillation by pacing in the region of Bachmann's bundle: results of a multicenter randomized trial. *J Cardiovasc Electrophysiol* 2001; **12**: 912–17.

129 Porciani MC, Musilli N, Sabini A *et al.* Interatrial septum pacing avoids the adverse effects on atrioventricular delay optimization in biventricular pacing. *Pacing Clin Electrophysiol* 2001; **24**: 539 [abstract].

130 Israel CW. Conflicting issues in permanent right atrial lead positioning. *Pacing Clin Electrophysiol* 2000; **23**: 1581–4.

131 Weretka S, Becker R, Hilbel T *et al.* Far-field R wave oversensing in a dual chamber arrhythmia management device: predisposing factors and practical implications. *Pacing Clin Electrophysiol* 2001; **24**: 1240–6.

132 Swerdlow CD. Supraventricular tachycardia–ventricular tachycardia discrimination algorithms in implantable cardioverter defibrillators: state-of-the-art review. *J Cardiovasc Electrophysiol* 2001; **12**: 606–12.

133 Nowak B, Kracker S, Rippin G *et al.* Effect of the atrial blanking time on the detection of atrial fibrillation in dual chamber pacing. *Pacing Clin Electrophysiol* 2001; **24**: 496–9.

134 Murphy JK, Haw JM, Pinski SL *et al.* Determinants of far-field R wave sensing in dual-chamber ICDs. *Pacing Clin Electrophysiol* 2002; **25**: 550 [abstract].

135 Bilitch M, Cosby RS, Cafferky EA. Ventricular fibrillation and competitive pacing. *N Engl J Med* 1967; **276**: 598–604.

136 Saeed M, Link MS, Mahapatra S *et al.* Analysis of intracardiac electrograms showing monomorphic ventricular tachycardia in patients with implantable cardioverter-defibrillators. *Am J Cardiol* 2000; **85**: 580–7.

137 Callans DJ, Hook BG, Marchlinski FE. Effect of rate and coupling interval on endocardial R wave amplitude variability in permanent ventricular sensing lead systems. *J Am Coll Cardiol* 1993; **22**: 746–50.

138 Brewer JE, Perttu JS, Kroll MW *et al.* Dual level sensing significantly improves automatic threshold control for R wave sensing in implantable defibrillators. *Pacing Clin Electrophysiol* 1996; **19**: 2051–9.

139 Hurwitz JL, Hook BG, Flores BT *et al.* Importance of abortive shock capability with electrogram storage in cardioverter-defibrillator devices. *J Am Coll Cardiol* 1993; **21**: 895–900.

140 Sra J, Akhtar M. Inappropriate shock delivery by implantable defibrillators with dual chamber pacing during nonsustained ventricular tachycardia in patients with heart block. *Pacing Clin Electrophysiol* 2000; **23**: 1054–6.

141 Mann DE, Kelly PA, Reiter MJ. Inappropriate shock therapy for nonsustained ventricular tachycardia in a dual chamber pacemaker defibrillator. *Pacing Clin Electrophysiol* 1998; **21**: 2005–6.

142 Shivkumar K, Feliciano Z, Boyle NG *et al.* Intradevice interaction in a dual chamber implantable cardioverter defibrillator preventing ventricular tachyarrhythmia detection. *J Cardiovasc Electrophysiol* 2000; **11**: 1285–8.

143 Glikson M, Beeman AL, Luria DM *et al.* Impaired detection of ventricular tachyarrhythmias by a rate-smoothing algorithm in dual-chamber implantable defibrillators: intradevice interactions. *J Cardiovasc Electrophysiol* 2002; **13**: 312–18.

144 Viskin S. A worrisome experience during testing of an implantable cardioverter-defibrillator (ICD). *J Cardiovasc Electrophysiol* 2001; **12**: 619 [letter].

145 Kopp DE, Lin AC, Burke MC *et al.* Adverse events with dual-chamber implantable cardioverter-defibrillators. *Pacing Clin Electrophysiol* 1999; **22**: 896 [abstract].

146 *GEM II DR System Reference Guide*. Minneapolis, MN: Medtronic, Inc., 1999: B-8.

147 Pinski SL, Haw J, Trohman RG. Usefulness of a dynamic postpace ventricular blanking period in dual-chamber, rate-responsive implantable defibrillators. *Pacing Clin Electrophysiol* 1999; **22**: 897 [abstract].

148 Ellenbogen KA, Edel T, Moore S *et al.* A prospective randomized-controlled trial of ventricular fibrillation detection time in a DDDR ventricular defibrillator. *Pacing Clin Electrophysiol* 2000; **23**: 1268–72. Erratum in: *Pacing Clin Electrophysiol* 2000; **23** (11 Pt I): viii.

149 Wasmer K, Tada H, Chough SP *et al.* Outcome of patients with ventricular dysfunction and a class I indication for pacing treated with a defibrillator. *Circulation* 2001; **104** (Suppl. II): II-784 [abstract].

150 Furman S. The future of the pacemaker. *Pacing Clin Electrophysiol* 2002; **25**: 1–2.

151 Pavia S, Perez-Lugones A, Lam C *et al.* Symptomatic deterioration post dual-chamber cardioverter-defibrillator implantation: a retrospective, observational study. *J Am Coll Cardiol* 2001; **37** (Suppl. A): 89A [abstract].

CHAPTER 18

Complexity of Follow-up in Multisite Pacing

Arnaud Lazarus

The first four-chamber pacing system to treat heart failure was successfully implanted 8 years ago to treat a patient with refractory congestive heart failure with a major interatrial and left intraventricular conduction delay [1]. The striking clinical benefit in this critically ill patient introduced the now widely accepted concept that multisite ventricular stimulation can improve the hemodynamics of patients with certain forms of heart failure, a process known as cardiac resynchronization [2–5]. Implantation of such devices requires a longer and more difficult procedure as well as more complex follow-up evaluation of the patient and device function.

Clinical monitoring

After device implantation, meticulous hemodynamic and electrophysiologic evaluation is essential because the patients are clinically fragile. Immediate postoperative telemetric electrocardiographic (ECG) monitoring allows detection of atrial or ventricular arrhythmias and initiation of treatment. The drug treatment of congestive heart failure is then gradually reappraised, with a possible reduction in the doses of diuretics, and changes in the prescription of angiotensin-converting enzyme inhibitors or beta-blockers, particularly in patients with pre-existing sinus node dysfunction. The pacemaker pocket merits greater surveillance because local complications seem more frequent than with conventional devices. A long implantation procedure, the need for anticoagulant therapy, the quasi-systematic use of a subclavian approach and in particular the greater volume of the implanted material account for the increased risk of local complications: hematoma (warfarin, aspirin); infection (long and sometimes complex procedures); and risk of skin erosion, especially with the use of a Y-connector that increases the volume of the implanted material. The follow-up of the patient with a conventional device focuses on technical considerations because the clinical evaluation of the patient is often performed by the referring physician. Multisite biventricular pacing does not permit dissociation of the clinical and electronic data, thereby increasing the time necessary for a follow-up visit. The latter requires systematic assessment of the functional status, appearance of symptoms suggesting progression of the underlying cardiomyopathy, signs of heart failure or paroxysmal arrhythmias, phrenic nerve stimulation, and search for electrical dysfunction of a more complicated pacing system. In addition, the stability of the left ventricular lead should be assessed with postoperative chest X-rays in multiple views.

Electrocardiography

The ECG characteristics of multisite pacing are detailed in Chapter 8. The ECG permits study and control of biventricular capture with the programmer, and analysis of the quality of electrical resynchronization. The limited effectiveness of the passive means of fixation of the left ventricular lead constitutes the principal cause of loss of capture or significant rises in the left ventricular pacing threshold by displacement, often early but sometimes late, or by rotation of the distal part of the lead. Sometimes, 'triple-site' ventricular capture by anodic stimulation starting from the proximal electrode of the right ventricular lead can confuse the electrocardiographic assessment of biventricular capture [6]. This phenomenon may occur with high pacing amplitudes in a bipolar configuration with a dual cathodal system using a single ventricular output.

Pacemaker parameters

Continual ventricular pacing and absence of spontaneous ventricular activity (except for ventricular premature beats) should be checked by the memory capability of the pacemaker. The percentage of ventricular pacing, except fusion beats, represents the delivery of effective therapy (biventricular pacing). In addition, the memory function may unveil the presence of clinically important chronotropic incompetence. The selection of the optimal hemodynamic atrioventricular delay, on sensed and paced P waves, is ideally carried out using Doppler echocardiography.

Concerning the initial settings of the pacing system, a significant ventricular pacing safety margin must be selected to overcome rises in the capture thresholds, related to an usual inflammatory reaction or micro- or macrodislodgement of the left ventricular lead. At present, dual cathodal systems do not allow individual testing of each ventricular lead. The use of pacing systems with separate ventricular channels, true 'triple chamber', will gradually replace dual cathodal devices with Y-connectors (external or incorporated into the header of the device), and will largely facilitate pacemaker analysis and individual programming of configurations, output and sensitivity. Phrenic stimulation must be sought diligently by high-output pacing and postural maneuvers. Reprogramming of the pacing parameters may occasionally correct phrenic nerve stimulation but repositioning of the left ventricular lead is often required. The quality of sensing must be checked, with selection of a high atrial sensitivity to diagnose a low-amplitude atrial arrhythmia, provided far-field R-wave sensing on the atrial channel is avoided.

Among the available algorithms, the mode-switching function should be used to deal with atrial tachyarrhythmias. However, arrhythmias seem less frequent with biventricular pacing, but their identification is significant. Paroxysmal episodes of atrial fibrillation cause hemodynamic impairment, not only by loss of atrial systole but also, in the event of spontaneous atrioventricular conduction, by loss of biventricular pacing with inhibition of ventricular pacing. Radiofrequency ablation of the atrioventricular junction is required if drug treatment is ineffectual, especially in the presence of a fast spontaneous ventricular rate during arrhythmia. In chronic atrial fibrillation patients, atrioventricular (AV) junction ablation is often mandatory to obtain permanent biventricular pacing. A biventricular implantable cardioverter defibrillator (ICD) should be considered in patients with serious ventricular arrhythmias. The same monitoring procedures apply to patients with biventricular ICDs.

Stimulation impedance

The advent of biventricular pacing for the treatment of congestive heart failure has created new complexity in the understanding of stimulation impedance [8].

Present pacing systems depend on Ohm's law: $V = IR$, $I = V/R$, $R = V/I$, where V is voltage, I is current and R is resistance or impedance.

Resistances in series: $R = R_1 + R_2$. The current is the same through both R_1 and R_2.

Resistances in parallel: $R = (R_1 R_2)/(R_1 + R_2)$. $R < R_1$ and $R < R_2$. The voltage across R_1 and R_2 is equal.

There are presently two systems for multisite pacing: split bipole and dual cathodal arrangements. Both use only one pacemaker port and require a Y-connector that may or may not be incorporated into the header of the pulse generator. Initial systems for biventricular pacing employed a split bipole with two separate unipolar leads (in series), one placed in the right ventricle and the other used for left ventricular stimulation. The pacing impedance during biventricular stimulation was then much higher than that for either electrode alone.

Until totally independent programmability is available for each lead, a divided pacemaker output or common dual cathodal system (simultaneous dual-site cathodal stimulation with the leads connected in parallel) is widely used. The parallel arrangement and the larger combined surface area of the right and left ventricular leads (compared to a single lead) result in a reduced stimulation impedance. Thus, the total lead impedance is likely to be low (in the range of 250–400 Ω) in a normally functioning biventricular system. A mechanical problem in one of the ventricular leads but not the other may not be readily detectable using standard impedance criteria. An open circuit (conductor fracture) involving one lead will not result in the very high impedances that are present with single-

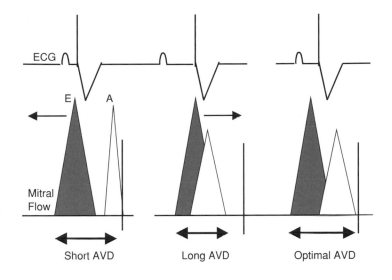

Figure 18.1 Determination of the hemodynamically optimal atrioventricular delay (AVD), providing the longest diastolic filling time without interruption of the A wave by the ventricular contraction that occurs with an excessively short AVD. An excessively long AVD generates a short filling time and fusion of the A and E waves.

chamber pacing. Rather, that lead will effectively be taken out of the system and the measured impedance will reflect the expected impedance for the intact ventricular lead. Hence, with an open circuit on one of the two ventricular leads, the measured impedance may rise to the normal range for a univentricular lead. The normally low impedance in a dual cathodal system may also complicate the diagnosis of an insulation failure in one of the leads. The low telemetered impedance that is associated with an insulation failure in a single-chamber lead may be in the 'normal' range during intact biventricular pacing.

Echocardiography

Echocardiography constitutes the most basic examination in the follow-up of patients with multisite devices and must be used systematically. Echocardiography follow-up has three objectives after implantation of a multisite pacing system.

1 *Setting of optimal pacemaker parameters.* With the majority of devices used today, the AV delay is the only hemodynamic parameter capable of optimization using echocardiography, as with conventional dual-chamber pacemakers [9]. The objective is to normalize the mitral flow pattern without fusion of E and A waves (too long AV delay), without interruption of the A wave by the ventricular contraction (too short AV delay), and with the longest filling time (Figure 18.1). In cases where a V–V delay can be programmed (devices with separate ventricular

channels, or conventional dual-chamber pacemakers in patients with chronic atrial fibrillation), the highest aortic ejection flow is selected [10].

2 *Quantification of mechanical and hemodynamic results.* The effect of cardiac resynchronization is analysed and quantified at three levels during biventricular pacing and compared to that of spontaneous rhythm using the atrioventricular, interventricular and intraventricular synchrony method:

(a) *Atrioventricular synchrony.* Doppler analysis of the transmitral flow shows in biventricular pacing mode an increase in the total diastolic filling time with resumption of the partial or complete fusion of E and A waves during spontaneous rhythm.

(b) *Interventricular asynchrony* (Figure 18.2). The pre-ejection delays (PEDs), measured from the beginning of the QRS complex to the beginning of the aortic and pulmonary ejection flows, are modified by pacing. Left ventricular pacing reduces the left PED, which is generally longer than that on the right. Then, when the leads are implanted at optimal sites, the interventricular delay diminishes, partly by reduction of the left PED together with stable or increased right PED. The phenomenon of right PED increase is related to the effect of right ventricular pacing as compared with spontaneous right ventricular activation, being less affected than on the left side in the case of left bundle branch block.

(c) *Intraventricular asynchrony* (Figure 18.3). The different segments of the left ventricle may

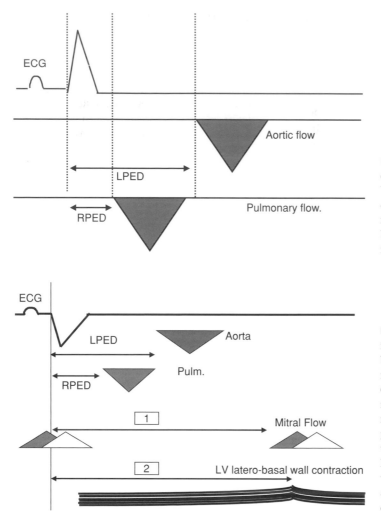

Figure 18.2 Left and right pre-ejection delays are easily measured from the beginning of the QRS complex to the onset of the aortic and pulmonary flows, respectively. The difference between these two values yields the interventricular delay.

Figure 18.3 Estimation of left intraventricular asynchrony by comparing two simple measurements: the delay from the QRS onset to the beginning of the mitral E wave, and the time delay from the QRS onset to the systolic peak of the left laterobasal wall using time–motion (TM) mode with a TM line positioned on the left laterobasal wall, at the level of the mitral annulus, in an apical four-chamber view.

not be activated synchronously because of intra-ventricular conduction disturbances. In this case, ventricular filling may begin when some segments usually the left laterobasal wall are still contracting. Measurement of the time delay between (i) the beginning of the QRS and the beginning of the mitral E wave (left ventricular filling) and (ii) the beginning of the QRS and the systolic peak of the left laterobasal (local systole) wall using time movement (TM) mode or Doppler tissue imaging then shows an abnormal overlap between those two opposite phases of myocardial function.

The sum of the abnormalities at these three different levels reflects the severity of the mechanical cardiac asynchrony and the effectiveness of optimized pacemaker settings in correcting these disturb-ances. One, two or the three levels can be involved in a patient, with various degrees of severity. Furthermore, in the intermediate and long-term follow-up, improvement in the left ejection fraction must be sought. The mechanical effect of resynchronization is also visible by assessing the changes in mitral and tricuspid regurgitation, with qualitative and quant-itative changes including modification of timing and axis of the regurgitated flows.

3 *Analysis of the cardiac susbstrate.* The basic status of underlying cardiac asynchrony must be analysed regularly to assess progression of disease and detect worsening conduction disturbances over time in advanced heart failure, because such changes may occasionally explain a deterioration of the patient's hemodynamic status.

Conventional echo Doppler techniques are adequate for a good assessment of multisite biventricular pacing for heart failure. Simple measurements give fast and easily reproducible quantifications of the different levels of mechanical asynchrony. This technique is widely accessible, with a low cost. However, new echocardiography refinements [11,12] such as Doppler tissue imaging, three-dimensional echo or color kinesis can provide more precise information. For example, Doppler tissue imaging allows a quantitative assessment of the ventricular segmental wall movements using an apical view. Real-time intramyocardial pulsed Doppler velocities are measured from multiple left and right ventricular sectors. Velocity profiles are then derived, allowing timing analysis and comparisons of different ventricular regions to quantify the degree of inter- and intraventricular asynchrony.

Echocardiography technicians should be trained in certain aspects of cardiac pacing, especially for the follow-up of patients with biventricular devices, so that they can manipulate the programmable indices during the postoperative follow-up examinations.

Cardiopulmonary exercise testing can be used to quantify the changes in functional capacity. The chronotropic function is analysed and, when applicable, the rate-responsive function is adapted. The 6-min walk test and the use of quality-of-life questionnaires are usually restricted to investigational studies.

All these specific procedures increase the time devoted to follow-up and merit specific training. However, they are essential to provide an optimal clinical benefit to the patient.

References

1 Cazeau S, Ritter P, Bakdach S *et al.* Four chamber pacing in dilated cardiomyopathy. *Pacing Clin Electrophysiol* 1994; **17** (Pt II): 1974–9.

2 Cazeau S, Ritter P, Lazarus A *et al.* Multisite pacing for end-stage heart failure: early experience. *Pacing Clin Electrophysiol* 1996; **19**: 1748–57.

3 Leclercq C, Cazeau S, Ritter P *et al.* A pilot experience with permanent biventricular pacing to treat advanced heart failure. *Am Heart J* 2000; **140**: 862–70.

4 Stellbrink C, Breithardt O, Franke A, Sack S, Bakker P, Auricchio A, on behalf of PATH-CHF Investigators, Pochet T, Salo R, Kramer A, Spinelli J, on behalf of CPI Guidant Congestive Heart Failure Research Group. Impact of cardiac resynchronization therapy using hemodynamically optimized pacing on left ventricular remodeling in patients with congestive heart failure and ventricular conduction disturbances. *J Am Coll Cardiol* 2001; **38**: 1957–65.

5 Cazeau S, Leclercq C, Lavergne T *et al.* for the Multisite Stimulation in Cardiomyopathies (MUSTIC) Study Investigators. Effects of multisite biventricular pacing in patients with heart failure and intraventricular conduction delay. *N Engl J Med* 2001; **344**: 873–80.

6 Steinhaus DM, Hayes DL, Curtis AB, Tang ASL. Anodal stimulation: a potential concern with biventricular pacing? [abstract 60]. *Pacing Clin Electrophysiol* 2001; **24** (4 Pt II): 553.

7 Cazeau S, Gras D, Lazarus A, Ritter P, Mugica J. Multisite stimulation for correction of cardiac asynchrony. *Heart* 2000; **84**: 579–81.

8 Barold SS, Levine PA. Significance of stimulation impedance in biventricular pacing. *J Interv Card Electrophysiol* 2002; **6**: 6.

9 Ritter P, Dib JC, Lelievre T *et al.* Quick determination of the optimal AV delay at rest in patients paced in DDD mode for complete AV block [abstract 163]. *Eur J Cardiac Pacing Electrophysiol* 1994; **4** (2): 39.

10 Sogaard P, Mortensen PT, Kim WY, Egeblad H. Sequential cardiac resynchronization with individual interventricular delay programming is superior to simultaneous cardiac resynchronization in patients with heart failure and bundle branch block. An InSync III study using three dimensional echocardiography and tissue velocity imaging [abstract 2032]. *Circulation* 2001; **104** (17): II-429.

11 Ansalone G, Giannantoni P, Ricci R, Trambaiolo P, Fedele F, Santini M. Doppler myocardial imaging to evaluate the effectiveness of pacing sites in patients receiveing biventricular pacing. *J Am Coll Cardiol* 2002; **39**: 489–99.

12 Kim WY, Søgaard P, Mortensen PT *et al.* Three dimensional echocardiography documents hemodynamic improvement by biventricular pacing in patients with severe heart failure. *Heart* 2001; **85**: 514–20.

CHAPTER 19

Electromagnetic Interference with Implantable Cardiac Devices

David L. Hayes

Introduction

Although pacemakers and implantable cardioverter defibrillators (ICDs) are subject to electromagnetic interference (EMI) from many sources, relatively few are capable of causing clinically significant interference. However, in the rapidly evolving technology-driven environment in which we live, new devices that could theoretically cause interference with implanted devices constantly appear both within and outside the hospital environment. It is important that the clinician caring for a patient with an implanted device be aware of these sources to provide appropriate education and protection for the patient. Therefore, even if there are few new threats for the patient with a pacemaker or ICD in 2003, a review of the known sources of EMI is important.

Most sources of EMI are non-biologic, but biologic sources of interference, such as myopotentials and extremes of temperature or irradiation, can also cause pulse generators to malfunction. In general, contemporary pacemakers and ICDs are effectively shielded against EMI, and the use of a bipolar sensing configuration has reduced the problem even further.

EMI enters an implanted pulse generator by conduction if the patient is in direct contact with the source or by radiation if the patient is in an electromagnetic field, with the pacemaker lead acting as an antenna [1]. Pacemakers and ICDs are protected from interference by shielding of the circuitry, which filters the incoming signal and reduces the distance between the electrodes to minimize the antenna. Contemporary pulse generators are protected from most sources of interference because the circuitry is shielded inside a stainless steel or titanium case. In addition, body tissues provide some protection by reflection or absorption of external radiation.

A bipolar sensing configuration is less susceptible to conducted and radiated interference because the distance between anode and cathode is smaller than that for unipolar leads. Bipolar sensing has largely eliminated myopotential inhibition and crosstalk as pacemaker problems. In addition, with bipolar sensing there is considerably less sensing of external electrical fields [2,3] and less effect from electrocautery during surgery [4].

Sensed interference is filtered by narrow bandpass filters to exclude non-cardiac signals (Figure 19.1). However, this still leaves signals in the 5–100-Hz range, which overlap the cardiac signal range and are not filtered. These signals can result in abnormal device behavior if they are interpreted as being cardiac events.

There are a number of possible device responses to external interference, including inappropriate inhibition of pacemaker output, inappropriate triggering of pacemaker output, asynchronous pacing, reprogramming to different parameters, and damage to the pacemaker circuitry.

Hospital environment

The hospital is the most common environment for potential sources of EMI that may cause significant interference with implantable devices.

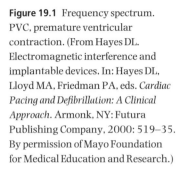

Figure 19.1 Frequency spectrum. PVC, premature ventricular contraction. (From Hayes DL. Electromagnetic interference and implantable devices. In: Hayes DL, Lloyd MA, Friedman PA, eds. *Cardiac Pacing and Defibrillation: A Clinical Approach*. Armonk, NY: Futura Publishing Company, 2000: 519–35. By permission of Mayo Foundation for Medical Education and Research.)

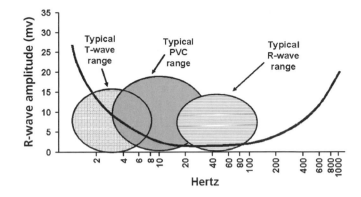

Electrocautery

Electrocautery continues to be one of the most common potential sources of EMI for patients with implanted devices [1,5,6]. Electrocautery involves the use of radiofrequency current to cut or coagulate tissues. It is usually applied in a unipolar configuration between the cauterizing instrument (the cathode) and the indifferent plate (the anode) attached at a distance to the patient's skin. Bipolar cautery uses a bipolar instrument for coagulation. The frequency is usually between 300 and 500 kHz (at frequencies of less than 200 kHz, muscle and nerve stimulation may occur) [1]. Cutting diathermy uses a modulated signal, so that bursts of energy are applied, whereas coagulation diathermy uses an unmodulated signal to heat the tissue. Coagulation diathermy is used in radiofrequency ablation of cardiac tissue for the treatment of arrhythmias.

The current generated by electrocautery is related to the distance and orientation of the cautery electrodes relative to the pacemaker and lead. High current is generated if the cautery cathode is close to the pacemaker, and particularly high currents are generated in the pacemaker if it lies between the two cautery electrodes.

Electrocautery can result in multiple clinical responses from an implanted device, including reprogramming, permanent damage to the circuitry, inhibition, reversion to a fall-back mode, noise reversion mode (Figure 19.2) and electrical reset. In addition, the electrocautery signal may induce currents in the pacing lead and cause local heating at the electrode, leading to myocardial damage with subsequent elevation of pacing or sensing thresholds, or both (Figure 19.3). Threshold alteration is often transient. In the patient with an ICD, electrocautery could result in inappropriate detection of what is interpreted to be a ventricular dysrhythmia or in failure to detect a ventricular arrhythmia.

To prevent inappropriate inhibition of the pacemaker, a magnet is often applied to the chest over the pacemaker during cautery to convert it to the asynchronous mode. This may be successful, but because in some pacemakers this procedure could theoretically make the device more susceptible to reprogramming by the electrocautery signal, it is controversial [6].

During surgery, pacemakers with rate-responsive functions may respond with rate increments caused by vibration sensed from intraoperative equipment or vibrations created by the surgical procedure. The electrocautery signal may overwhelm the impedance-measuring circuit of a minute-ventilation rate-responsive pacemaker and cause pacing at the upper rate limit. Minute-ventilation rate-responsive pacemakers may also be susceptible to upper rate limit pacing if a specific type of impedance monitoring is used intraoperatively or postoperatively, and positive pressure ventilation may result in inappropriate rate response [1,7,8].

Patients with pacemakers who are to undergo surgery in which electrocautery may be used should be assessed preoperatively (Table 19.1) to determine the programmed settings and whether the patient is pacemaker dependent. In patients with ICDs, the 'therapies' should be programmed 'off' for the duration of the surgical procedure to avoid inappropriate detection of EMI as a ventricular dysrhythmia. The patient must be continuously monitored from the time therapies are programmed 'off' until they are reactivated.

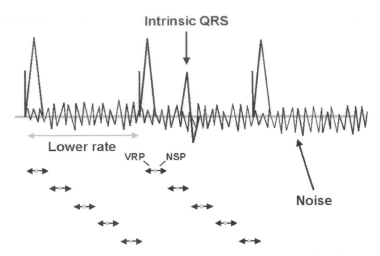

Figure 19.2 Response of a VVI pacemaker to noise. There is no sensing during the ventricular refractory period (VRP). Noise is detected in the noise-sampling period (NSP) immediately after the VRP and causes restarting of the VRP. In the next NSP, noise is again detected, and the VRP is again restarted. This continues until the lower rate interval (LRI) times out, and a ventricular pacing pulse is delivered. Because the sensing channel is refractory throughout the LRI, the intrinsic cardiac beat (R) is not sensed, and pacing is asynchronous. (From Hayes DL. Electromagnetic interference and implantable devices. In: Hayes DL, Lloyd MA, Friedman PA, eds. *Cardiac Pacing and Defibrillation: A Clinical Approach.* Armonk, NY: Futura Publishing Company, 2000: 519–35. By permission of Mayo Foundation for Medical Education and Research.)

Apex-anterior   ## Apex-posterior

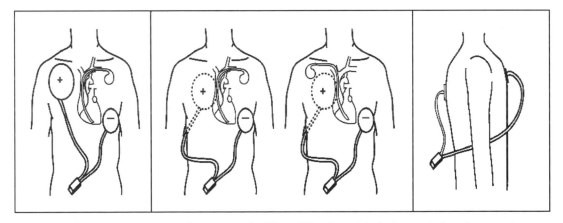

Figure 19.3 Schematic representation of positioning of paddles or R2 pads to minimize damage to the pulse generator and pacemaker lead. (From Hayes DL. Electromagnetic interference and implantable devices. In: Hayes DL, Lloyd MA, Friedman PA, eds. *Cardiac Pacing and Defibrillation: A Clinical Approach.* Armonk, NY: Futura Publishing Company, 2000: 519–35. By permission of Mayo Foundation for Medical Education and Research.)

In the operating room, it is most important that the indifferent plate of the electrocautery device be placed at a distance from the pulse generator, usually on the thigh, and that good contact be ensured. The effect of electrocautery may be difficult to assess because it causes interference on the electrocardio-gram (ECG) monitor. Other methods of assessing cardiac rhythm should be used; for example, pulse oximetry or arterial blood pressure monitoring.

Cautery should be used with caution in the vicinity of the pulse generator and its leads. The cathode should be kept as far from the pulse generator as

Table 19.1 Perioperative management with use of electrocautery in patients who have implanted cardiac devices.

Preoperatively
Identify pacemaker and determine 'reset' mode
Check pacemaker program, telemetry, thresholds, battery status
Deactivate rate response and, if applicable, Vario function
Record pacemaker information

Intraoperatively
Position the indifferent plate for electrocautery away from pacemaker so that
    pacemaker is not between electrocautery electrodes
Monitor pulse or oximeter (electrocardiogram is obscured by artifacts)
Have programmer readily available
Use bipolar cautery when possible
Do not use cautery near pacemaker
Use cautery in short bursts
Reprogram, if necessary, if reset mode is hemodynamically unstable
Rarely, consider use of VVT mode if necessary

Postoperatively
Check pacemaker program, telemetry, thresholds
Reprogram if necessary

possible, the lowest possible amplitude should be used, and the surgeon should deliver only brief bursts.

During electrocautery, pulse generator function and cardiac rhythm should be carefully assessed. The most likely response is that of transient inhibition or asynchronous pacing, which should cause no significant hemodynamic problem. If persistent pacemaker inhibition occurs, a magnet can be applied to the pacemaker during electrocautery.

Postoperatively, it is critical that the pulse generator be interrogated and reprogrammed to the original settings if any changes have occurred. Ideally, thresholds should be reassessed and compared with preoperative values. If any problems are encountered when the pacemaker is interrogated or reprogrammed to its original settings, the manufacturer should be consulted to determine whether malfunction has occurred.

Defibrillation

External transthoracic defibrillation produces the largest amount of electrical energy delivered in the vicinity of an implanted device and has the potential to damage both the pulse generator and the cardiac tissue in contact with the lead [1,6]. The device is protected from damage from high defibrillation energies by special circuitry that electronically regulates the voltage entering the circuit and should prevent high currents from being conducted via the

lead to the myocardium. However, the extremely high energies can overwhelm this protection and cause damage to the implanted device or the heart. Internal defibrillation via epicardial or subcutaneous patches or intracardiac defibrillation electrodes delivers smaller amounts of energy but may also interfere with device function. As previously noted, devices with bipolar sensing configuration are less susceptible to interference from defibrillation.

The degree of damage seems to be related to the distance of the defibrillation paddles from the pulse generator. The paddles used for defibrillation should be placed as far as possible from the generator and, when possible, an anterior–posterior configuration is preferred (Figure 19.3). In the anterior–anterior configuration, the paddles should be 10 cm away from the pulse generator if possible. After defibrillation, the device should be interrogated and the programmed parameters compared with those before defibrillation–cardioversion. A transient rise in threshold should be managed by increasing the energy output if necessary (Figure 19.4). Rarely, a prolonged, severe increase in threshold occurs, necessitating lead replacement.

Catheter ablation

Nearly all ablations are now performed with radiofrequency current, which is the same as that used for coagulation electrocautery, that is, unmodulated

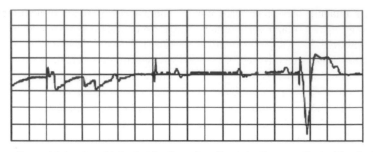

Figure 19.4 Electrocardiographic tracing obtained at the time of cardioversion from a patient with a dual-chamber pacemaker. The patient was relatively pacemaker dependent. After delivery of the external shock, there is profound asystole. Subsequently the patient had markedly increased ventricular pacing thresholds, which returned to baseline about 48 h after cardioversion. (From Hayes DL, Wang PJ, eds. *Cardiac Pacemakers and Implantable Defibrillators: A Multi-Volume Workbook*, Vol. 4. *ICDs and Pacemakers*. Armonk, NY: Futura Publishing Company, 2000: 37. By permission of Blackwell Publishing.)

radiofrequency current at a frequency of 400–500 kHz. Effects similar to those of surgical electro-cautery have been reported, including inappropriate inhibition, asynchronous pacing and resetting to back-up mode [9,10]. Radiofrequency ablation has been carried out safely in the presence of implanted pulse generators and does not appear to result in any significant myocardial damage at the site of the pacemaker electrode.

Before radiofrequency ablation is done, the implanted pulse generator should be interrogated and programmed settings recorded. A programmer should be available during the radiofrequency procedure. After the procedure, the device should be reinterrogated and reprogrammed if necessary.

Magnetic resonance imaging

In magnetic resonance imaging (MRI), a large magnetic field is generated by an electromagnet and is modulated by a radiofrequency electrical signal. Newer MRI scanners have magnets as strong as 3.0 tesla.

When a pacemaker is near an MRI scanner with the electromagnet 'on', the reed switch closes and asynchronous pacing occurs. Although there may be competition with the underlying cardiac rhythm, it does not commonly cause a clinical problem.

Measuring the effect of MRI on pacemakers and ICDs is difficult because the radiofrequency pulses cause ECG artifacts. However, several studies of pacemakers in dogs have demonstrated the potential adverse effects. In some pacemakers, the only effect was asynchronous pacing [11]. In other pacemakers, cardiac pacing at the same frequency or a multiple of the frequency of the radiofrequency current occurred; for example, if MRI was operating at 200 ms, pacing rates at 300 b.p.m. were observed in some dogs [11,12]. The radiofrequency signal is detected by the leads acting as an antenna and is then amplified by the pacemaker circuitry to produce sufficient energy to pace the heart.

Reported problems with pacemakers in MRI scanners include magnet-activated asynchronous pacing, inhibition by the radiofrequency signal, rapid pacing induced by the radiofrequency signal [13,14], discomfort at the pacemaker pocket, and death [14]. Reported deaths have presumably been secondary to rapid pacing that led to hemodynamic collapse or induction of ventricular tachycardia or ventricular fibrillation. It is difficult to know with any certainty how many deaths or potentially life-threatening complications have occurred, but the number is not insignificant. Transient reed switch malfunction has also been seen [11]. Investigators have also demonstrated MRI-induced heating of the conductor coil and electrode tip in an animal model [14]. Such heating could result in damage at the electrode–myocardium interface. Clinically, the results could be an increase in pacing and sensing thresholds, complete failure to capture, and a discrete area of myocardial damage. Temporary pacemakers are also subject to interference from MRI, and a patient actively requiring temporary pacing should not be considered for MRI.

As of 2003, MRI should still be considered contraindicated in patients with an implanted device. Several approaches have been used in an effort to accomplish MRI in a patient with an implanted device when other imaging modalities were not adequate for making a specific diagnosis. Methods, concerns and precautions for the patient with a device undergoing MRI have been reported, but this author does not advocate any of these practices.

If MRI is undertaken in a patient with an implanted device, the patient should be fully informed of the potential complications and the discussion should be documented in the patient's clinical record. Any patient considered for MRI must not be dependent on the pacemaker; that is, must be able to undergo the study without any pacing support. Also, patients must have cardiac monitoring beginning at the time the pacemaker is reprogrammed to yield non-capture and continuing throughout the procedure.

There have been reports of programming the pacemaker to a non-pacing mode, i.e. OOO or ODO, or programming the energy output settings, i.e. voltage amplitude and pulse width, to subthreshold values to prevent capture [15]. Even if the pacemaker is rendered ineffectual for capture, risks from MRI are not precluded. With the programming described, MRI theoretically could still couple with the implanted lead or leads and result in rapid pacing and subsequent adverse outcomes. In addition, MRI-induced heating of the conductor coil and electrode tip theoretically could still occur.

MRI has also been performed after explantation of the permanent pacemaker. If this is considered, explantation must be done with careful sterile technique. The patient should be informed that even with the best technique, the incidence of infection increases with manipulation of the pacemaker pocket. If the device is explanted, the incision should be closed in a normal fashion and the incision 'dressed' until the device is reimplanted. The patient should be continuously monitored during the time the device is not in place or operational. If the implanted device is not at replacement indicators and a new device cannot be justified, two options have been used. The implant suite in which the device has been explanted can be left intact but the room 'closed' to any other procedures or even personnel 'traffic' until the patient is returned to the room for reimplantation of the device. After the device has been explanted, it should be wiped with an antibiotic solution by the physician or a 'sterile' scrub assistant, wrapped in a sterile towel or gauze,

and placed on the instrument table, which is then covered until the patient is returned to the room for reimplantation. If the implant room cannot be left unused until the patient returns for reimplantation, the patient's device could be resterilized by accepted techniques, packaged in a sterile manner, and then reimplanted the next day.

In addition to being told that explantation of the implanted device increases the risk of infection, the patient should understand that the indwelling lead or leads can be a source of adverse effects, as previously described. This author does not advocate lead extraction in an effort to perform MRI.

Extracorporeal shock wave lithotripsy

Extracorporeal shock wave lithotripsy (ESWL) is a non-invasive treatment for nephrolithiasis and cholelithiasis that delivers multiple, focused hydraulic shocks, generated by an underwater spark gap, to a patient lying in a water bath. The shock is focused on the stones by an ellipsoidal metal reflector. Because the shock wave can produce ventricular extrasystoles, it is synchronized to the R wave.

ESWL is safe to use with implanted pulse generators, provided that the shock is given synchronously with the ECG and that dual-chamber pacemakers have safety pacing enabled. In the pacemaker-dependent patient, it is recommended that a dual-chamber pacemaker be programmed to the VVI, VOO or DOO pacing mode to avoid ventricular inhibition [16]. Programming of a DDD pulse generator to the VVI, VOO or DOO mode also avoids rare instances of irregularities of pacing rate, supraventricular arrhythmias that could be tracked or induced, and triggering of the ventricular output by electromechanical interference.

ESWL has not been known to cause any damage to the pacemaker, except that if an activity-sensing pacemaker is placed at the focal point of the ESWL, the piezoelectric crystal could be shattered [17]. Patients with rate-adaptive pacemakers that have piezoelectric crystal activity can probably undergo lithotripsy safely if the device is implanted in the thorax, but lithotripsy should be avoided in these patients if the device is located in the abdomen. Patients with ICDs should have the ICD therapeutic capability deactivated during ESWL. While the therapies are 'off', the patient must be on continuous cardiac monitoring.

Transcutaneous electrical nerve stimulation

Transcutaneous electrical nerve stimulation (TENS) is a widely used method for the relief of acute and chronic pain from musculoskeletal and neurologic problems. A TENS unit consists of several electrodes placed on the skin and connected to a pulse generator that applies pulses of between 1 and 200 V and 0–60 mA at a frequency of 20–110 Hz. The output and frequency of the unit can be adjusted by the patient to provide maximum relief of pain.

The repetition frequency of the TENS output is similar to the normal range of heart rates, so it would be expected that TENS pulses could cause pacemaker inhibition. Although an older study of 51 patients with pacemakers showed no inhibition during TENS stimulation [18], instances of asymptomatic inhibition of pacemaker output by TENS have been reported [19,20]. Interference is most likely to occur in significantly older pacemakers and pacemakers in the unipolar sensing configuration.

TENS can probably be used safely in most patients with bipolar pacemakers or ICDs. However, it is reasonable to take special precautions in patients who are pacemaker dependent or have ICDs and monitor them during initial TENS application. If TENS results in interference in pacemaker-dependent patients or is detected as ventricular activity in patients with ICDs, TENS should be avoided. If patients with unipolar pacemakers have interference with use of TENS, the testing can be repeated after reprogramming the sensitivity to a less sensitive value or programming the device to a bipolar configuration if it is polarity programmable and bipolar leads are in place.

Dental equipment

Dental ultrasound equipment may cause inhibition or asynchronous pacing in older pulse generators, but this reaction appears to be uncommon with contemporary devices [21]. Repetitive activation of other dental equipment may cause inhibition [22]. Dental drilling can cause sufficient vibration to increase the pacing rate of an activity-sensing pacemaker.

Therapeutic radiation

The dose of radiation used in diagnostic X-ray procedures does not affect pulse generator function either acutely or cumulatively. Therapeutic radiation can cause failure in contemporary implanted devices [23–25].

The amount of therapeutic radiation that causes device failure is unpredictable and may involve changes in sensitivity, amplitude or pulse width; loss of telemetry; failure of output; or runaway rates. If dysfunction occurs, replacement of the device is required. Although some changes may resolve in hours to days, the long-term reliability of the pulse generator is suspect, and it should be replaced. It should be emphasized that radiation therapy to any part of the body away from the site of the pulse generator should not cause a problem with the pulse generator, but the pulse generator should be shielded to avoid scatter.

Centers that perform therapeutic radiation should have a protocol for patients with implanted devices [26]. Before radiation begins, the pacemaker should be identified and evaluated. The most common clinical situation is development of malignant breast cancer on the ipsilateral side in a patient with a permanent pacemaker or ICD. The pulse generator must be moved out of the field of radiation because shielding the device would result in suboptimal radiation therapy. The pulse generator can be explanted and a new system implanted on the contralateral side. Alternatively, it is often possible to explant the device and tunnel the existing permanent lead or leads through the subcutaneous tissues to the contralateral side. A new subcutaneous pocket is formed on the contralateral side and the pulse generator reattached to the now-tunneled lead or leads and reimplanted.

Electroconvulsive therapy

Electroconvulsive therapy is safe in relation to the function of implanted devices, because the high impedance of body tissues keeps all but a minimal amount of electricity from reaching the heart [1]. Because seizures possibly could cause sufficient myopotentials to result in pacemaker inhibition or ventricular tracking, ECG monitoring and interrogation of the implanted device are advisable. In unipolar pacemakers, seizure activity may generate sufficient myopotentials to result in inhibition or ventricular tracking.

Diathermy

Short-wave diathermy consists of therapeutic application of current directly to the skin. Diathermy can be a source of interference and should be avoided near the implantation site, because its high frequency has the potential to inhibit the pulse generator or damage its circuitry by excessive heating.

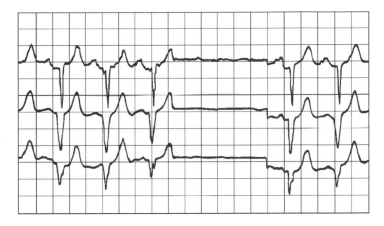

Figure 19.5 Electrocardiographic tracings from an ambulatory tracing in a pacemaker-dependent patient working in close contact with an induction oven. What appears to have been some interference consists of artifacts generated by the equipment. Both pulse and pacemaker-generated electrograms verified normal function of the device throughout this period.

Non-hospital environment

Conventional wisdom has been to advise patients with implanted devices to avoid 'arc welding' and close contact with combustion engines. However, as previously noted, pacemakers of unipolar sensing configuration remain more susceptible to EMI than pacemakers in a bipolar sensing configuration. For patients whose livelihood involves equipment with potential for EMI, bipolar sensing configuration should be used routinely.

Industrial environments with significant potential for clinically significant EMI with implantable devices include those in which industrial-strength welding equipment (exceeding 500 A), degaussing equipment and induction ovens are used. If a patient works in one of these environments or potentially some other even more obscure environment that suggests significant potential for EMI, the work environment should be carefully evaluated. If the patient is pacemaker dependent, consideration should be given to on-site assessment of the work environment. In some cases, the device manufacturer may be able to assist in this assessment. If

the patient is not pacemaker dependent, assessment may be achieved by ambulatory monitoring during exposure to the environment or by review of patient-triggered event records stored within the pacemaker (Figure 19.5).

From a practical standpoint, most patients who do 'arc welding' use low-amperage equipment for hobby welding. If the patient uses welding equipment in the 100–150 A range, significant EMI is unlikely to occur [27]. However, before giving a patient permission to return to this activity, the clinician caring for the patient with an implanted device must consider the type of hardware implanted as well as the dependency status.

Testing methods have been designed to allow exposure of the patient with a pacemaker or ICD to progressively stronger fields of EMI. Although this testing is not practical for the individual patient, studies [27,28] have determined levels of interference at a variety of programmed sensitivities (Table 19.2). This information could be applied to an individual patient if readings of EMI strengths in the work environment were obtainable.

Potential sources of EMI in the non-industrial and

Table 19.2 Electromagnetic interference levels capable of pacemaker interference in work environments.

Sensitivity setting (mV)	Atrial*		Ventricular*	
	Unipolar	Bipolar	Unipolar	Bipolar
0.5	4509	17 984	1720	14 240
0.75	5744	20 000	NA	NA
1.0	7679	20 000	4705	18 100
1.5	10 143	20 000	NA	NA
2.0	11 790	20 000	7454	19 630
3.0	15 034	20 000	10 003	20 000

NA, not available.
* Values in milligauss units.

home environments are capable of one-beat inhibition of the pacemaker (Table 19.3). However, it would be unusual for any of these sources to cause EMI of clinical significance. It is also unlikely that any of the devices in Table 19.3 can produce sustained interference with an ICD that becomes clinically significant. However, anecdotal reports exist [29–33]. Clinicians must now consider what effect inhibition would have on the patient with a cardiac resynchronization device. Single-beat inhibition probably would not have any significant impact. However, inhibition of a cardiac resynchronization

Table 19.3 Potential sources of electromagnetic interference.*

Source	Pacemaker damage	Total inhibition	One-beat inhibition	Asynchrony, noise	Rate increase
Acupuncture	No	Yes	Yes	Yes	No
Airport detector	No	No	Yes	No	No
Antitheft equipment	?	?	Yes	Yes	?
Arc welder	No	Yes	Yes	Yes	No
Cardioversion	Yes	No	No	Yes	Yes
Cautery, coagulation	Yes	Yes	Yes	Yes	Yes†‡
CB radio	No	No	Yes	No	No
Cellular phone	No	Yes	Yes	Yes	Yes
CT scanner	No	No	No	No	No
Defibrillation	Yes	No	No	Yes	Yes
Diathermy	Yes	Yes	Yes	Yes	Yes
ECT, EST	No	Yes	Yes	Yes	Yes‡
Electric blanket	No	No	Yes§	No	No
Electric drill	No	No	Yes§	No	No
Electric shaver	No	No	Yes§	No	No
Electric switch	No	No	Yes§	No	No
Electrolysis	No	No	Yes	Yes	No
Electrotome	No	No	Yes§	No	No
Ham radio	No	No	Yes	No	No
Heating pad	No	No	No	Yes	No
Lithotripsy	Yes‡	Yes§	Yes§	Yes§	Yes//
Metal detector	No	No	Yes§	No	No
Microwave	No	No	No	No	No
MRI	?	No	Yes	Yes	Yes
PET scanner	?	No	No	No	No
Power line	No	No	No	Yes	No
Radar	No	No	Yes§	No	No
Radiation, Dx	No	No	No	No	Yes
Radiation, Rx	Yes	No	No	No	Yes
RF ablation	Yes	Yes	No	No	Yes
TENS	No	Yes	No	Yes	Yes
TV remote control	No	No	No	No	No
Ultrasound, Dx	No	No	No	No	No

CB, citizens' band; CT, computed tomography; Dx, diagnostic; ECT, electroconvulsive therapy; EST, electroshock therapy; MRI, magnetic resonance imaging; PET, positron emission tomography; RF, radiofrequency; Rx, therapeutic; TENS, transcutaneous electrical nerve stimulation; TV, television.

* Not an all-inclusive list. There are case reports and anecdotal information on single-beat inhibition from other environmental sources.

† Impedance-based pulse generators.

‡ Piezoelectric crystal-based pulse generators.

§ Remote potential for interference.

// DDD mode only.

device could lead to alteration in the timing cycles for the device and, in turn, to longer episodes of inhibition and ineffective resynchronization support.

Although few sources are capable of causing clinically significant EMI resulting in pacemaker malfunction, the potential for interference from cellular phones and electronic article surveillance equipment has been of interest because of their widespread use. Before these are discussed in detail, several other potential sources, some of historical importance only, merit mention.

One of the most common questions still asked by pacemaker recipients today is whether they can use a microwave oven. In many areas, signs are still posted warning the patient with a pacemaker not to use a microwave oven. The original warnings were put in place because ineffective microwave shielding and less effective shielding of early pacemakers created the potential for pacemaker interference. Because of better shielding of both microwave ovens and device circuitry, the ovens are no longer a significant source of interference.

Metal detectors are frequently mentioned as a potential problem, and warning signs are often seen at airport security stations. The issue becomes greater in this era of heightened security, especially airport security. A study of patients wearing ambulatory ECG monitors who passed through metal detector gates while their pacemakers were programmed to the most sensitive programmable option showed no effect on pacing [34], although asynchronous pacing or inhibition could occur for one or two beats without ill effect to the patient. The major reason for discussing metal detectors with patients who have an implanted device is that the metal device may 'set off' the detector. Patients should be advised to present their device identification card to security personnel before proceeding through the metal detector. These patients are likely to be escorted around the metal detector and manually searched. A number of new types of detectors and security measures are being introduced. At this time, no specific information can be offered on new types of security technology and the effects on implanted devices. The best advice for now is to have the patient present an identification card.

Electronic article surveillance equipment

Antitheft devices (electronic article surveillance [EAS] equipment) in many retail stores and libraries consist of a tag or marker that is sensed by an electromagnetic field as the person walks through or by a 'gate.' Most systems consist of a 'deactivator' that is removed or deactivated before the item is taken from the store or library. This allows the customer to purchase an item and leave the store without activating an alarm. These electronic antitheft devices consist of multiple technologic processes that generate electromagnetic fields in various ranges. The devices use the radiofrequency range of 2–10 mHz, magnetic material in the range of 50–100 kHz, pulsed systems at various frequencies, and electromagnetic fields in the microwave range. In a study of 33 patients with 35 implanted devices (18 pacemakers and 17 ICDs) exposed to six different EAS detectors (three radiofrequency, one magnetoacoustic and two magnetic), no reprogramming of or damage to pulse generators was noted [35]. Sixteen of the pacemakers demonstrated noise reversion or inhibition when exposed to a magnetoacoustic system at a close range (± 45 cm). Reprogramming the sensitivity of the pacemaker could not abolish this effect. In addition, one epicardial unipolar pacemaker exhibited inhibition or noise reversion in each magnetic device. No EMI effects on any of the ICDs were demonstrated. No EMI was detected in any patient during exposure to the radiofrequency system.

Although a case report stated that a patient with an ICD received inappropriate shocks because the device oversensed the pulsed electromagnetic signal from an EAS detector [36], a large study of patients with ICDs did not demonstrate any significant adverse effects from EAS equipment unless exposure was prolonged (more than 2 min) [37].

At this time, it is reasonable to advise patients to pass rapidly through any obvious EAS equipment and avoid leaning on or standing 'near' the EAS detector: that is, 'Don't linger, don't lean' [38,39].

Cellular phones

A number of studies have investigated the potential of cellular phones to interfere with pacemakers or ICDs [40–46]. An early case report described injury to a pacemaker-dependent patient using a digital cellular phone [42].

In a multicenter study [43], 980 patients were tested with as many as six cellular phones for 5533 phone exposures. In this study, a highly variable incidence of interference was observed. The overall incidence, 20%, was high, but to quote this single percentage out of context would be misleading clinically. Interference at the 'normal' position on the ear was very low, and none was clinically significant, supporting the safety of 'normal' use. The incidences of interference and, specifically, clinically significant interference were also highly variable by combination of phone type, pacemaker manufacturer and pacemaker model. Eliminating a single cellular phone that is not commercially available from the analysis decreased the incidences of interference and clinically significant interference significantly to 13.1% and 2.8%, respectively.

Although symptoms occurred during 7.2% of the phone exposures, most were due to palpitations. The incidences of interference were highly variable by pacemaker manufacturer. Even for a given manufacturer, incidences differed by pacemaker model, reflecting the effect of design on susceptibility to interference.

The highest incidence of interference occurred when the cellular phone was directly over the pacemaker. Although this situation might exist if an activated phone were carried in a pocket directly over the pacemaker, this position is certainly not 'normal' for use of the phone and could be consciously avoided. As stated earlier, minimal interference was found at the ear position. Most adverse effects are eliminated if the phone is kept 8–10 cm from the implanted device.

Even though specific pacemaker and ICD design changes, such as feedthrough filters, have significantly reduced interference rates, the potential remains that new phone technologies could result in interference with implantable cardiac devices. Therefore, new wireless technologies will require subsequent testing.

Clinical advice

Nearly all patients can be reassured that EMI will not affect their pacemakers during the course of daily life. Patients in specialized industrial environments should be assessed individually. Improvements in pacemaker and ICD shielding should continue to minimize clinical concerns. However, the potential for EMI should never be taken lightly, and appropriate screening and monitoring should be performed to avoid adverse clinical outcomes. In addition, despite improvements in pulse generator shielding, emerging technologic advances result in new challenges for the patient with an implanted arrhythmia control device. Assessment of newer technologies for potential interference to the patient with a pacemaker or ICD must continue to be performed [47,48].

References

1 Hayes DL, Strathmore NF. Electromagnetic interference with implantable devices. In: Ellenbogen KA, Kay GN, Wilkoff BL. *Clinical Cardiac Pacing and Defibrillation*, 2nd edn. Philadelphia: W. B. Saunders Company, 2000: 939–52.

2 Toivonen L, Valjus J, Hongisto M, Metso R. The influence of elevated 50 Hz electric and magnetic fields on implanted cardiac pacemakers: the role of the lead configuration and programming of the sensitivity. *Pacing Clin Electrophysiol* 1991; **14**: 2114–22.

3 Astridge PS, Kaye GC, Whitworth S, Kelly P, Camm AJ, Perrins EJ. The response of implanted dual chamber pacemakers to 50 Hz extraneous electrical interference. *Pacing Clin Electrophysiol* 1993; **16**: 1966–74.

4 Roman-Gonzalez J, Hyberger LK, Hayes DL. Is electrocautery still a clinically significant problem with contemporary technology? [abstract]. *Pacing Clin Electrophysiol* 2001; **24**: 709.

5 Pinski SL, Trohman RG. Interference with cardiac pacing. *Cardiol Clin* 2000; **18**: 219–39.

6 Atlee JL, Bernstein AD. Cardiac rhythm management devices (part II): perioperative management. *Anesthesiology* 2001; **95**: 1492–1506.

7 Andersen C, Madsen GM. Rate-responsive pacemakers and anaesthesia: a consideration of possible implications. *Anaesthesia* 1990; **45**: 472–6.

8 Thiagarajah S, Azar I, Agres M, Lear E. Pacemaker malfunction associated with positive-pressure ventilation. *Anesthesiology* 1983; **58**: 565–6.

9 Pfeiffer D, Tebbenjohanns J, Schumacher B, Jung W, Luderitz B. Pacemaker function during radiofrequency ablation. *Pacing Clin Electrophysiol* 1995; **18**: 1037–44.

10 Ellenbogen KA, Wood MA, Stambler BS. Acute effects of radiofrequency ablation of atrial arrhythmias on implanted permanent pacing systems. *Pacing Clin Electrophysiol* 1996; **19**: 1287–95.

11 Holmes DR Jr, Hayes DL, Gray JE, Merideth J. The effects of magnetic resonance imaging on implantable pulse generators. *Pacing Clin Electrophysiol* 1986; **9**: 360–70.

12 Hayes DL, Holmes DR Jr, Gray JE. Effect of 1.5 tesla nuclear magnetic resonance imaging scanner on

implanted permanent pacemakers. *J Am Coll Cardiol* 1987; **10**: 782–6.

13 Gimbel JR, Lorig RJ, Wilkoff BL. Safe magnetic resonance imaging of pacemaker patients [abstract]. *J Am Coll Cardiol* 1995; **25** Special Issue: 11A.

14 Achenbach S, Moshage W, Diem B, Bieberle T, Schibgilla V, Bachmann K. Effects of magnetic resonance imaging on cardiac pacemakers and electrodes. *Am Heart J* 1997; **134**: 467–73.

15 Barold SS, Zipes DP. Cardiac pacemakers and antiarrhythmic devices. In: Braunwald E, ed. *Heart Disease: A Textbook of Cardiovascular Medicine*, 5th edn. Philadelphia: W. B. Saunders Company, 1997: 705–41.

16 Langberg J, Abber J, Thuroff JW, Griffin JC. The effects of extracorporeal shock wave lithotripsy on pacemaker function. *Pacing Clin Electrophysiol* 1987; **10**: 1142–6.

17 Cooper D, Wilkoff B, Masterson M *et al.* Effects of extracorporeal shock wave lithotripsy on cardiac pacemakers and its safety in patients with implanted cardiac pacemakers. *Pacing Clin Electrophysiol* 1988; **11**: 1607–16.

18 Rasmussen MJ, Hayes DL, Vlietstra RE, Thorsteinsson G. Can transcutaneous electrical nerve stimulation be safely used in patients with permanent cardiac pacemakers? *Mayo Clin Proc* 1988; **63**: 443–5.

19 O'Flaherty D, Wardill M, Adams AP. Inadvertent suppression of a fixed rate ventricular pacemaker using a peripheral nerve stimulator. *Anaesthesia* 1993; **48**: 687–9.

20 Chen D, Philip M, Philip PA, Monga TN. Cardiac pacemaker inhibition by transcutaneous electrical nerve stimulation. *Arch Phys Med Rehabil* 1990; **71**: 27–30.

21 Agarval A, Hewson J, Redding V. Ultrasound dental scalers and demand pacing [abstract]. *Pacing Clin Electrophysiol* 1988; **11**: 853.

22 Rahn R, Zegelman M, Kreuzer J. The influence of dental treatment on the Activitrax [abstract]. *Pacing Clin Electrophysiol* 1988; **11**: 852.

23 Rodriguez F, Filimonov A, Henning A, Coughlin C, Greenberg M. Radiation-induced effects in multiprogrammable pacemakers and implantable defibrillators. *Pacing Clin Electrophysiol* 1991; **14**: 2143–53.

24 Last A. Radiotherapy in patients with cardiac pacemakers. *Br J Radiol* 1998; **71**: 4–10.

25 Souliman SK, Christie J. Pacemaker failure induced by radiotherapy. *Pacing Clin Electrophysiol* 1994; **17**: 270–3.

26 Marbach JR, Sontag MR, Van Dyk J, Wolbarst AB. Management of radiation oncology patients with implanted cardiac pacemakers: report of AAPM Task Group No. 34. American Association of Physicists in Medicine. *Med Phys* 1994; **21**: 85–90.

27 Marco D, Eisinger G, Hayes DL. Testing of work environments for electromagnetic interference. *Pacing Clin Electrophysiol* 1992; **15**: 2016–22.

28 Hubmann M, Ruppert T, Eichhorn KF, Grzeganek A, David E, Hardt R. A standardized method for evaluation of pacemaker safety in the work place: a case evaluation. *Prog Biomed Res* 2000; **5**: 489–92.

29 Seifert T, Block M, Borggrefe M, Breithardt G. Erroneous discharge of an implantable cardioverter defibrillator caused by an electric razor. *Pacing Clin Electrophysiol* 1995; **18**: 1592–4.

30 Man KC, Davidson T, Langberg JJ, Morady F, Kalbfleisch SJ. Interference from a hand held radiofrequency remote control causing discharge of an implantable defibrillator. *Pacing Clin Electrophysiol* 1993; **16**: 1756–8.

31 Sabate X, Moure C, Nicolas J, Sedo M, Navarro X. Washing machine associated 50 Hz detected as ventricular fibrillation by an implanted cardioverter defibrillator. *Pacing Clin Electrophysiol* 2001; **24**: 1281–3.

32 Putzke JJ, Ideker RE. Environmental interference and interactions with implantable cardioverter-defibrillator functions. *Card Electrophysiol Rev* 2001; **5**: 115–17.

33 Goldschlager N, Epstein A, Friedman P, Gang E, Krol R, Olshansky B, North American Society of Pacing and Electrophysiology (NASPE) Practice Guideline Committee. Environmental and drug effects on patients with pacemakers and implantable cardioverter/defibrillators: a practical guide to patient treatment. *Arch Intern Med* 2001; **161**: 649–55.

34 Copperman Y, Zarfati D, Laniado S. The effect of metal detector gates on implanted permanent pacemakers. *Pacing Clin Electrophysiol* 1988; **11**: 1386–7.

35 McIvor ME, Reddinger J, Floden E, Sheppard RC. Study of pacemaker and implantable cardioverter defibrillator triggering by electronic article surveillance devices (SPICED TEAS). *Pacing Clin Electrophysiol* 1998; **21**: 1847–61.

36 Santucci PA, Haw J, Trohman RG, Pinski SL. Interference with an implantable defibrillator by an electronic antitheft-surveillance device. *N Engl J Med* 1998; **339**: 1371–4.

37 Groh WJ, Boschee SA, Engelstein ED *et al.* Interactions between electronic article surveillance systems and implantable cardioverter-defibrillators. *Circulation* 1999; **100**: 387–92.

38 Harthorne JW. Pacemakers and store security devices. *Cardiol Rev* 2001; **9**: 10–17.

39 Burlington DB. Important information on antitheft and metal detector systems and pacemakers, ICDs, and spinal cord stimulators. U.S. Food and Drug Administration—Center for Devices and Radiological

Health [Online] 1998, September 28. Retrieved May 6, 2002 from the World Wide Web: http://www. fda.gov/cdrh/safety.html.

40 Hayes DL, Carrillo RG, Findlay GK, Embrey M. State of the science: pacemaker and defibrillator interference from wireless communication devices. *Pacing Clin Electrophysiol* 1996; **19**: 1419–30.

41 Irnich W, Batz L, Muller R, Tobisch R. Electromagnetic interference of pacemakers by mobile phones. *Pacing Clin Electrophysiol* 1996; **19**: 1431–46.

42 Yesil M, Bayata S, Postaci N, Aydin C. Pacemaker inhibition and asystole in a pacemaker dependent patient. *Pacing Clin Electrophysiol* 1995; **18**: 1963.

43 Hayes DL, Wang PJ, Reynolds DW *et al.* Interference with cardiac pacemakers by cellular telephones. *N Engl J Med* 1997; **336**: 1473–9.

44 Sanmartin M, Fernandez Lozano I, Marquez J *et al.* The absence of interference between GSM mobile telephones and implantable defibrillators: an in-vivo study. Groupe Systemes Mobiles [Spanish]. *Rev Esp Cardiol* 1997; **50**: 715–19.

45 Fetter JG, Ivans V, Benditt DG, Collins J. Digital cellular telephone interaction with implantable cardioverter-defibrillators. *J Am Coll Cardiol* 1998; **31**: 623–8.

46 Grant FH, Schlegel RE. Effects of an increased air gap on the in vitro interaction of wireless phones with cardiac pacemakers. *Bioelectromagnetics* 2000; **21**: 485–90.

47 Hayes DL, Charboneau JW, Lewis BD, Asirvatham SJ, Dupuy DE, Lexvold NY. Radiofrequency treatment of hepatic neoplasms in patients with permanent pacemakers. *Mayo Clin Proc* 2001; **76**: 950–2.

48 Tan K-S, Seregelyi J, Cule D, Bouchard P, Hinberg I, Wu Y. Electromagnetic interference from digital television signals on medical devices. *J Clin Eng* 2001; **26**: 140–4.

Index